The State of the Art in Endodontics

The State of the Art in Endodontics

Editors

Massimo Amato
Giuseppe Pantaleo
Alfredo Iandolo

MDPI • Basel • Beijing • Wuhan • Barcelona • Belgrade • Manchester • Tokyo • Cluj • Tianjin

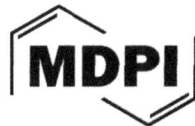

Editors

Massimo Amato
Department of Medicine,
Surgery and Dentistry,
Scuola Medica Salernitana,
University of Salerno,
84126 Salerno, Italy

Giuseppe Pantaleo
Department of Medicine,
Surgery and Dentistry,
Scuola Medica Salernitana,
University of Salerno,
84126 Salerno, Italy

Alfredo Iandolo
Faculty of Dentistry,
University of Salerno,
84084 Salerno, Italy

Editorial Office
MDPI
St. Alban-Anlage 66
4052 Basel, Switzerland

This is a reprint of articles from the Special Issue published online in the open access journal *Journal of Clinical Medicine* (ISSN 2077-0383) (available at: https://www.mdpi.com/journal/jcm/special_issues/2021_Endodontics).

For citation purposes, cite each article independently as indicated on the article page online and as indicated below:

LastName, A.A.; LastName, B.B.; LastName, C.C. Article Title. *Journal Name* **Year**, *Volume Number*, Page Range.

ISBN 978-3-0365-4795-4 (Hbk)
ISBN 978-3-0365-4796-1 (PDF)

© 2022 by the authors. Articles in this book are Open Access and distributed under the Creative Commons Attribution (CC BY) license, which allows users to download, copy and build upon published articles, as long as the author and publisher are properly credited, which ensures maximum dissemination and a wider impact of our publications.

The book as a whole is distributed by MDPI under the terms and conditions of the Creative Commons license CC BY-NC-ND.

Contents

Alfredo Iandolo, Alessandra Amato, Dina Abdellatif, Giuseppe Pantaleo and Massimo Amato
Special Issue "The State of the Art in Endodontics"
Reprinted from: *J. Clin. Med.* **2022**, *11*, 2329, doi:10.3390/jcm11092329 1

Vicente Faus-Matoses, Vicente Faus-Llácer, Celia Ruiz-Sánchez, Sharon Jaramillo-Vásconez, Ignacio Faus-Matoses, Benjamín Martín-Biedma and Álvaro Zubizarreta-Macho
Effect of Rotational Speed on the Resistance of NiTi Alloy Endodontic Rotary Files to Cyclic Fatigue—An In Vitro Study
Reprinted from: *J. Clin. Med.* **2022**, *11*, 3143, doi:10.3390/jcm11113143 5

Victor Roda-Casanova, Antonio Pérez-González, Alvaro Zubizarreta-Macho, Vicente Faus-Matoses
Influence of Cross-Section and Pitch on the Mechanical Response of NiTi Endodontic Files under Bending and Torsional Conditions—A Finite Element Analysis
Reprinted from: *J. Clin. Med.* **2022**, *11*, 2642, doi:10.3390/jcm11092642 17

Mohmed Isaqali Karobari, Sohaib Arshad, Tahir Yusuf Noorani, Naveed Ahmed, Syed Nahid Basheer, Syed Wali Peeran, Anand Marya, Charu Mohan Marya, Pietro Messina and Giuseppe Alessandro Scardina
Root and Root Canal Configuration Characterization Using Microcomputed Tomography: A Systematic Review
Reprinted from: *J. Clin. Med.* **2022**, *11*, 2287, doi:10.3390/jcm11092287 37

Mario Alovisi, Damiano Pasqualini, Narcisa Mandras, Janira Roana, Pietro Costamagna, Allegra Comba, Roberta Cavalli, Anna Luganini, Alfredo Iandolo, Lorenza Cavallo, Nicola Scotti and Elio Berutti
Confocal Laser Scanner Evaluation of Bactericidal Effect of Chitosan Nanodroplets Loaded with Benzalkonium Chloride
Reprinted from: *J. Clin. Med.* **2022**, *11*, 1650, doi:10.3390/jcm11061650 71

Elena Riad Deglow, Nayra Zurima Lazo Torres, David Gutiérrez Muñoz, María Bufalá Pérez, Agustín Galparsoro Catalán, Álvaro Zubizarreta-Macho, Francesc Abella Sans and Sofía Hernández Montero
Influence of Static Navigation Technique on the Accuracy of Autotransplanted Teeth in Surgically Created Sockets
Reprinted from: *J. Clin. Med.* **2022**, *11*, 1012, doi:10.3390/jcm11041012 79

Julien Beauquis, Hugo M. Setbon, Charles Dassargues, Pierre Carsin, Sam Aryanpour, Jean-Pierre Van Nieuwenhuysen and Julian G. Leprince
Short-Term Pain Evolution and Treatment Success of Pulpotomy as Irreversible Pulpitis Permanent Treatment: A Non-Randomized Clinical Study
Reprinted from: *J. Clin. Med.* **2022**, *11*, 787, doi:10.3390/jcm11030787 91

Vicente Faus-Llácer, Dalia Pulido Ouardi, Ignacio Faus-Matoses, Celia Ruiz-Sánchez, Álvaro Zubizarreta-Macho, Anabella María Reyes Ortiz and Vicente Faus-Matoses
Comparative Analysis of Root Canal Dentin Removal Capacity of Two NiTi Endodontic Reciprocating Systems for the Root Canal Treatment of Primary Molar Teeth. An In Vitro Study
Reprinted from: *J. Clin. Med.* **2022**, *11*, 338, doi:10.3390/jcm11020338 105

Victor Roda-Casanova, Antonio Pérez-González, Álvaro Zubizarreta-Macho and Vicente Faus-Matoses
Fatigue Analysis of NiTi Rotary Endodontic Files through Finite Element Simulation: Effect of Root Canal Geometry on Fatigue Life
Reprinted from: *J. Clin. Med.* **2021**, *10*, 5692, doi:10.3390/jcm10235692 . . . . **115**

Saulius Drukteinis, Goda Bilvinaite, Hagay Shemesh, Paulius Tusas and Vytaute Peciuliene
The Effect of Ultrasonic Agitation on the Porosity Distribution in Apically Perforated Root Canals Filled with Different Bioceramic Materials and Techniques: A Micro-CT Assessment
Reprinted from: *J. Clin. Med.* **2021**, *10*, 4977, doi:10.3390/jcm10214977 . . . . **131**

Vicente Faus-Llácer, Nirmine Hamoud-Kharrat, María Teresa Marhuenda Ramos, Ignacio Faus-Matoses, Álvaro Zubizarreta-Macho, Celia Ruiz Sánchez and Vicente Faus-Matoses
Influence of the Geometrical Cross-Section Design on the Dynamic Cyclic Fatigue Resistance of NiTi Endodontic Rotary Files—An In Vitro Study
Reprinted from: *J. Clin. Med.* **2021**, *10*, 4713, doi:10.3390/jcm10204713 . . . . **143**

Álvaro Zubizarreta-Macho, Roberta Tosin, Fabio Tosin, Pilar Velasco Bohórquez, Lara San Hipólito Marín, José María Montiel-Company, Jesús Mena-Álvarez and Sofía Hernández Montero
Influence of Guided Tissue Regeneration Techniques on the Success Rate of Healing of Surgical Endodontic Treatment: A Systematic Review and Network Meta-Analysis
Reprinted from: *J. Clin. Med.* **2022**, *11*, 1062, doi:10.3390/jcm11041062 . . . . **155**

Luísa Bandeira Lopes, Catarina Calvão, Filipa Salema Vieira, João Albernaz Neves, José João Mendes, Vanessa Machado and João Botelho
Vital and Nonvital Pulp Therapy in Primary Dentition: An Umbrella Review
Reprinted from: *J. Clin. Med.* **2022**, *11*, 85, doi:10.3390/jcm11010085 . . . . **171**

Elina Mekhdieva, Massimo Del Fabbro, Mario Alovisi, Allegra Comba, Nicola Scotti, Margherita Tumedei, Massimo Carossa, Elio Berutti and Damiano Pasqualini
Postoperative Pain following Root Canal Filling with Bioceramic vs. Traditional Filling Techniques: A Systematic Review and Meta-Analysis of Randomized Controlled Trials
Reprinted from: *J. Clin. Med.* **2021**, *10*, 4509, doi:10.3390/jcm10194509 . . . . **183**

Pratima Panda, Lora Mishra, Shashirekha Govind, Saurav Panda and Barbara Lapinska
Clinical Outcome and Comparison of Regenerative and Apexification Intervention in Young Immature Necrotic Teeth—A Systematic Review and Meta-Analysis
Reprinted from: *J. Clin. Med.* **2022**, *11*, 3909, doi:10.3390/jcm11133909 . . . . **193**

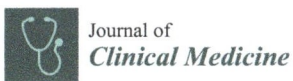

Editorial

Special Issue "The State of the Art in Endodontics"

Alfredo Iandolo [1,*], Alessandra Amato [1], Dina Abdellatif [2], Giuseppe Pantaleo [1] and Massimo Amato [1]

[1] Department of Conservative and Endodontics, Faculty of Dentistry, University of Salerno, 84084 Salerno, Italy; aale.amato@gmail.com (A.A.); giuseppepantaleo88@gmail.com (G.P.); maxamato1@gmail.com (M.A.)
[2] Department of Endodontics, Faculty of Dentistry, University of Alexandria, Alexandria 21545, Egypt; dinaabdellatif81@gmail.com
* Correspondence: aiandolo@unisa.it

Currently, the term "modern endodontics" is used more often due to contemporary applied science and original materials that have been developed in recent years. Various instruments and devices were developed to simplify and improve our endodontic treatments. For instance, these include operating microscopes, ultrasonic devices, different lasers, modified alloys for rotating Ni-Ti files, powerful irrigation strategies, the latest irrigant solutions, newly developed materials for filling root canals, 3D (three dimensional) radiography, and several more [1]. Furthermore, difficult root canal treatments can be performed safely when these advanced techniques are employed, consequently ensuring adequate therapy for patients and saving teeth that would otherwise be condemned for extraction. General practitioners and endodontists, who are equally important, should be aware of and apply these advanced techniques in their daily work.

The current Special Issue, "The State of the Art in Endodontics", in the *Journal of Clinical Medicine*, is dedicated to collecting high-quality scientific contributions that mainly focus on modern technologies and protocols.

Presently, with the introduction of 3D radiography and CBCT in endodontics, more precise correct diagnoses can be achieved. For example, it is possible to anticipate complex anatomies, identify root fractures, make a differential diagnosis between external and internal resorptions, and identify small periapical lesions that are not perceptible with traditional radiology [1,2]. All of these aspects can improve the prognosis of the treatment to be carried out.

After reaching a correct diagnosis, endodontic treatment begins by the preparation of an access cavity. In recent years, the concept of minimally invasive endodontics has been advancing progressively. This concept begins with access cavities.

By creating conservative cavities, it is possible to save more dental tissue and avoid the risk of fracture [3].

Once the access cavity is prepared and all root canals have been identified, the subsequent shaping phase can be begun.

Two studies in the current Special Issue studied the shaping phase during endodontic treatment [4,5]. Nickel–titanium (NiTi) endodontic rotary files allow clinicians to maintain the original anatomy of root canals, especially in curved canals. Consequently, the possibility of conceivable mishaps during the mechanical preparation of a root canal system is diminished. The innovation of the heat treatment process during the manufacturing of Ni-Ti files allows for modifications in the physical properties of the NiTi rotating instrument. For instance, this treatment increases cyclic fatigue resistance and helps the files to conform to diverse curves and angles in a root canal. Research has illustrated the utilization of a single rotary instrument in a reciprocation action when treating primary teeth and reported considerable advantages in pedodontics. For example, the therapy time was reduced, the liability for iatrogenic mistakes was also diminished, and cross-contamination between patients was prevented [6,7].

It has been reported that the shaping phase alone, regardless of the file used, cannot reach the whole of the complex endodontic space. Manual and rotating files can only be used in the central portion of the root canal. Files cannot reach lateral anatomies such as isthmuses, lateral canals, loops, deltas, and similar. For this reason, the cleaning phase is important and is considered a fundamental step to adequately eliminating bacteria and necrotic tissue [8].

Furthermore, minimally invasive shaping protocols in the form of using rotary files that are small in size and taper promote more efficient irrigation protocols and safer, more conservative endodontic treatments [9].

Sodium hypochlorite (NaOCl) is considered the most common irrigant used during the cleaning phase owing to its high tissue dissolution ability and prominent antimicrobial action [10].

Several techniques can be applied to utilize the action and effect of NaoCl. A recently introduced technique, internal heating, combined with ultrasonic activation, can also achieve excellent results in the case of conservative shaping [8,11].

Numerous additional antimicrobial solutions were suggested for use in root canal chemical cleaning, such as benzalkonium chloride (BAK) and chlorhexidine (CHX) [12,13].

In our current Special Issue, new research evaluated the antibacterial effect and depth of penetration of a chitosan nanodroplet (ND) solution packed with benzalkonium chloride (BAK) inside dentinal tubules [14]. The study showed that BAK induces structural disorganization, the loss of cytoplasmic membrane integrity, and has damaging impacts on microorganisms [15]. Additionally, when BAK is used in solution concentrated up to 5%, it is believed to offer antibacterial effects and durable outcomes as it inhibits the proteases of microorganisms [15].

In this research, the NaOCl solution showed the highest antimicrobial efficacy, but nanodroplets with BAK seemed to have an identical effect to CHX, with a high depth of efficacy.

After finishing the shaping and cleaning step, the obturation phase occurs next in the endodontic space.

In recent years, new sealers with excellent properties, such as biosealers, have also been developed, in addition to the invention of new techniques for use in the obturation phase [16]. The major features of these new sealers are their increased PH, greater antibacterial activity, decreased setting time, biocompatibility, and micro-expansion in the root canal.

In the current Special Issue [17], a new technique was evaluated that employs ultrasonic tips to apply sealer in the root canal.

Ultrasonic devices have been effectively employed in the field of endodontics in recent decades for most of the endodontic steps, including root canal obturation [18].

Many studies showed that the application of ultrasonic energy on sealers during the root canal filling procedure can boost the sealer's penetration inside the dentinal tubules and enhance the boundary connection between the obturation material and the root canal wall [17]. In addition, ultrasonic energy can rearrange the sealer particles and eradicate the trapped air, hence decreasing the porosity.

Utilizing micro-CT analysis, the study evaluated the effect of direct ultrasonic activation on the porosity diffusion in biosealer in root canal filling. Within the limits of this in vitro study, they concluded that none of the obturation procedures could offer pore-free endodontic obturation in the apical 5 mm.

After the completion of the obturation phase, up to 40% of patients may report postoperative pain [19].

Postoperative pain can remain for some time after the treatment and can be intense according to multiple prognostic aspects. The factor that corresponds the most to postoperative pain is the obturation technique; this can be in the form of a cold lateral, single cone, or warm vertical compaction technique. Moreover, the sealer was found to play an important role in postoperative pain, with the most traditionally used being resin-based or zinc-oxide eugenol sealers [19].

In this Special Issue, using a systematic review and meta-analysis, Mekhdieva et al. reported the impact of using the biosealer filling technique in comparison to conventional obturation processes on postoperative pain in adult patients following endodontic treatment [20].

Mekhdieva et al. proposed that the biosealer obturation method may have a positive effect on postoperative pain. Concurrently, it was reported that many factors affected the flare-up of pain, for example, if analgesics were administered, the pulp status, and the number of visits when using biosealer compared with resin-based sealer. Nevertheless, additional well-designed clinical studies are warranted to augment their results due to several restrictions in their analyses.

In conclusion, the knowledge and the application of modern technologies and the continuous search for and development of new techniques and endodontic materials are crucial to making root canal treatment safer and more efficient.

As the Guest Editors, we would like to sincerely appreciate and thank the reviewers for their insightful remarks and the *JCM* team's support. Ultimately, we heartily thank all of the contributing authors for their valuable input.

Funding: This editorial received no external funding.

Conflicts of Interest: The authors declare no conflict of interest.

References

1. Iandolo, A.; Iandolo, G.; Malvano, M.; Pantaleo, G.; Simeone, M. Modern technologies in endodontics. *G. Ital. Endod.* **2016**, *30*, 2–9. [CrossRef]
2. Patel, S.; Brown, J.; Pimentel, T.; Kelly, R.D.; Abella, F.; Durack, C. Cone beam computed tomography in Endodontics—A review of the literature. *Int. Endod. J.* **2019**, *52*, 1138–1152. [CrossRef] [PubMed]
3. Plotino, G.; Grande, N.M.; Isufi, A.; Ioppolo, P.; Pedullà, E.; Bedini, R.; Gambarini, G.; Testarelli, L. Fracture Strength of Endodontically Treated Teeth with Different Access Cavity Designs. *J. Endod.* **2017**, *43*, 995–1000. [CrossRef]
4. Faus-Llácer, V.; Ouardi, D.P.; Faus-Matoses, I.; Ruiz-Sánchez, C.; Zubizarreta-Macho, A.; Reyes Ortiz, A.M.; Faus-Matoses, V. Comparative Analysis of Root Canal Dentin Removal Capacity of Two NiTi Endodontic Reciprocating Systems for the Root Canal Treatment of Primary Molar Teeth. An In Vitro Study. *J. Clin. Med.* **2022**, *11*, 338. [CrossRef] [PubMed]
5. Roda-Casanova, V.; Pérez-González, A.; Zubizarreta-Macho, A.; Faus-Matoses, V. Fatigue Analysis of NiTi Rotary Endodontic Files through Finite Element Simulation: Effect of Root Canal Geometry on Fatigue Life. *J. Clin. Med.* **2021**, *10*, 5692. [CrossRef] [PubMed]
6. Prabhakar, A.R.; Yavagal, C.; Dixit, K.; Naik, S.V. Reciprocating vs. Rotary Instrumentation in Pediatric Endodontics: Cone Beam Computed Tomographic Analysis of Deciduous Root Canals using Two Single-file Systems. *Int. J. Clin. Pediatr. Dent.* **2016**, *9*, 45–49. [CrossRef] [PubMed]
7. Katge, F.; Patil, D.; Poojari, M.; Pimpale, J.; Shitoot, A.; Rusawat, B. Comparison of instrumentation time and cleaning efficacy of manual instrumentation, rotary systems and reciprocating systems in primary teeth: An in vitro study. *J. Indian Soc. Pedod. Prev. Dent.* **2014**, *32*, 311–316. [CrossRef] [PubMed]
8. Iandolo, A.; Simeone, M.; Orefice, S.; Rengo, S. 3D cleaning, a perfected technique: Thermal profile assessment of heated NaOCl. *G. Ital. Endod.* **2017**, *31*, 58–61. [CrossRef]
9. Iandolo, A.; Abdellatif, D.; Pantaleo, G.; Sammartino, P.; Amato, A. Conservative shaping combined with three-dimensional cleaning can be a powerful tool: Case series. *J. Conserv. Dent.* **2020**, *23*, 648–652. [CrossRef] [PubMed]
10. Fedorowicz, Z.; Nasser, M.; Sequeira-Byron, P.; de Souza, R.F.; Carter, B.; Heft, M. Irrigants for non-surgical root canal treatment in mature permanent teeth. *Cochrane Database Syst. Rev.* **2012**, *12*, 9–17. [CrossRef] [PubMed]
11. Yared, G.; Ramli, G.A. Ex vivo ability of a noninstrumentation technique to disinfect oval-shaped canals. *J. Conserv. Dent.* **2020**, *23*, 10–14. [CrossRef] [PubMed]
12. Mohammadi, Z.; Abbott, P.V. The properties and applications of chlorhexidine in endodontics. *Int. Endod. J.* **2009**, *42*, 288–302. [CrossRef] [PubMed]
13. Bukiet, F.; Couderc, G.; Camps, J.; Tassery, H.; Cuisinier, F.; About, I.; Charrier, A.; Candoni, N. Wetting properties and critical micellar concentration of benzalkonium chloride mixed in sodium hypochlorite. *J. Endod.* **2012**, *38*, 1525–1529. [CrossRef] [PubMed]
14. Alovisi, M.; Pasqualini, D.; Mandras, N.; Roana, J.; Costamagna, P.; Comba, A.; Cavalli, R.; Luganini, A.; Iandolo, A.; Cavallo, L.; et al. Confocal Laser Scanner Evaluation of Bactericidal Effect of Chitosan Nanodroplets Loaded with Benzalkonium Chloride. *J. Clin. Med.* **2022**, *11*, 1650. [CrossRef] [PubMed]

15. Arias-Moliz, M.T.; Ruiz-Linares, M.; Cassar, G.; Ferrer-Luque, C.M.; Baca, P.; Ordinola-Zapata, R.; Camilleri, J. The effect of benzalkonium chloride additions to AH Plus sealer. Antimicrobial, physical and chemical properties. *J. Dent.* **2015**, *43*, 846–854. [CrossRef] [PubMed]
16. Abdellatif, D.; Amato, A.; Calapaj, M.; Pisano, M.; Iandolo, A. A novel modified obturation technique using biosealers: An ex vivo study. *J. Conserv. Dent.* **2021**, *24*, 369–373. [PubMed]
17. Drukteinis, S.; Bilvinaite, G.; Shemesh, H.; Tusas, P.; Peciuliene, V. The Effect of Ultrasonic Agitation on the Porosity Distribution in Apically Perforated Root Canals Filled with Different Bioceramic Materials and Techniques: A Micro-CT Assessment. *J. Clin. Med.* **2021**, *10*, 4977. [CrossRef] [PubMed]
18. da Silva Machado, A.P.; de Souza, A.C.C.C.; Gonçalves, T.L.; Marques, A.A.F.; da Fonseca Roberti Garcia, L.; Bortoluzzi, E.A.; de Carvalho, F.M.A. Does the ultrasonic activation of sealer hinder the root canal retreatment? *Clin. Oral Investig.* **2021**, *25*, 4401–4406. [CrossRef] [PubMed]
19. Nosrat, A.; Dianat, O.; Verma, P.; Nixdorf, D.R.; Law, A.S. Postoperative Pain: An Analysis on Evolution of Research in Half-Century. *J. Endod.* **2020**, *47*, 358–365. [CrossRef] [PubMed]
20. Mekhdieva, E.; Del Fabbro, M.; Alovisi, M.; Comba, A.; Scotti, N.; Tumedei, M.; Carossa, M.; Berutti, E.; Pasqualini, D. Postoperative Pain following Root Canal Filling with Bioceramic vs. Traditional Filling Techniques: A Systematic Review and Meta-Analysis of Randomized Controlled Trials. *J. Clin. Med.* **2021**, *10*, 4509. [CrossRef] [PubMed]

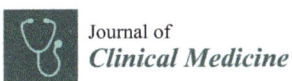

Article

Effect of Rotational Speed on the Resistance of NiTi Alloy Endodontic Rotary Files to Cyclic Fatigue—An In Vitro Study

Vicente Faus-Matoses [1], Vicente Faus-Llácer [1], Celia Ruiz-Sánchez [1], Sharon Jaramillo-Vásconez [1], Ignacio Faus-Matoses [1,*], Benjamín Martín-Biedma [2] and Álvaro Zubizarreta-Macho [3,4]

1. Department of Stomatology, Faculty of Medicine and Dentistry, University of Valencia, 46010 Valencia, Spain; vicente.faus@uv.es (V.F.-M.); fausvj@uv.es (V.F.-L.); ceruizsan@gmail.com (C.R.-S.); sjavas@alumni.uv.es (S.J.-V.)
2. Department of Surgery and Medical-Surgical Specialties, School of Medicine and Dentistry, Universidad de Santiago de Compostela, 15705 Santiago de Compostela, Spain; benjamin.martin@usc.es
3. Department of Implant Surgery, Faculty of Health Sciences, Alfonso X El Sabio University, 28691 Madrid, Spain; amacho@uax.es
4. Department of Surgery, Faculty of Medicine and Dentistry, University of Salamanca, 37008 Salamanca, Spain
* Correspondence: ignacio.faus@uv.es

Abstract: The present study aims to evaluate and contrast the function of the rotational speed of NiTi alloy endodontic rotary files on how resistant they are to dynamic cyclic fatigue. Methods: A total of 150 NiTi alloy endodontic rotary files with similar geometrical design and metallurgical properties were randomly divided into study groups: Group A: 200 rpm (n = 30); Group B: 350 rpm (n = 30); Group C: 500 rpm (n = 30); Group D: reciprocating movement at 350 rpm with 120° counterclockwise and 30° clockwise motion (350 rpm+) (n = 30); and Group E: reciprocating movement at 400 rpm with 120° counterclockwise and 30° clockwise motion (400 rpm+) (n = 30). A dynamic device was designed to carry out dynamic cyclic fatigue tests using artificial root canal systems made from stainless steel with an apical diameter of 250 µm, 5 mm radius of curvature, 60° curvature angle, and 6% taper, and 20 mm in length. A Weibull statistical analysis and ANOVA test were used to analyze the results. Results: The ANOVA analysis showed differences in time to failure among all the study groups that were of statistical significance ($p < 0.001$). Conclusions: NiTi alloy endodontic rotary files using reciprocating movement at 350 rpm with 120° counterclockwise and 30° clockwise motion exhibit greater resistance to dynamic cyclic fatigue than files used with a reciprocating movement at 400 rpm with 120° counterclockwise and 30° clockwise motion, continuous rotational speed at 200 rpm, continuous rotational speed at 350 rpm, or continuous rotational speed at 500 rpm; it is therefore advisable to use reciprocating movements at a low speed.

Keywords: continuous rotation; cyclic fatigue; endodontics; endodontic rotary file; reciprocating; speed; resistance

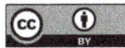

1. Introduction

Chemical disinfection and mechanical instrumentation of the root canal system are crucial in the prevention of apical periodontitis that arises due to treatment, or to cure it if already established [1]. However, the failure of nickel–titanium (NiTi) alloy endodontic rotary files remains a major dilemma for endodontists during root canal treatment, despite the NiTi alloy undergoing continuous chemical and mechanical enhancements by manufacturers so as to help prevent complications during endodontic therapy [2]. The fracture of NiTi alloy endodontic rotary files can be caused by torsional fatigue, cyclic fatigue, or some combination thereof [3]. Torsional failure happens when the end of a NiTi alloy endodontic rotary file has become trapped on one of the root canal walls while the instrument is still rotating, causing the file to fracture once the elasticity of the material has been exceeded [4,5]. Flexural bending fatigue is caused by the repeated application of compression and traction cycles that the NiTi alloy endodontic rotary file experiences at the site of maximum curvature of the root canal; these stresses subsequently lead to plastic deformation, which can result in unexpected file fracture [3,6].

Several studies have reported that a fractured fragment of the NiTi alloy endodontic rotary file may block the curved canal, negatively affecting the treatment outcome, as disinfecting agents can no longer reach the infected root canal areas [1,7,8]. Additionally, root canal systems that have not been properly disinfected may have a lower likelihood of healing in teeth with periapical lesions [9].

Several additional factors have been linked to the fracture of NiTi alloy endodontic rotary files, including instruments with a cross-section design [10], taper and apical diameter [11], flute length, pitch, and helix angle [12]. In addition, the dynamics of the instrument, such as torque [13] and canal geometry [8], as well as the manufacturing process, whether electropolishing, heat treatment, or ion implantation [14], can influence the risk of fracture.

It remains unclear whether or not rotational speed affects the resistance to cyclic fatigue of NiTi alloy endodontic rotary files. Yared et al. and Martín et al. have found that rotational speed does indeed influence the prevalence of fracture in NiTi alloy endodontic rotary files [15,16]. However, Pruett et al. showed that rotational speed had no significant impact on the risk of fracture of NiTi alloy endodontic rotary files [8]. Additionally, some studies have reported that reciprocating motion may overextend the cyclic fatigue life of NiTi alloy endodontic files in comparison to continuous motion [17,18].

The present study aims to evaluate and assess the effect of the rotational speed of NiTi alloy endodontic rotary files on their resistance to dynamic cyclic fatigue, with a null hypothesis (H_0) postulating that rotational speed has no effect on how resistant NiTi alloy endodontic rotary files are to dynamic cyclic fatigue.

2. Materials and Methods

2.1. Study Design

One hundred and fifty (150) sterile, brand new endodontic rotary files with a parallelogram cross-section design, 6% taper, and 250 μm apical diameter (Ref.: IRE 02506, D, Endogal, Galician Endodontics Company, Lugo, Spain) were randomly distributed among different study groups: Group A: continuous rotational speed at 200 rpm (200 rpm) (n = 30); Group B: continuous rotational speed at 350 rpm (350 rpm) (n = 30); Group C: continuous rotational speed at 500 rpm (500 rpm) (n = 30); Group D: reciprocating movement at 350 rpm with 120° counterclockwise and 30° clockwise motion (350 rpm+) (n = 30); and Group E: reciprocating movement at 400 rpm with 120° counterclockwise and 30° clockwise motion (400 rpm+) (n = 30). The final total of experimental units included was 150, with these being assigned to one of the five study groups in keeping with the proportions determined by the researchers. The power was set at 80% and testing the null hypothesis H_0 resulted in an effect size of 0.606. A single-factor ANOVA test for independent samples was used to make equal the mean values of the five groups, and the significance level was set at 5%. A microscope (OPMI pico, Zeiss, Oberkochen, Germany) was used to examine all NiTi alloy endodontic rotary files (Ref.: IRE 02506, D, Endogal, Galician Endodontics Company, Lugo, Spain) prior to use, with no files discarded. Between January and July 2022, this controlled experiment was conducted at the Department of Stomatology of the Faculty of Medicine and Dentistry at the University of Valencia (Valencia, Spain).

2.2. Analysis with Scanning Electron Microscopy

A scanning electron microscope (SEM) (HITACHI S-4800, Fukuoka, Japan) was used at ×30 and ×600 for the initial inspection of the NiTi alloy endodontic rotary files (Ref.: IRE 02506, D, Endogal, Galician Endodontics Company, Lugo, Spain). This analysis was conducted at the Central Support Service for Experimental Research of the University of Valencia in Burjassot, Spain. The analysis was carried out with the following exposure parameters: 20 kV acceleration voltage; magnification from 100× to 6500×; and resolution ranging from −1.0 nm at 15 kV to 2.0 nm at 1 kV. Researchers did this to evaluate the surface characteristics and ensure there were no manufacturing surface defects.

2.3. Analysis with Energy-Dispersive X-ray Spectroscopy

In addition, energy-dispersive X-ray spectroscopy (EDX) was also used to analyze all the NiTi alloy endodontic rotary files (Ref.: IRE 02506, D, Endogal, Galician Endodontics Company, Lugo, Spain). This was conducted at the Central Support Service for Experimental Research at the University of Valencia in Burjassot, Spain. This inspection used these exposure parameters: 20 kV acceleration voltage; magnification from 100× to 6500×; and resolution ranging from −1.0 nm at 15 kV to 2.0 nm at 1 kV. These parameters were used to assess the elemental makeup of the chemicals in the files used to test their resistance to static fatigue. The researchers also evaluated the atomic weight percent, taking measurements from three different sections (apical third, medium third, and coronal third of the NiTi alloy endodontic files).

2.4. Experimental Model Simulating Dynamic Cyclic Fatigue

The researchers conducted tests of resistance to dynamic cyclic fatigue at room temperature (20 °C) to evaluate the mechanical behavior of the instruments, according to Martins et al. [19], using the aforementioned customized device (Utility Model Patent No. ES1219520) [20]. CAD/CAE 2D/3D software (Midas FX+®, Brunleys, Milton Keynes, UK) was used to design the structure of the device, which was subsequently created with 3D-printing software (ProJet® 6000 3D Systems©, Rock Hill, SC, USA) (Figure 1).

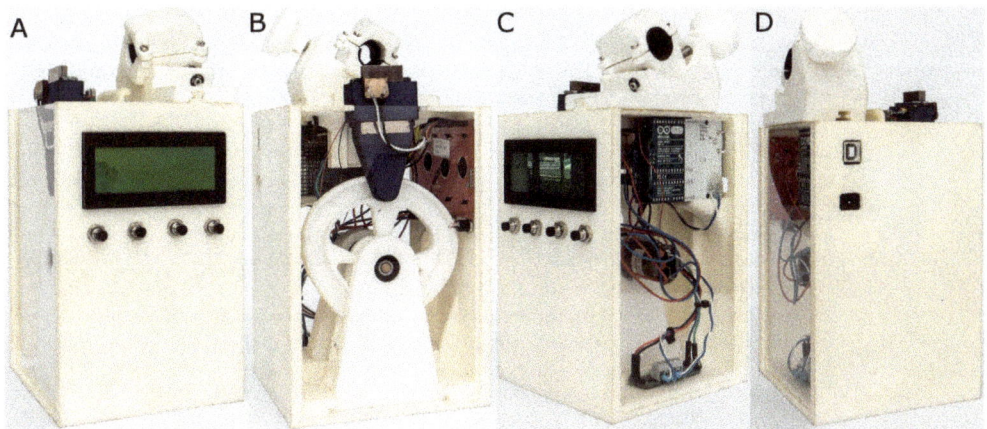

Figure 1. (**A**) Front, (**B**) back, (**C**) right, and (**D**) left sides of the dynamic cyclic fatigue device.

The customized artificial root canals were performed using Schneider's measuring technique, with a curvature of 60° [21] and a 5 mm curvature radius. The inverse engineering software used for this purpose was CAD/CAE 2D/3D. Molybdenum wire-cut technology (Cocchiola S.A., Buenos Aires, Argentina) was used with electrical discharge machining (EDM) to create the artificial root canal from stainless steel. Researchers also ensured that the NiTi files were flush with the walls of the artificial root canal. This newly created artificial canal was then positioned on its support, and a light-dependent resistor (LDR) sensor (Ref.: C000025, Arduino LLC®, Ivrea, Italy) placed at the apex of the canal was used to identify any failures in the endodontic rotary instruments (Ref.: IRE 02506, D, Endogal, Galician Endodontics Company, Lugo, Spain). This device works by measuring the light source continuously generated by a very strong white LED (20,000 mcd) (Ref.: 12.675/5/b/c/20k, Batuled, Coslada, Spain). The LED was positioned opposite the artificial root canal. An LED LDR sensor (Ref.: C000025, Arduino LLC®) at 50 ms was used to interpret the LED signals so as to identify the precise time of failure.

A roller bearing system (Ref.: MR104ZZ, FAG, Schaeffler Herzogenaurach, Herzogenaurach, Germany) was used to apply the movement direction and speed indicated by the operator (Ref.: DRV8835, Pololu® Corporation, Las Vegas, NV, USA) and created by the brushed DC gear motor (Ref.: 1589, Pololu® Corporation, Las Vegas, NV, USA) to the artificial support. The support was maneuvered in an exclusively axial motion with the help of a linear guide (Ref.: HGH35C 10249-1 001 MA, HIWIN Technologies Corp. Taichung, Taiwan). A torque-controlled motor and 6:1 reduction handpiece (X-Smart plus, Dentsply Maillefer, Baillagues, Switzerland) were used in conjunction with the NiTi endodontic rotary files.

A frequency of 60 pecks per minute was used for the NiTi endodontic files within the dynamic cyclic fatigue device, following the parameters of a prior study [19]. Researchers also applied a high-flow synthetic oil (Singer All-Purpose Oil; Singer Corp., Barcelona, Spain) to help prevent friction between the NiTi endodontic files and the walls of the artificial root canal; this oil is specifically formulated for the lubrication of mechanical parts.

The files were all used until failure. The researchers recorded and evaluated both the length of time and the number of cycles the files took to fracture.

2.5. Statistical Tests

Statistical analysis of all variables was performed using SAS 9.4 (SAS Institute Inc., Cary, NC, USA). The mean value and SD were used to express the descriptive statistics of the quantitative variables. The researchers then used an ANOVA test to perform a comparative analysis of the number of cycles to failure and the time to failure (in seconds). In 2-to-2 comparisons, the Tukey method was used to determine the *p*-values and correct any Type I errors. The researchers also calculated the Weibull modulus and Weibull characteristic strength. Statistical significance was defined as $p < 0.05$.

3. Results

Scanning electron microscopy (SEM) analysis of the NiTi alloy endodontic rotary files did not detect any structural alterations or accumulated organic matter. Additionally, due to the laser machining process used to make them, the manufacturing lines were parallel to each other and perpendicular to the longitudinal axis of the files. The distance and width between these manufacturing lines were indicators of the precision and intensity of the laser machining manufacturing process. The laser machining process also resulted in tubular porosity that was observed in the files. Additionally, tubular porosity was visible in all of the NiTi alloy endodontic rotary files as a result of the combination of other chemical elements with the Ti alloys (Figure 2).

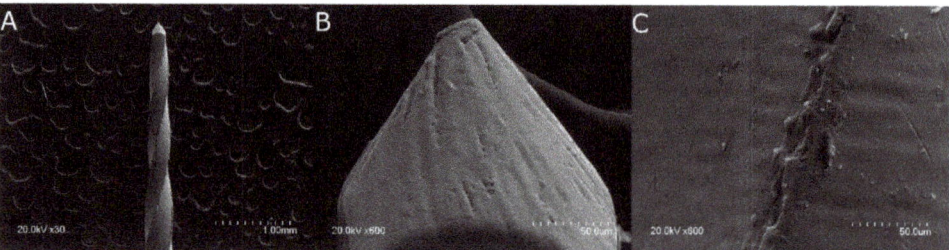

Figure 2. (**A**) SEM images of the full-length NiTi alloy endodontic rotary files (Ref.: IRE 02506, D, Endogal, Galician Endodontics Company, Lugo, Spain) at ×30, (**B**) and specifically of the end of the file at ×600 and (**C**) the surface of the file at ×600.

EDX micro-analysis of the NiTi alloy endodontic rotary files was performed at three different locations at 20 kV, enabling a thorough and precise analysis of the composition of the NiTi alloy endodontic rotary files. Through EDX micro-analysis at 20 kV, the NiTi alloy endodontic rotary files were found to comprise Ti (37.59–34.52 wt.%) and Ni (34.19–38.81 wt.%), although O and C were also observed (Figure 3).

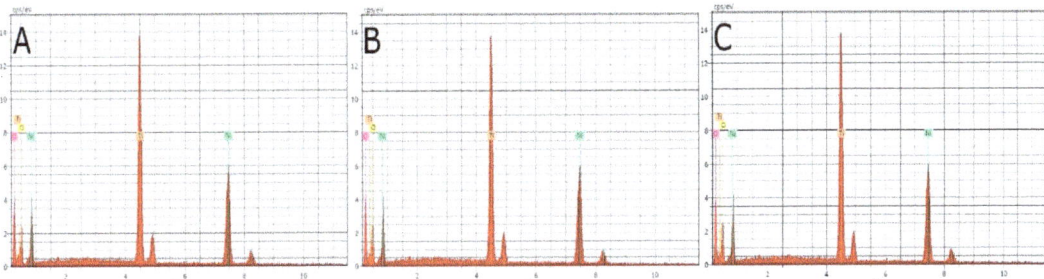

Figure 3. EDX micro-analysis of the NiTi alloy endodontic rotary files at locations (**A**) 1, (**B**) 2, and (**C**) 3.

Table 1 and Figure 4 show the mean and SD values of the time to failure (in seconds) across all study groups.

Table 1. Descriptive analysis of time to failure (seconds).

Study Group	n	Mean	SD	Minimum	Maximum
200 rpm	30	364.30 [a]	6.71	352.38	375.49
350 rpm	30	282.42 [b]	7.19	261.90	293.71
500 rpm	30	143.84 [c]	5.70	132.08	152.39
350 rpm+	30	590.38 [d]	11.19	561.37	608.08
400 rpm+	30	488.44 [e]	12.93	462.19	512.33

[a,b,c,d,e] Statistically significant differences among groups ($p < 0.05$).

The ANOVA analysis found there were differences of statistical significance among all of the study groups with regard to the time to failure ($p < 0.001$) (Figure 5). The results of the time to failure could be applied to the "number of cycles to failure" since all of the NiTi endodontic files were used at a frequency of 60 pecks per minute within the dynamic cyclic fatigue device.

The Weibull statistics scale distribution parameter (η) identified differences of statistical significance among all of the study groups with regard to the time to failure ($p < 0.001$) (Table 2, Figure 5). The Weibull statistics shape distribution parameter (β) revealed differences great enough to be statistically significant with regard to time to failure between the 200 rpm and 400 rpm+ groups ($p = 0.0236$), the 500 rpm and 350 rpm+ groups ($p = 0.0003$), the 350 rpm+ and 400 rpm+ groups ($p = 0.0154$), the 350 rpm and 500 rpm groups ($p = 0.0152$), and the 200 rpm and 500 rpm groups ($p = 0.0005$). However, there were not enough differences observed in the time to failure between the 350 rpm and 400 rpm+ groups ($p = 0.2283$), the 500 rpm and 400 rpm groups ($p = 0.1908$), the 200 rpm and 350 rpm+ groups ($p = 0.08925$), the 350 rpm and 350 rpm+ groups ($p = 0.2492$), and the 200 rpm and 350 rpm groups ($p = 0.3123$) to be statistically significant (Table 2, Figure 5). In short, the NiTi alloy endodontic rotary systems exhibited very predictable behavior, as it took about the same amount of time for the majority of the endodontic rotary files within each study group to reach the point of failure. The more gradual slope seen when using the NiTi endodontic rotary files at 350 rpm+ would indicate that this behavior is easier to predict than other kinematics. The NiTi alloy endodontic rotary files at 350 rpm+ were shown to be the most resistant to cyclic fatigue, followed by the NiTi alloy endodontic rotary files at 400 rpm+, 200 rpm, 350 rpm, and 500 rpm.

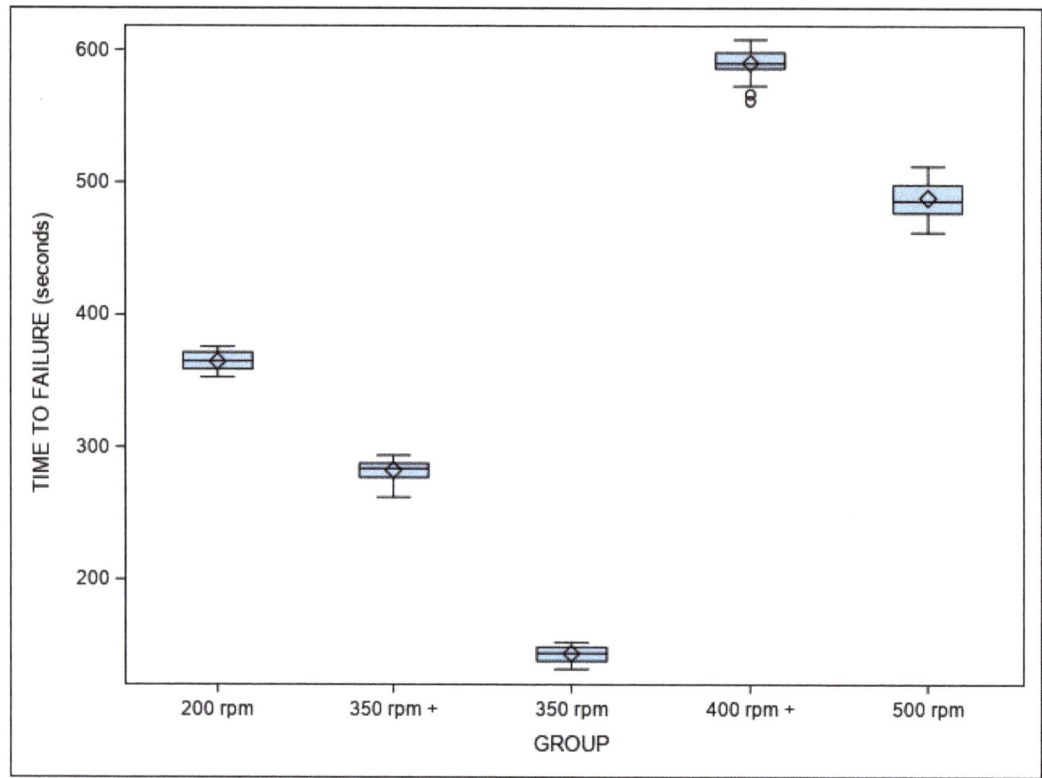

Figure 4. Box plot of time to failure. The median value of the respective study groups is represented by the horizontal line in each box. ◊—Box plot mean value. O—Extrema value.

Table 2. Weibull statistics for the time to failure across the study groups.

Study Group	Weibull Shape (β)				Weibull Scale (η)			
	Estimate	St Error	Lower	Upper	Estimate	St Error	Lower	Upper
200 rpm	61.9124	8.8223	46.8258	81.8598	367.5283	1.1471	365.2868	369.7836
350 rpm	50.3905	7.3394	37.8766	67.0388	285.6319	1.0898	283.5039	287.7759
500 rpm	30.5162	4.4688	22.9024	40.6611	146.4785	0.9251	144.6765	40.6611
350 rpm+	63.6086	8.9083	48.3399	83.7000	595.4815	1.8047	591.9549	599.0291
400 rpm+	39.6357	5.3913	30.3603	51.7449	494.7559	2.4189	490.0376	499.5197

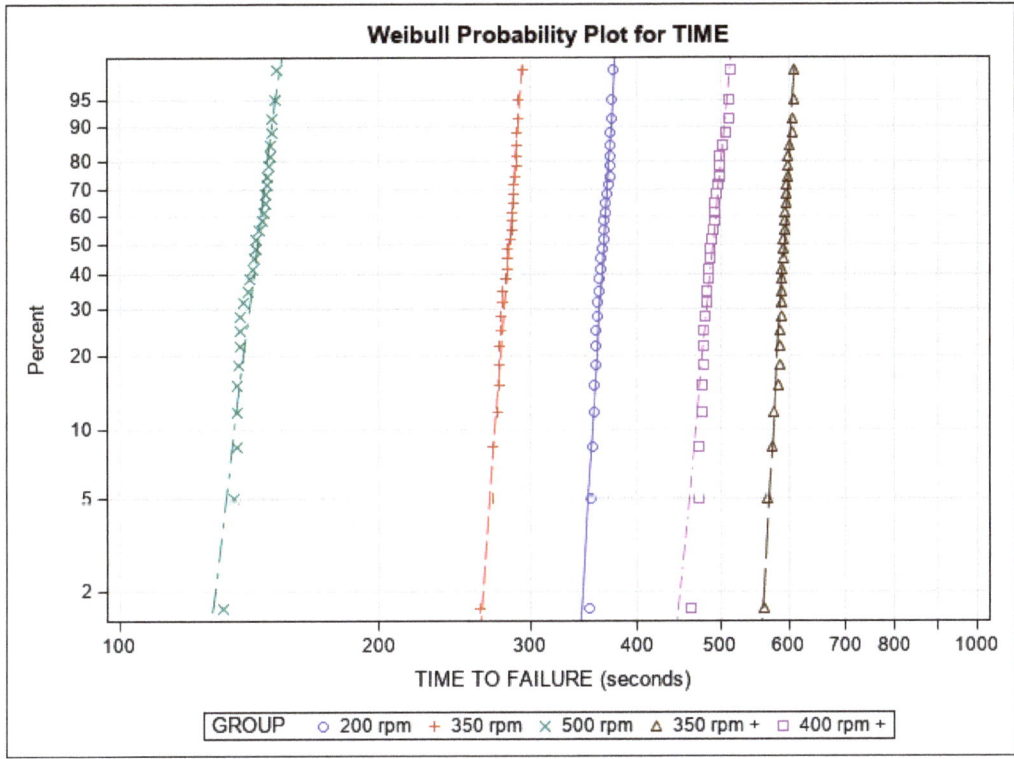

Figure 5. Weibull probability plot displaying time to failure across study groups.

4. Discussion

The findings of the present study do not accept the null hypothesis (H_0), which postulates that rotational speed does not affect the dynamic fatigue resistance of NiTi alloy endodontic rotary files.

The present study used the same NiTi alloy endodontic instruments in rotary and reciprocating kinematic motion since the manufacturer reported that the geometrical design of the NiTi alloy endodontic files allows for its use in both kinematic movements; therefore, manufacturers recommend its use with both continuous and reciprocating rotations. Furthermore, other instrumentation systems can be used with continuous or reciprocating rotation, and it is necessary to have a motor in which the angles can be adjusted. Clear examples can be found in the studies of Yared 2008 [22] and De Deus 2010 [17], where they used instruments that cut clockwise in a reciprocating mode.

Previous studies have analyzed the effects of rotational speed on the number of cycles to fracture of rotary NiTi instruments. Lopes et al. subjected ProTaper Universal instruments F3 and F4 to 300 and 600 rpm; however, the speed values selected were too distant, a cylindrical tube was used as the artificial root canal, and the fracture detection of the NiTi alloy endodontic rotary files was subjective and therefore imprecise. Furthermore, they did not carry out any additional measurement methods [23]. Additionally, some reviews have been conducted with the aim of analyzing the mechanical and metallurgical behavior of endodontic instruments under different testing conditions and methodologies [24–26].

The results derived from the present study indicate that the resistance of NiTi alloy endodontic rotary files to cyclic fatigue is inversely proportional to the rotational speed. In addition, reciprocating movements were shown to be more resistant to cyclic fatigue when compared with continuous rotational movements. Moreover, the results derived from the present study present a direct application to the clinical setting, since the reciprocating systems provided higher resistance to cyclic fatigue, followed by the lower values of rotational speed. Therefore, clinicians should choose reciprocating motion systems or reduce the rotational speed of the endodontic torque-controlled motor if the NiTi endodontic rotary or reciprocating file is expected to experience high cyclic fatigue, particularly in root canal systems with a pronounced angle and/or curvature radius.

Specification #28 of the American Dental Association/American National Standards Institute (ADA/ANSI) outlines tests used to measure how flexible stainless steel hand files are, as well as their strength under torsion. These same tests were also adopted under ISO 3630/1, which is meant for instruments with a 0.02 ISO taper. Currently, there are still no specifications or international standards with regard to testing the resistance of endodontic rotary instruments to cyclic fatigue [27]. The ideal model would entail curved canals being instrumented in natural teeth. That being said, each tooth can only be used once with these tests, and instrumentation causes changes to the shape of the root canal, rendering it impossible to establish standardized experimental conditions. Therefore, various methods and devices have been used to analyze the in vitro resistance of NiTi rotary endodontic instruments to cyclic fatigue fractures [28]. Cyclic fatigue is considered a dynamic event itself since the movement of the NiTi alloy endodontic rotary or reciprocating instruments inside the root canal system gives it dynamism. Cyclic fatigue tests have been carried out in a static model under well-controlled experimental conditions; however, the novel pecking movement of the endodontic handpiece of the present cyclic fatigue device provides an additional dynamic movement more representative of the in-and-out motion made by the operator. That being said, studies have shown that the number of cycles to failure is significantly higher in the dynamic model, regardless of the brand or manufacturing processes [29–31]. In the static testing model, there is no up-and-down movement applied to the instrument, causing stresses to accumulate at a fixed point. With the dynamic model, however, these stresses are spread out along the full length of the instrument, thereby increasing its cyclic fatigue resistance [23]. Furthermore, researchers have found that the up-and-down motion should not exceed 1, 2, or 3 mm/s in the dynamic testing model so as to simulate clinical conditions [24]. An automatic detection system can be used to identify the precise point of failure of endodontic rotary files [19]. Given this, the present study used an anatomically based artificial root canal design in accordance with Schneider's method [20], using a 60° curvature angle and radius of 5 mm, and modifying the geometry to adapt to the NiTi endodontic rotary files used in this study [11].

The findings of this study corroborate the findings of Kim et al., who found that the Reciproc R25 and WaveOne Primary heat-treated NiTi alloy endodontic reciprocating files were more resistant to torsion and cyclic fatigue when compared with ProTaper F2 NiTi alloy endodontic rotary files used under continuous rotation [32]. Similarly, De Deus et al. found that the ProTaper F2 NiTi alloy endodontic rotary file also exhibited significantly greater resistance to cyclic fatigue when employed using reciprocating movement rather than continuous rotational motion [17]. Furthermore, several other studies have emphasized the increase in the lifespan of NiTi alloy endodontic rotary files when using reciprocating movement as opposed to continuous rotational motion [33,34]. That being said, there are several studies that have analyzed the impact of rotational speed on how resistant NiTi alloy endodontic rotary files are to cyclic fatigue, although the findings remain controversial. Lopes et al. found that the ProFile NiTi alloy endodontic rotary instrument exhibited greater susceptibility to accidental fracture at higher rotational speeds, and they found that the total number of cycles to failure was about 30% lower in ProTaper instruments when the rotational speed was increased from 300 to 600 rpm [23]. On the other hand, Martin et al. reported that unexpected fracture of NiTi alloy endodontic rotary instruments was correlated with the rotational speed, as the ProTaper NiTi alloy endodontic rotary instrument was more susceptible to fracture at 350 rpm than at 250 or 150 rpm [16]. However, Gao et al. reported no statistically significant differences ($p > 0.05$) between files that had similar NiTi alloys and apical diameters when used at different rotational speeds [35]. The discrepancies in these findings may be due to differing study designs, NiTi alloys, or geometrical designs of the instruments under study. Additionally, not only the asymmetric oscillatory counterclockwise motion (reciprocation motion) but also the asymmetric oscillatory clockwise motion can be used with any rotary instrument. Martins et al. evaluated the cyclic fatigue resistance of three replicate rotary instruments compared with their original brand systems using continuous rotation and optimum torque reverse kinematics. They reported that reciprocating files showed greater resistance to cyclic fatigue than continuous rotation files, and the replicas showed higher cyclic fatigue resistance than the original brand instruments and higher transition temperatures to the austenitic phase [36].

The results found by Ray et al. were corroborated by those obtained in the present study using an analysis of dynamic cyclic fatigue when employing a standardized axial movement, increasing the durability of NiTi alloy endodontic rotary instruments subjected to cyclic fatigue in comparison with the results observed in static cyclic fatigue devices [37]. Most studies comparing dynamic and static cyclic fatigue appliances have concluded endodontic rotary instruments exhibited a time to fracture roughly 20–40% longer when undergoing dynamic cyclic fatigue than the time to fracture found in studies of static cyclic fatigue, with this also being more similar to the clinical setting [38–40].

The cyclic fatigue testing was performed in a room temperature setting, according to the results by La Rosa et al., who showed that studies at body temperature impaired the cyclic fatigue resistance of most files [41]. In addition, Plotino et al. reported that the surrounding temperature affected the NiTi crystalline phase transformation, significantly decreasing the cyclic fatigue resistance at body temperature [42].

Regrettably, the limitations of this study precluded analyzing any additional kinematic movements, under both reciprocating and continuous rotation movements. Future studies ought to include more NiTi alloys, apical diameters, pitch, helix angles, manufacturing processes, and tapers. Furthermore, due to difficulties with the standardization of samples, the present study was not conducted in a clinical setting. However, the present study provided multimethod research, including SEM, EDX, and an accurate dynamic cyclic fatigue device, increasing the knowledge of the mechanical behavior of NiTi endodontic rotary files under different kinematic conditions.

5. Conclusions

NiTi alloy endodontic rotary files used with a reciprocating movement at 350 rpm with 120° counterclockwise and 30° clockwise motion were more resistant to dynamic cyclic fatigue than those used with a reciprocating movement at 400 rpm with 120° counterclockwise and 30° clockwise motion, continuous rotational speed at 200 rpm, continuous rotational speed at 350 rpm, and continuous rotational speed at 500 rpm. It is therefore advisable to use reciprocating movements at a low speed.

Author Contributions: Conceptualization, V.F.-M., S.J.-V.; data acquisition, V.F.-L.; design, I.F.-M.; review and editing, B.M.-B.; Formal analysis, C.R.-S.; all statistical analyses, Á.Z.-M. All authors have read and agreed to the published version of the manuscript.

Funding: This research did not receive any external funding.

Institutional Review Board Statement: Not applicable.

Informed Consent Statement: Not applicable.

Data Availability Statement: Information available upon request, subject to relevant restrictions (such as privacy or ethical).

Conflicts of Interest: The authors declare no conflict of interest.

References

1. Siqueira, J.F., Jr.; Rôças, I.N.; Ricucci, D.; Hülsmann, M. Causes and management of post-treatment apical periodontitis. *Br. Dent. J.* **2014**, *216*, 305–312. [CrossRef] [PubMed]
2. Bergmans, L.; Van Cleynenbreugel, J.; Wevers, M.; Lambrechts, P. Mechanical root canal preparation with NiTi rotary instruments: Rationale, performance and safety. Status report for the American Journal of Dentistry. *Am. J. Dent.* **2001**, *14*, 324–333.
3. Sattapan, B.; Nervo, G.J.; Palamara, J.E.; Messer, H.H. Defects in rotary nickel-titanium files after clinical use. *J. Endod.* **2000**, *26*, 161–165. [CrossRef] [PubMed]
4. Peters, O.A.; Barbakow, F. Dynamic torque and apical forces of ProFile.04 rotary instruments during preparation of curved canals. *Int. Endod. J.* **2002**, *35*, 379–389. [CrossRef]
5. Varghese, N.O.; Pillai, R.; Sujathen, U.N.; Sainudeen, S.; Antony, A.; Paul, S. Resistance to torsional failure and cyclic fatigue resistance of ProTaper Next, WaveOne, and Mtwo files in continuous and reciprocating motion: An in vitro study. *J. Conserv. Dent.* **2016**, *19*, 225–230. [CrossRef] [PubMed]
6. Kuhn, G.; Tavernier, B.; Jordan, L. Influence of structure on nickel-titanium endodontic instruments failure. *J. Endod.* **2001**, *27*, 516–520. [CrossRef]
7. Cheung, G.S. Instrument fracture: Mechanisms, removal of fragments, and clinical outcomes. *Endod. Top.* **2007**, *16*, 1–26. [CrossRef]
8. Pruett, J.P.; Clement, D.J.; Carnes, D.L., Jr. Cyclic fatigue testing of nickel-titanium endodontic instruments. *J. Endod.* **1997**, *23*, 77–85. [CrossRef]
9. Sjogren, U.; Hagglund, B.; Sundqvist, G.; Wing, K. Factors affecting the long-term results of endodontic treatment. *J. Endod.* **1990**, *16*, 498–504. [CrossRef]
10. Faus-Llácer, V.; Hamoud-Kharrat, N.; Marhuenda Ramos, M.T.; Faus-Matoses, I.; Zubizarreta-Macho, Á.; Ruiz Sánchez, C.; Faus-Matoses, V. Influence of the Geometrical Cross-Section Design on the Dynamic Cyclic Fatigue Resistance of NiTi Endodontic Rotary Files-An In Vitro Study. *J. Clin. Med.* **2021**, *10*, 4713. [CrossRef]
11. Faus-Llácer, V.; Kharrat, N.H.; Ruiz-Sánchez, C.; Faus-Matoses, I.; Zubizarreta-Macho, Á.; Faus-Matoses, V. The Effect of Taper and Apical Diameter on the Cyclic Fatigue Resistance of Rotary Endodontic Files Using an Experimental Electronic Device. *Appl. Sci.* **2021**, *11*, 863. [CrossRef]
12. Kwak, S.W.; Ha, J.H.; Lee, C.J.; El Abed, R.; Abu-Tahun, I.H.; Kim, H.C. Effects of Pitch Length and Heat Treatment on the Mechanical Properties of the Glide Path Preparation Instruments. *J. Endod.* **2016**, *42*, 788–792. [CrossRef]
13. Gambarini, G. Cyclic fatigue of nickel-titanium rotary instruments after clinical use with low- and high-torque endodontic motors. *J. Endod.* **2001**, *27*, 772–774. [CrossRef]
14. Gutmann, J.L.; Gao, Y. Alteration in the inherent metallic and surface properties of nickel-titanium root canal instruments to enhance performance, durability and safety: A focused review. *Int. Endod. J.* **2012**, *45*, 113–128. [CrossRef] [PubMed]
15. Yared, G.M.; Bou Dagher, F.E.; Machtou, P. Cyclic fatigue of Profile rotary instruments after simulated clinical use. *Int. Endod. J.* **1999**, *32*, 115–119. [CrossRef] [PubMed]
16. Martín, B.; Zelada, G.; Varela, P.; Bahillo, J.G.; Magán, F.; Ahn, S.; Rodríguez, C. Factors influencing the fracture of nickel-titanium rotary instruments. *Int. Endod. J.* **2003**, *36*, 262–266. [CrossRef]
17. De-Deus, G.; Moreira, E.J.; Lopes, H.P.; Elias, C.N. Extended cyclic fatigue life of F2 ProTaper instruments used in reciprocating movement. *Int. Endod. J.* **2010**, *43*, 1063–1068. [CrossRef]
18. Pedullà, E.; Grande, N.M.; Plotino, G.; Gambarini, G.; Rapisarda, E. Influence of continuous or reciprocating motion on cyclic fatigue resistance of 4 different nickel-titanium rotary instruments. *J. Endod.* **2013**, *39*, 258–261. [CrossRef]
19. Martins, J.N.R.; Silva, E.J.N.L.; Marques, D.; Belladonna, F.; Simões-Carvalho, M.; Vieira, V.T.L.; Antunes, H.S.; Braz Fernandes, F.M.B.; Versiani, M.A. Design, metallurgical features, mechanical performance and canal preparation of six reciprocating instruments. *Int. Endod. J.* **2021**, *54*, 1623–1637. [CrossRef]
20. Zubizarreta-Macho, A.; Mena Álvarez, J.; Albadalejo Martínez, A.; Segura-Egea, J.J.; Caviedes Brucheli, J.; Agustín-Panadero, R.; López Píriz, R.; Alonso-Ezpeleta, O. Influence of the pecking motion on the cyclic fatigue resistance of endodontic rotary files. *J. Clin. Med.* **2020**, *9*, 45. [CrossRef]
21. Schneider, S.W. A comparison of canal preparations in straight and curved root canals. *Oral Surg. Oral Med. Oral Pathol.* **1971**, *32*, 271–275. [CrossRef]
22. Yared, G. Canal preparation using only one Ni-Ti rotary instrument: Preliminary observations. *Int. Endod. J.* **2008**, *41*, 339–344. [CrossRef]
23. Lopes, H.P.; Ferreira, A.A.; Elias, C.N.; Moreira, E.J.; de Oliveira, J.C.; Siqueira, J.F., Jr. Influence of rotational speed on the cyclic fatigue of rotary nickel-titanium endodontic instruments. *J. Endod.* **2009**, *35*, 1013–1016. [CrossRef]
24. Zanza, A.; D'Angelo, M.; Reda, R.; Gambarini, G.; Testarelli, L.; Di Nardo, D. An Update on Nickel-Titanium Rotary Instruments in Endodontics: Mechanical Characteristics, Testing and Future Perspective-An Overview. *Bioengineering* **2021**, *16*, 218. [CrossRef]
25. Schäfer, E.; Bürklein, S.; Donnermeyer, D. A critical analysis of research methods and experimental models to study the physical properties of NiTi instruments and their fracture characteristics. *Int. Endod. J.* **2022**, *55*, 72–94. [CrossRef]
26. Ferreira, F.; Adeodato, C.; Barbosa, I.; Aboud, L.; Scelza, P.; Zaccaro Scelza, M. Movement kinematics and cyclic fatigue of NiTi rotary instruments: A systematic review. *Int. Endod. J.* **2017**, *50*, 143–152. [CrossRef]

27. ANSI/ADA Specification N° 28-2002. *Root Canal Files and Reamers, Type K for Hand Use*; American Dental Association: Chicago, IL, USA, 2002.
28. Plotino, G.; Grande, N.M.; Cordaro, M.; Testarelli, L.; Gambarini, G. A review of cyclic fatigue testing of nickel-titanium rotary instruments. *J. Endod.* **2009**, *35*, 1469–1476. [CrossRef]
29. Rodrigues, R.C.; Lopes, H.P.; Elias, C.N.; Amaral, G.; Vieira, V.T.; De Martin, A.S. Influence of different manufacturing methods on the cyclic fatigue of rotary nickel-titanium endodontic instruments. *J. Endod.* **2011**, *37*, 1553–1557. [CrossRef]
30. Li, U.M.; Lee, B.S.; Shih, C.T.; Lan, W.H.; Lin, C.P. Cyclic fatigue of endodontic nickel titanium rotary instruments: Static and dynamic tests. *J. Endod.* **2002**, *28*, 448–451. [CrossRef]
31. Lopes, H.P.; Elias, C.N.; Vieira, M.V.; Siqueira, J.F., Jr.; Mangelli, M.; Lopes, W.S.; Vieira, V.T.; Alves, F.R.; Oliveira, J.C.; Soares, T.G. Fatigue Life of Reciproc and Mtwo instruments subjected to static and dynamic tests. *J. Endod.* **2013**, *39*, 693–696. [CrossRef]
32. Kim, H.C.; Kwak, S.W.; Cheung, G.S.; Ko, D.H.; Chung, S.M.; Lee, W. Cyclic fatigue and torsional resistance of two new nickel-titanium instruments used in reciprocation motion: Reciproc versus WaveOne. *J. Endod.* **2012**, *38*, 541–544. [CrossRef]
33. Varela-Patiño, P.; Ibañez-Párraga, A.; Rivas-Mundiña, B.; Cantatore, G.; Otero, X.L.; Martin-Biedma, B. Alternating versus continuous rotation: A comparative study of the effect on instrument life. *J. Endod.* **2010**, *36*, 157–159. [CrossRef]
34. You, S.Y.; Bae, K.S.; Baek, S.H.; Kum, K.Y.; Shon, W.J.; Lee, W. Lifespan of one nickel-titanium rotary file with reciprocating motion in curved root canals. *J. Endod.* **2010**, *36*, 1991–1994. [CrossRef]
35. Gao, Y.; Shotton, V.; Wilkinson, K.; Phillips, G.; Johnson, W.B. Effects of raw material and rotational speed on the cyclic fatigue of ProFile Vortex rotary instruments. *J. Endod.* **2010**, *36*, 1205–1209. [CrossRef]
36. Martins, J.N.R.; Nogueira Leal Silva, E.J.; Marques, D.; Ginjeira, A.; Braz Fernandes, F.M.; De Deus, G.; Versiani, M.A. Influence of Kinematics on the Cyclic Fatigue Resistance of Replicalike and Original Brand Rotary Instruments. *J. Endod.* **2020**, *46*, 1136–1143. [CrossRef]
37. Ray, J.J.; Kirkpatrick, T.C.; Rutledge, R.E. Cyclic fatigue of EndoSequence and K3 rotary files in a dynamic model. *J. Endod.* **2007**, *33*, 1469–1472. [CrossRef]
38. Gambarini, G.; Galli, M.; Di Nardo, D.; Seracchiani, M.; Donfrancesco, O.; Testarelli, L. Differences in cyclic fatigue lifespan between two different heat treated NiTi endodontic rotary instruments: WaveOne Gold vs. *EdgeOne Fire. J. Clin. Exp. Dent.* **2019**, *11*, e609–e613. [CrossRef]
39. Lopes, H.P.; Britto, I.M.; Elias, C.N.; Machado de Oliveira, J.C.; Neves, M.A.; Moreira, E.J.; Siqueira, J.F., Jr. Cyclic fatigue resistance of ProTaper Universal instruments when subjected to static and dynamic tests. *Oral Surg. Oral Med. Oral Pathol. Oral Radiol. Endod.* **2010**, *110*, 401–404. [CrossRef]
40. De-Deus, G.; Leal Vieira, V.T.; Nogueira da Silva, E.J.; Lopes, H.; Elias, C.N.; Moreira, E.J. Bending resistance and dynamic and static cyclic fatigue life of Reciproc and WaveOne large instruments. *J. Endod.* **2014**, *40*, 575–579. [CrossRef]
41. La Rosa, G.R.M.; Shumakova, V.; Isola, G.; Indelicato, F.; Bugea, C.; Pedullà, E. Evaluation of the Cyclic Fatigue of Two Single Files at Body and Room Temperature with Different Radii of Curvature. *Materials* **2021**, *14*, 2256. [CrossRef]
42. Plotino, G.; Grande, N.M.; Mercadé Bellido, M.; Testarelli, L.; Gambarini, G. Influence of Temperature on Cyclic Fatigue Resistance of ProTaper Gold and ProTaper Universal Rotary Files. *J. Endod.* **2017**, *43*, 200–202. [CrossRef] [PubMed]

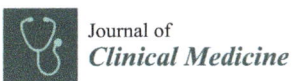

Article

Influence of Cross-Section and Pitch on the Mechanical Response of NiTi Endodontic Files under Bending and Torsional Conditions—A Finite Element Analysis

Victor Roda-Casanova [1], Antonio Pérez-González [1], Alvaro Zubizarreta-Macho [2,3,*] and Vicente Faus-Matoses [4]

[1] Department of Mechanical Engineering and Construction, Universitat Jaume I, 12071 Castelló de la Plana, Spain; vroda@uji.es (V.R.-C.); aperez@uji.es (A.P.-G.)
[2] Department of Dentistry, Alfonso X el Sabio University, 28691 Madrid, Spain
[3] Department of Orthodontics, University of Salamanca, 37008 Salamanca, Spain
[4] Department of Stomatology, Faculty of Medicine and Dentistry, University of Valencia, 46010 Valencia, Spain; vfaus@clinicafaus.com
* Correspondence: amacho@uax.es

Abstract: In this article, the effects of cross-section and pitch on the mechanical response of NiTi endodontic files is studied by means of finite element analyses. The study was conducted over a set of eight endodontic rotary files, whose geometry was obtained from combinations of two cross-sections (square and triangular) and four pitches. Each file was subjected to bending and torsional analyses, simulating the testing conditions indicated in the ISO 3630 Standard, in order to assess their stiffness and mechanical strength. The results indicate that endodontic files with a square cross-section have double the stiffness of those with triangular cross-sections, both in terms of bending and torsion. For both loading modes, endodontic files with a triangular cross-section can undergo larger deformations before overload failure than those with a square cross-section: up to 20% more in bending and 40% in torsion. Moreover, under equivalent boundary conditions, endodontic files with triangular cross-sections present a higher fatigue life than those with square cross-sections: up to more than 300% higher for small pitches. The effect of pitch on the stiffness and strength of the file is smaller than that of the cross-section shape, but smaller pitches could be beneficial when using a triangular cross-section, as they increase the bending flexibility, fatigue life, and torsion stiffness. These results suggest a clinical recommendation for the use of files with a triangular-shaped cross-section and a small pitch in order to minimize ledging and maximize fatigue life. Finally, in this study, we reveal the sensitivity of the orientation of files with respect to the bending direction, which must be taken into account when designing, reporting, and interpreting test results under such loading conditions.

Keywords: endodontic file; cross-section; pitch; flexural bending; torsion; stress distribution; finite element analysis

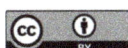

1. Introduction

The introduction of nickel–titanium alloy (NiTi) for the manufacturing of root canal instruments entailed a great revolution in the field of endodontics, as the consequent endodontic files decreased the incidence of iatrogenic complications [1,2]. However, despite the continuous mechanical and chemical improvements made by manufacturers, the failure of endodontic files during root canal treatments remains a concern for clinicians [3], as the incidence of their fracture still ranges from 0.09% to 5% [4,5].

The fracture of rotary instruments occurs mainly due to two different mechanisms, usually referred to as torsion overload and flexural fatigue [6,7]. On one hand, the torsion overload failure mechanism corresponds to a static failure that typically occurs when the tip of the endodontic file becomes blocked in the root canal whilst the instrument continues rotating [8]. In static failure, the file fails because the stress value reaches the elastic limit of the material, such that the file undergoes permanent deformation and finally fractures. On the other hand, flexural fatigue is a failure mechanism produced mainly by the alternating compressive and tensile stresses and strains that appear in any point of a file rotating inside a curved root canal [8,9]. This type of fatigue failure results in a sudden fracture of the file after a certain number of rotations, even if the stress levels are far below the elastic limit of the material, due to the nucleation and progression of small cracks in some stressed sections of the file. Thus, bending and torsion are essential conditions to evaluate the mechanical behavior of endodontic instruments [10]. The unexpected failure of NiTi endodontic files may condition the outcome of the root canal treatment by blocking the advancement of disinfecting agents beyond the fractured instrument [11–13], which may lead to subsequent pulp necrosis and the formation of periapical lesions [14], or decrease the success rate of root canal treatment of teeth with periapical pathology [15]. In addition, extraction of the fractured NiTi endodontic rotary file from the root canal system requires root dentin removal to provide access to the fractured instruments [16]. This causes a loss of dentin tissue, which can negatively affect the structural integrity of the tooth [17]. Furthermore, it can lead to root perforation and increase the risk of vertical root fracture, especially in the apical third [16]. For these reasons, a better understanding of the independent and combined effects of the different parameters that affect these failure mechanisms is desirable, and additional research must be addressed to this end.

Several works have been conducted to analyze the influence of both the NiTi alloy [18] and the geometrical parameters on the torsional and bending resistance of endodontic instruments. Both the chemical composition and crystalline structure of the NiTi alloy have been studied, and it has been shown that they highly influence the strength of the endodontic file [19]. In particular, endodontic rotary systems with a higher concentration of the martensitic phase and manufactured using electropolishing, ion implantation, cryogenic treatment, and heat treatments improve the mechanical behavior of NiTi endodontic rotary files, increasing their cyclic fatigue resistance. The geometric parameters of the endodontic files have also been reported to influence the instrument's performance, including the taper and apical diameter [20], cross-section design [21,22], flute length, helix angle, and pitch [23]. The influence of these variables has been analyzed using static and dynamic custom-made cyclic fatigue testing devices, which have not been submitted to a standardization normative, and do not allow for independently assessing the influence of each geometric parameter associated with flexural fatigue or torsional overload. There are other standardized testing devices, such as those described in ISO 3630-1:2008 [24], which allow for the independent assessment of both torsional and bending phenomena, although their capability to reproduce the actual operating conditions of endodontic files has not yet been verified.

Computer simulation has proven to be an interesting tool for studying the failure of endodontic rotary files. In the simplest cases, analytical methods can be used for such a purpose, which are usually based on the small strain theory of elasticity. In this line, Zhang et al. [25] have analyzed the mechanical behavior of NiTi endodontic files under torsional and bending loads. Tsao et al. [26] have developed analytical models to study the flexibility of NiTi instruments subjected to bending loads. These analytical models have the advantage of being fast and easy to implement, but their capabilities to consider non-linear behaviors (i.e., material non-linearity) or complex loading scenarios are limited. These limitations can be overcome by using numerical methods such as the finite element method.

The ability of the finite element method to reproduce the results obtained from experimental tests using endodontic rotary files has been proven in several works [7,10,27–29], whose main conclusions have been summarized in a recent bibliographical review [30]. This review concluded that the finite element method is a reliable tool for evaluating the behavior of NiTi rotary instruments, and has the advantage of reducing instrument development time and costs. Another important advantage of the finite element method is that it also allows us to assess aspects of the mechanical behavior of the instruments, such as the stress distribution, which are difficult to obtain in laboratory tests [10]. The finite element method has been previously used to analyze the influence of cross-section design and pitch on the stiffness and stress distribution under bending and torsional conditions [10,31–37]. Appendix B collects detailed information about these previous studies, including their main conclusions and limitations. Some of these studies have used proprietary file models, such as ProTaper, ProFile, Mtwo, and others, which hampers the independent evaluation of parameters such as cross-section geometry, cross-section area, or pitch [10,32–35]. Other studies have used theoretical file models to avoid this problem, but with some limitations; for example, in [36], the authors analyzed four different cross-sections and three pitch values under torsion, but did not provide detailed information about the material model for the shape memory alloy (SMA) of the files or about the quality of the finite element mesh. In another study, Versluis et al. [33] analyzed the effects of pitch and cross-section geometry on flexural stiffness and stresses using a representative SMA material model. However, the boundary conditions were specified differently to those in ISO 3630-1:2008 [24] and the bending applied was low, leading to maximum von Mises stresses below the initial stress for transformation from austenite to martensite, and, thus, the effect of the super-elasticity of the files was not analyzed; furthermore, torsion behavior was not included in the study. In [37], the effect of cross-section geometry and pitch on the 'screw-in' tendency of the files was analyzed, but a linear material model was used for the file. A more recent study investigated different geometric options for the sides of a triangle shaped cross section (straight, convex, and concave), as well as the use of files with combinations of these geometries along the file [31], but the pitch effect was not analyzed.

Some of these finite element models are limited in their accuracy, in terms of representing the correct geometry and boundary conditions of the endodontic files, or use simplified material models that are incapable of representing their actual mechanical response under load. In this study, we address all of these partial limitations of previous studies by undertaking a comprehensive analysis of the effects of pitch and cross-section using an accurate finite element model that allows us to simulate the testing conditions of the ISO3630 Standard to the best extent possible. The method used to obtain the parametric geometrical representation of the endodontic instrument and the corresponding finite element mesh has been proposed in our previous work [38]. The use of an accurate numerical model in these tests can foster improvements in new generations of more resistant and flexible endodontic files, reducing the need for expensive and time-consuming experiments in the early design stages. From a clinical perspective, these improvements are expected to reduce the risk of failure of endodontic instruments, thus preventing clinical complications.

The aim of this study was to analyze and compare the effects of the cross-section and the pitch on the mechanical response (in terms of strength and stiffness) of NiTi endodontic files under bending and torsional conditions, similar to those indicated in the ISO 3630 Standard [24], using the finite element method. The study was conducted using a set of eight different endodontic rotary files whose geometries were obtained from combinations of two cross-sections (triangular and square) and four pitches (1 mm, 2 mm, 4 mm, and 8 mm). Under these conditions, the following individual objectives were pursued: (i) to develop a finite element model which reproduces the experimental tests conducted in the ISO 3630 Standard; (ii) to conduct a bending analysis of the selected endodontic rotary files, in order to predict the stiffness and strength of the files under static and cyclic loading conditions; and (iii) to conduct a torsional analysis of the selected endodontic rotary files, in order to predict the stiffness and the strength of the files under static loading conditions.

2. Materials and Methods

For this study, different endodontic instruments were analyzed using numerical simulation with finite elements. Figure 1 shows the geometries of the eight endodontic files considered. The different geometries were obtained by varying the cross-section (square and triangular) and the pitch ($p_z = \{1\,\text{mm}, 2\,\text{mm}, 4\,\text{mm}, 8\,\text{mm}\}$) of the files. All of them had a total length of $L_{total} = 25$ mm, the length of their active part was $L_a = 16$ mm, and their tip and shaft diameters were $d_a = 0.25$ mm and $d_{sh} = 1.20$ mm, respectively. The taper of the endodontic files was 6%.

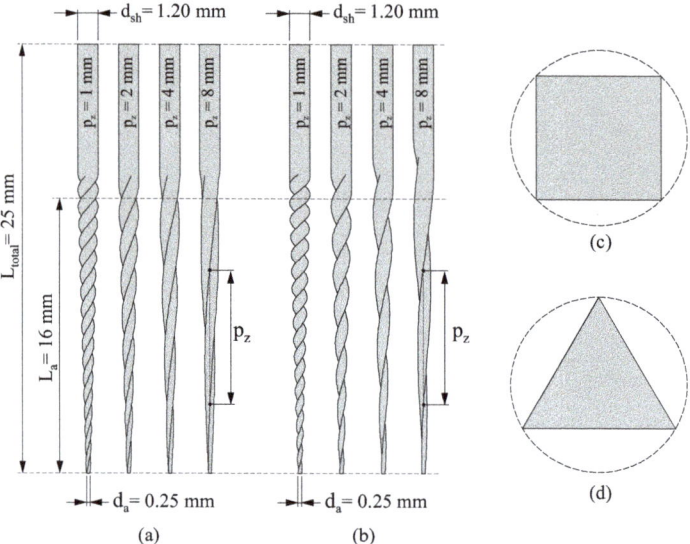

Figure 1. Geometries of the analyzed endodontic files: endodontic files with square cross-section (**a**); endodontic files with triangular cross-section (**b**); normalized square cross-section (**c**); and normalized triangular cross-section (**d**).

The material for all the files was considered to be NiTi, which exhibits a super-elastic stress–strain curve, as shown in Figure 2. Here, E_A and E_M represent the Young's moduli of austenite and martensite, respectively. The beginning and end of the loading phase transformation are denoted by σ_L^S and σ_L^E, respectively, whereas the beginning and the end of the unloading transformation phase are denoted by σ_U^S and σ_U^E. Finally, ε_L represents the uni-axial transformation strain, and σ_{ME}^E indicates the end of the martensitic elastic regime.

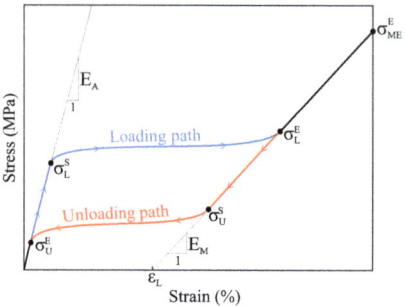

Figure 2. Sample stress–strain curve for NiTi material.

2.1. Devices for Experimental Bending and Torsion Analysis

Endodontic files are usually tested in terms of bending and torsional loads, and the typical standardized procedure for these tests has been described in the ISO 3630 Standard [24], as summarized in Figure 3. For the torsion analysis (Figure 3a), the last 3 mm at the tip of the endodontic file are inserted inside a clamping jaw. After checking that the endodontic file is properly fixed and aligned with the axis of rotation, the top of the file is rigidly connected to the torsion device. This torsion device is increasingly rotated at angle θ_z, and the torsional moment M_z is measured using a torquemeter attached to the clamping jaw. The test ends with the failure of the endodontic file. At this point, the maximum rotated angle $\theta_{z,max}$ and maximum torsional moment $M_{z,max}$ are registered.

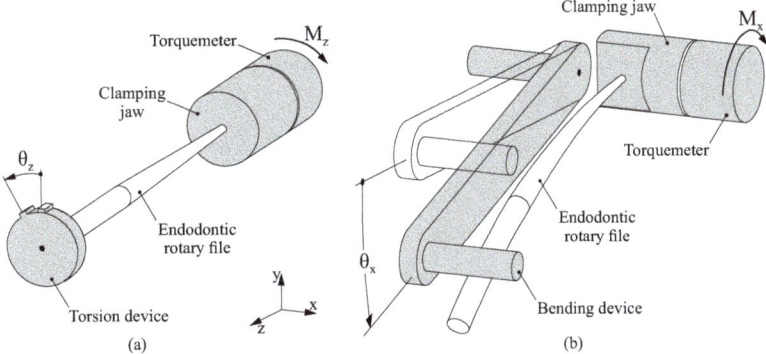

Figure 3. Devices used for torsion (**a**) and bending (**b**) analyses.

In a similar way, in the bending analysis (Figure 3b), the last 3 mm at the tip of the endodontic file are inserted inside a clamping jaw. After checking that the endodontic file is properly fixed and aligned with the axis of rotation, the bending device is positioned until it contacts the endodontic file. Then, the bending device is increasingly rotated at angle θ_x, and the bending moment M_x is measured using a torquemeter attached to the clamping jaw. The test ends with the failure of the endodontic file. At this point, the maximum rotated angle $\theta_{x,max}$ and maximum bending moment $M_{x,max}$ are registered.

2.2. Definition of the Finite Element Model for the NiTi Endodontic File

Figure 4 shows an example of the finite element model created for the endodontic file simulation experiments, as described in Section 2.1. Here, only the portion of the endodontic file subjected to stresses and strains was considered in the analysis (i.e., the part of the endodontic file inserted into the clamping jaw was not included in the finite element model). The geometry of the endodontic file was generated and then discretized into quadratic finite element tetrahedrons following the meshing procedure developed in our previous work [38]. Using this procedure, the finite element mesh of a endodontic file was automatically built from its geometrical parameters (d_{sh}, d_a, L_a, L_{total}, and p_z, as shown in Figure 1) and the average element size.

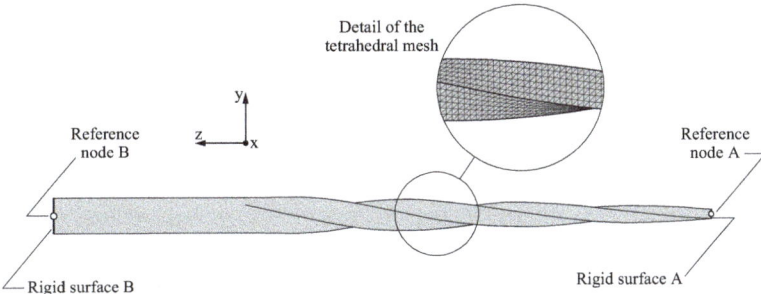

Figure 4. Definition of the finite element model.

To select the average element size, a mesh sensitivity study was conducted in our previous work [38] for a finite element model of an endodontic file with similar geometry, element type, boundary, and loading conditions, as described in Figure 4. In this study, the variations in the maximum element energy error and energy norm error with respect to the average element size were observed, and it was concluded that an average element size equal to 0.1 mm provided a good compromise between accuracy and computational cost. For these reasons, this average element size was used to perform this study, resulting in a finite element model with 89,295 nodes and 58,749 elements.

The super-elastic behavior of the NiTi alloy used to manufacture the endodontic files was modeled using the material model developed by Auricchio [39]. The material properties that characterize this material model were extracted from [10], and are shown in Table 1.

Table 1. Material properties to characterize the super-elastic behavior of NiTi alloy. Reprinted/adapted with permission from Ref. [10]. 2014, Elsevier.

Parameter	Variable	Magnitude
Young's modulus of austenite	E_A	42,530 MPa
Austenite Poisson's ratio	ν_A	0.33
Young's modulus of martensite	E_M	12,828 MPa
Martensite Poisson's ratio	ν_M	0.33
Uni-axial transformation strain	ε_L	6%
Slope of the stress–temperature curve for loading	$(\delta\sigma/\delta T)_L$	6.7
Start of transformation loading	σ_L^S	492 MPa
End of transformation loading	σ_L^E	630 MPa
Reference temperature	T_0	22 °C
Slope of the stress–temperature curve for unloading	$(\delta\sigma/\delta T)_U$	6.7
Start of transformation unloading	σ_U^S	192 MPa
End of transformation unloading	σ_U^E	97 MPa
End of martensitic elastic regime	σ_{ME}^E	1200 MPa

The surface at the fixed end of the endodontic file was defined as a rigid surface (denoted as rigid surface A in Figure 4). This rigid surface was rigidly connected to reference node A, which was used to introduce the boundary conditions for the finite element model. To simulate the effect of the clamping jaw over the endodontic file, all of the degrees of freedom of reference node A were restricted. At the other side of the file, the top surface was also defined as a rigid surface (denoted as rigid surface B in Figure 4). This rigid surface was rigidly connected to reference node B, which was used to define the loading conditions of the model. Two different loading conditions were considered in the analyses, one for the bending analysis and the other for the torsional analysis:

- In the bending analysis, an increasing displacement was imposed at reference node B in the negative direction of the y-axis, until the maximum von Mises stress along the endodontic file σ_{max} reached the end of the martensitic elastic regime. As the results of the bending analyses are sensitive to the orientation of the endodontic file with respect to the bending direction, the analysis was conducted in 24 different angular positions, given by a rotation $\varphi_z = \{0°, 15°, 30°, \ldots, 360°\}$ of the endodontic file with respect to the z-axis.
- In the torsional analysis, an increasing rotation was imposed at reference node B along the positive direction of z-axis, until the maximum von Mises stress along the endodontic file σ_{max} reached the end of the martensitic elastic regime. Here, the results of the analysis do not depend on the orientation of the file.

The finite element model was solved through transient analysis using the large displacements formulation, which was conducted using the ABAQUS software. Hence, material and geometric non-linearities were considered in the study. In each one of these analyses, the rotation at reference node B (θ_x for bending analysis and θ_z for torsional analysis) and the reaction moment at reference node A (M_x for bending analysis and M_z for torsional analysis) were registered for each analysis frame. The maximum von Mises stress and the maximum principal strain were also retrieved for each analysis frame, using the method indicated in Appendix A.1, in order to minimize possible numerical singularities in the model. Finally, the bending fatigue life was estimated following the method described in Appendix A.2, based on the Coffin–Manson relation, considering the material properties indicated in Table 2.

Table 2. Material properties used to characterize the fatigue behavior of NiTi alloy [28,40].

Parameter	Variable	Magnitude
Fatigue ductility coefficient	ε'_F	0.68
Fatigue strength coefficient	σ'_F	705 MPa
Fatigue ductility exponent	c	−0.6
Fatigue strength exponent	b	−0.06
Modulus of elasticity	E	42.5 GPa

3. Results

3.1. Bending Analysis

Figure 5 shows the von Mises stress plot for the bending analysis of two representative endodontic files with pitch $p_z = 4$ mm and analysis angular position given by $\varphi_z = 0°$, for the analysis frame in which the maximum von Mises stress in the model reaches the end of the loading transformation phase ($\sigma_{max} = \sigma_L^E$). Figure 5a shows the von Mises stress plot over an endodontic file with square cross-section and Figure 5b shows the von Mises stress plot over an endodontic file with triangular cross-section. The figure shows that, under these boundary conditions, the highest stresses were located in the apical third of the file.

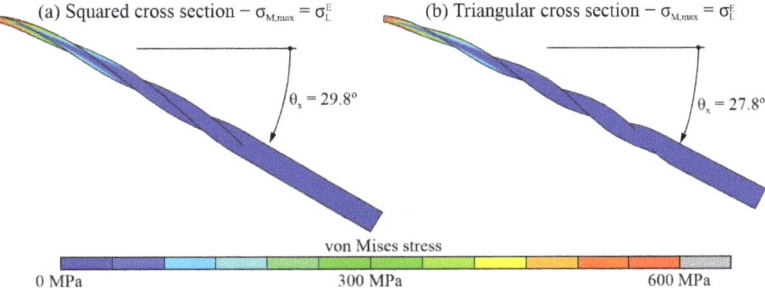

Figure 5. The von Mises stress plots for the bending analysis of endodontic files with $p_z = 4$ mm and $\varphi = 0°$.

Figure 6 shows the relationship between the rotation θ_x and the reaction bending moment M_x obtained from the bending analysis of the endodontic files with square (Figure 6a) and triangular (Figure 6b) cross-sections and pitch $p_z = 4$ mm. Here, the abscissa axis shows the rotation of the reference node B along the x-axis, while the ordinate axis shows the reaction bending moment at reference node A. The figure also shows the points where the maximum von Mises stress in the finite element model reaches the start of the phase transformation, the end of the phase transformation, and the end of the martensitic elastic regime. The curves in the figure exhibit a significant decrease in the slope for a rotation close to 20°, corresponding to a change in the stiffness of the file, as the transformation from austenite to martensite progresses in part of the file. As the bending response of an endodontic file is dependent on its orientation (given by the angle φ_z), different curves were obtained for each cross-section. For clarity, only the lower and upper curves are shown for each case, along with another intermediate representative curve. The figures also show the cross-section orientation at the encastré for each case.

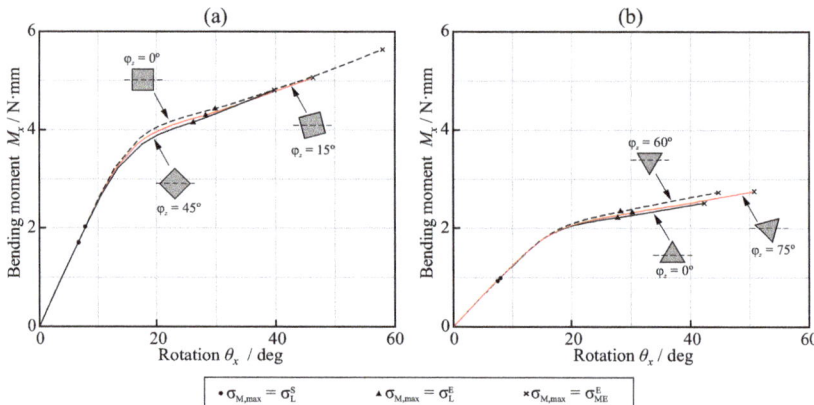

Figure 6. Bending moment–rotation relationships for the bending analysis of endodontic files with $p_z = 4$ mm: squared cross-section (**a**) and triangular cross-section (**b**).

Figure 7 shows the bending overload failure mechanism evaluation, which occurs when the maximum von Mises stress in the endodontic file reaches the end of the martensitic elastic regime ($\sigma_{max} = \sigma_{ME}^{E}$). On one hand, Figure 7a shows, for each considered pitch and cross-section, the rotation that needs to be applied at the free end of the endodontic files to reach the end of the martensitic elastic regime in the bending analysis. On the other hand, Figure 7b shows, for each considered pitch and cross-section, the maximum bending moment that can be applied at the free end of the endodontic files before they reach the end of the martensitic elastic regime in the bending analysis. As different angular positions were evaluated for each cross-section and pitch, the results shown are the range between the minimum and maximum obtained values. The bold lines represent the mean value within this range.

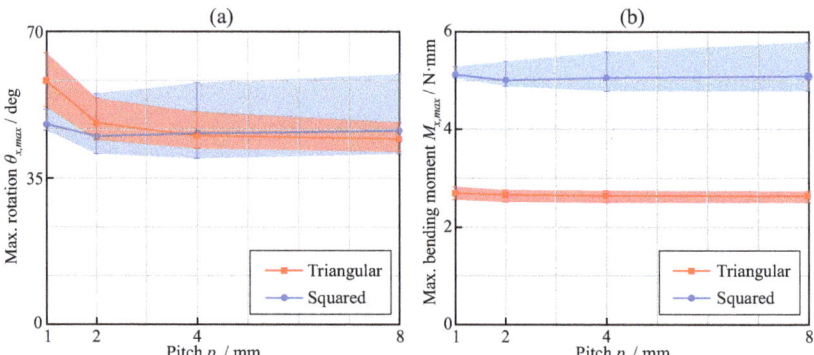

Figure 7. Bending analysis: effect of the pitch on the maximum rotation (**a**) and maximum applied torque (**b**) when the end of the martensitic elastic regime is reached.

Figure 7a shows that the maximum rotation was, on average, quite similar for triangular and square cross-sections when the pitch value was larger than 3 mm. For these pitch values, it was nearly independent of the pitch, but with a slight tendency to increase with the pitch when using a square cross-section and to decrease when using a triangular cross-section. For pitches below 3 mm, files with triangular cross-sections exhibited larger rotations than files with square cross-sections. From Figure 7b, it can be observed that the moment required to bend the square cross-section to failure was almost twice that for the triangular cross-section. The results shown in Figure 7a,b indicate that square cross-sections are more sensitive to the orientation of the file (φ_z) than triangular cross-sections, as the results exhibited larger variability.

Figure 8 shows the bending stiffness of the endodontic rotary files for the austenite and transformation phases. The stiffness in the austenite phase was calculated as the slope of the bending moment–rotation curve before σ_L^S, while that in the transformation phase was calculated as the slope of the bending moment–rotation curve between σ_L^E and σ_{ME}^E. In general, it was observed that the stiffness of the endodontic files with square cross-sections was larger than that of the files with triangular cross-sections, both in the austenite and transformation phases. Moreover, the sensitivity to the orientation of the files with square cross-sections was larger than that of those with triangular cross-sections, especially in the austenite phase. The effect of the pitch on the stiffness was negligible for pitches larger than 3 mm. With smaller pitches, a reduction in the stiffness was observed, except for the austenite phase with the square cross-section.

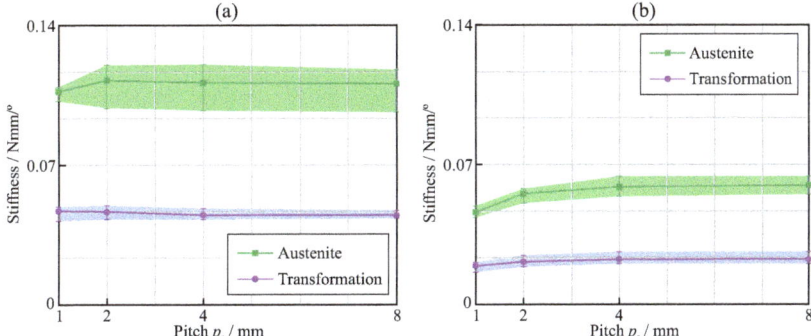

Figure 8. Bending analysis: bending stiffness of the endodontic rotary files with (**a**) square and (**b**) triangular cross-section.

Finally, Figure 9 shows the evaluation of the expected fatigue life of the endodontic files when cyclically subjected to a purely reversed bending, which produced a rotation of $\theta_x = 20°$ at the free end of the file. As explained in Appendix A.2, the bending fatigue life depends on the maximum principal strain in the file. Figure 9a shows the maximum principal strain predicted by the finite element model as a function of the pitch, for both square and triangular cross-sections. In both cases, the effect of file orientation with respect to the bending moment was significant, and the effect of the pitch was noted especially for pitches smaller than near 3 mm, for which a decrease in the strain was observed. For the square cross-section, the increase was almost linear; meanwhile, for the triangular cross-section, this increase approximated a logarithmic function. Figure 9b shows the number of cycles that the endodontic files could bear before bending fatigue failure, calculated from the maximum principal strains using the Coffin–Manson relation. It was observed that endodontic files with triangular cross-sections can withstand a larger number of cycles than those with square cross-sections, especially for small pitches.

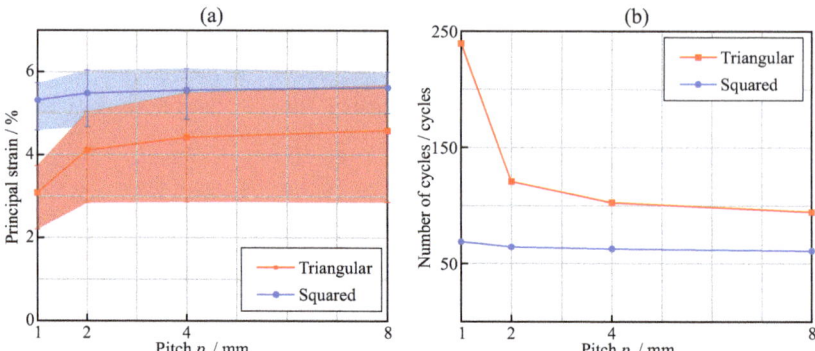

Figure 9. Bending analysis: effect of the pitch on the maximum principal strain (**a**) and the expected number of cycles (**b**) when the rotated angle is $\theta_x = 20°$.

3.2. Torsional Analysis

Figure 10 shows the von Mises stress plot for the torsional analysis of the endodontic files with square (Figure 10a) and triangular (Figure 10b) cross-sections and pitch $p_z = 4$ mm, for the analysis frames in which the maximum von Mises stress in the model reached the end of the loading transformation phase ($\sigma_{max} = \sigma_L^E$). As in the case of the bending analysis, the highest stresses were located near the apical part of the file.

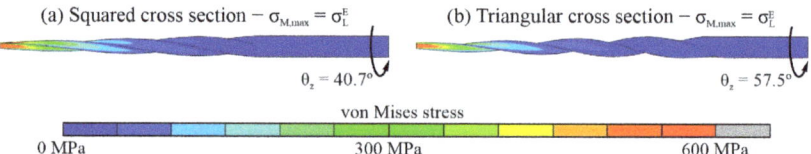

Figure 10. The von Mises stress plots for the torsional analysis of endodontic files with $p_z = 4$ mm.

Figure 11 shows the relationship between the rotation θ_z and the reaction torque M_z, obtained from the torsional analysis of the endodontic files with square (Figure 11a) and triangular (Figure 11b) cross-sections. Here, the abscissa axis shows the rotation of reference node B along the z-axis, while the ordinate axis shows the reaction torsional moment measured at reference node A. The figure also shows the points where the maximum von Mises stress in the finite element model reaches the start of the phase transformation, the end of the phase transformation, and the end of the martensitic elastic regime.

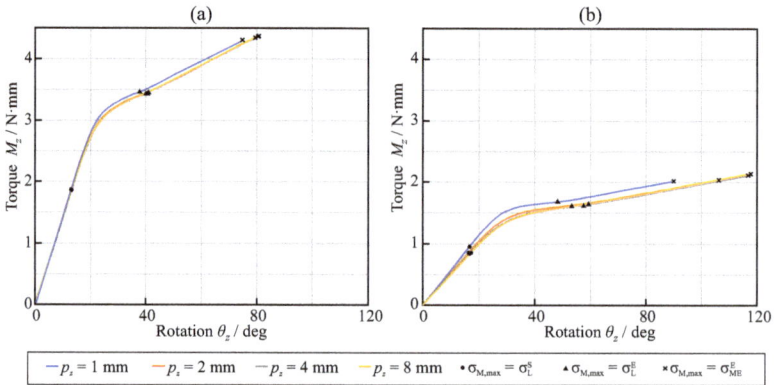

Figure 11. Torque–rotation relationships for the torsional analysis of endodontic files with different axial pitch: squared cross-section (**a**) and triangular cross-section (**b**).

Figure 12a shows, for each considered pitch and cross-section, the maximum rotation that needed to be applied at the free end of the endodontic files so that they reached the end of the martensitic elastic regime in the torsional analysis. The results show that the triangular cross-section was able to bear larger rotations before plastic deformation than the square cross-section. The rotation before failure was nearly independent of the pitch with the square cross-section, whereas it increased with the pitch for the triangular cross-section and pitch values between 1 mm and 4 mm. Figure 12b shows, for each considered pitch and cross-section, the maximum torque that could be applied at the free end of endodontic files before they reached the end of the martensitic elastic regime in the torsional analysis. It was observed that a square cross-section was able to bear almost double the torsional moment of the triangular cross-section. The strength of the files was independent of the pitch for these loading conditions.

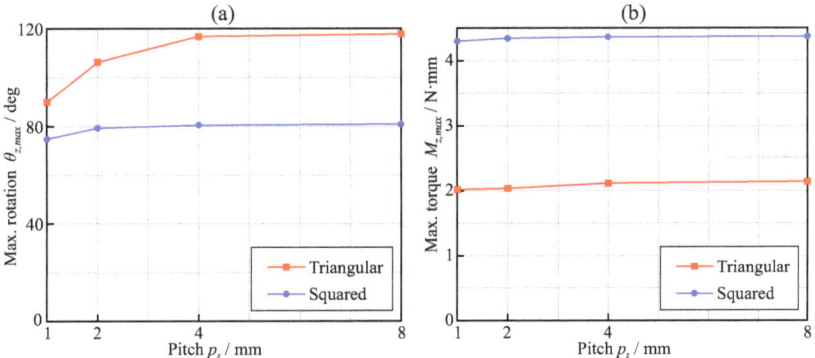

Figure 12. Torsional analysis: effect of the pitch on the applied torque (**a**) and rotation (**b**) when the end of the martensitic elastic regime is reached.

Finally, Figure 13 shows the torsional stiffness of the endodontic rotary files for the austenite and transformation phases. The stiffness in the austenite phase was calculated as the slope of the torque–rotation curve before σ_L^S, while the stiffness in the transformation phase was calculated as the slope of the torque–rotation curve between σ_L^E and σ_{ME}^E. In general, it was observed that the stiffness of the endodontic files with a square cross-section was larger than that of those with a triangular cross-section, both in the austenite and transformation phases.

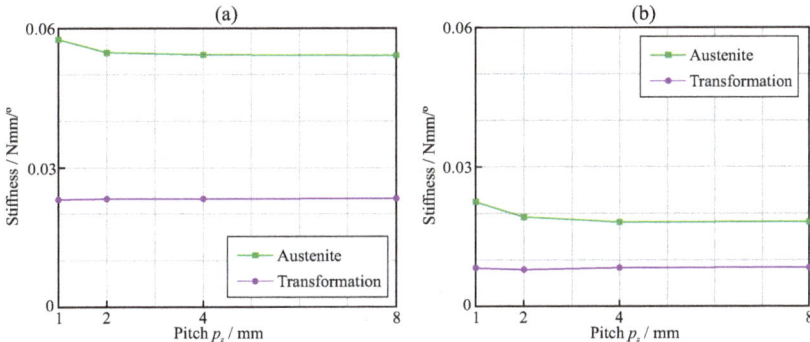

Figure 13. Torsional analysis: torsion stiffness of the endodontic rotary files with (**a**) square and (**b**) triangular cross-section.

4. Discussion

In this study, we applied an accurate non-linear finite element model to better understand the effects of the cross-section and pitch of NiTi endodontic files on their mechanical response under bending and torsion loads, according to the ISO 3630 Standard. Finite element analysis has been shown to be a good tool for this type of analysis, providing information about the stress distribution and circumventing experimental variability limitations [24]. Previous research using simulation with the same or similar objectives was first thoroughly analyzed, and the main conclusions and limitations of these studies are summarized in Appendix B, as a reference for further research. The importance of this research is supported by fact that the failure of endodontic files during root canal treatments remains a serious concern for clinicians.

The results of this study demonstrated that, for equal file diameter and taper, the cross-section shape, either triangular or square, has a greater effect than the pitch on the flexural and torsional stiffness of the file. The use of a square cross-section more than doubled the stiffness, compared to that of the triangular cross-section, as explained by the greater second moment of the area of the cross-section. The effect of pitch on stiffness was only appreciable for pitches lower than 3 mm, and was more important for triangular than for square cross-sections. When a NiTi file is bent or twisted, according to the conditions of ISO 3630, the super-elastic behavior of the material appears—which is evident from a significant decrease in the stiffness of the file—as a result of the progression of the transformation from the austenite to martensite phase in the most stressed areas of the file (see Figures 6 and 11). Our results indicate that, for a file with a shaft diameter of 1.2 mm and 6% taper, this change in stiffness appears when the rotation of the shank end section, with respect to the tip end section, is approximately 20° in bending or 30° in torsion. The stiffness of the file decreases by a factor greater than 2 after this transformation point (Figures 8 and 13). The file pitch has the opposite effect on the stiffness for torsion and bending: decreasing the pitch reduces the flexural stiffness, but increases the torsional stiffness. This effect is common for triangular and square cross-sections in the austenite phase, but it is less clear in the transformation phase, where the stiffness is less affected by pitch. This result is in agreement with those obtained in [33,36] for bending and torsion, respectively. As indicated in [33], pitch reduction could benefit both cutting efficiency, due to the higher torsional stiffness, and better adaptation to the canal shape, due to lower bending stiffness.

The obtained stress distributions (Figures 5 and 10) indicate that, for the boundary conditions imposed by the ISO 3630 Standard, the highest stresses were located near the tip of the file (where it is clamped), both in terms of bending and torsion and for both cross-section shapes. The stresses in the proximal part of the file were negligible when the stress corresponding to the end of the loading transformation phase ($\sigma_{max} = \sigma_L^E$) was reached in the tip of the file. This can be explained by the smaller section at the tip and, in the case of bending, by the higher bending moment in this area.

Static failure under bending was obtained for comparable rotations—close to 40° for pitch greater than 3 mm and ranging between 40° and 60°, depending on the pitch—for both triangular and square cross-sections (see Figure 7a). However, the bending moment necessary to reach this bending (and, thus, the reaction in the clamp) was quite different, given the difference in stiffness between the cross-section shapes (Figure 7b). This implies greater reaction forces (close to double) in the root canal with the square cross-section than with the triangular cross-section, for comparable bending deformations. The effect of the pitch on bending strength was only significant for pitches below 3 mm, where a progressive reduction in strain was observed when the pitch decreased (Figure 9a). This allows for bending of the file to a greater deformation before failure for small pitches, with a corresponding higher expected fatigue life for the same bending deformation (Figure 9b). This effect was especially observed for the triangular cross-section and, to a lesser extent, for the square cross-section. The analysis carried out to estimate the fatigue life also showed that, for the same pitch, the triangular cross-section had a higher expected life than the square cross-section, in agreement with [36], the difference being remarkable for the smallest pitch analyzed (1 mm), for which the expected life may be more than three times longer.

Our results showed that the orientation of the bending moment, with respect to the cross-section, had a significant effect on the results, changing the results by up to 19.1° and 0.97 N·mm for the square cross-section and up to 13.0° and 0.27 N·mm for the triangular cross-section. This should be taken into account when designing, reporting, and interpreting experimental bending tests according to ISO 3630.

On the other hand, for torsion, the triangular cross-section files could be rotated to a higher angle before failure than those with a square cross-section, as can be observed from Figure 12. However, due to the difference in stiffness, this failure was reached for a torque less than half that for the square cross-section. The effect of the pitch was opposite to that observed in bending, with a reduction in the pitch leading to a lower strength, as shown by the lower possible rotation before failure, which was also in agreement with the results in [36].

From a clinical perspective, the results obtained in this study suggest that the use of a triangular-shaped cross-section with small pitch for endodontic files could be better for the safe shaping of curved root canals, as its lower stiffness would produce less reaction forces in the channel, thus reducing the possibility of ledging and canal transportation. At the same time, files with a triangular cross-section and 1 mm pitch could exhibit a fatigue life more than double that of files with higher pitches or with a square cross-section. This is accompanied by a lower rotational stiffness, which could be beneficial for improving cutting efficiency [36]. The use of a smaller pitch can only partially compensate for this lower torsional stiffness of the triangular cross-section.

The results obtained in this simulation study refer to the boundary conditions established for the tests described in ISO 3630; however, it should be noted that the stress distribution within the file in these tests is not always comparable to the clinical situation, as the bending of the file is also constrained by contact with the canal walls, resulting in a different deformation, depending on the root curvature. As shown in [38], in a curved canal, the maximum strain is usually located near the highest curvature of the curved root canal axis and the fatigue life is clearly dependent on the radius of curvature. Under the conditions of ISO 3630, the highest curvature of the deformed file is close to the tip, so the conclusions in this study are especially valid for root canals with the highest curvature located near the apical end.

Finally, this work has certain limitations that deserve to be mentioned. This investigation was conducted through theoretical studies, by means of finite element analyses of endodontic rotary files; as such, no experimental tests were conducted. Regarding the investigated endodontic file geometries, all of them had uniform parameters (pitch and cross-section) throughout their entire length, even though there exist endodontic instruments in which these parameters vary through their active length. Finally, the bending fatigue life of the endodontic instruments was assessed considering a fully reversed fatigue phenomenon corresponding to a continuous rotation motion of the file within the root canal. The study of the bending fatigue under other types of motion (e.g., reciprocating and adaptive motions) is left for future research.

5. Conclusions

In this study, we simulated the mechanical response of NiTi rotary endodontic files with different cross-sections and pitches using an accurate finite element model under bending and torsion according to the conditions of the ISO 3630 Standard.

From the results obtained, we can conclude that, with equivalent shaft diameter and taper, endodontic files with a square-shaped cross-section have more than double the stiffness of those with a triangular-shaped cross-section under both bending and torsion. The effect of the pitch on stiffness was less significant, but the use of a pitch lower than 3 mm made the files more flexible for bending and stiffer for torsion when using a triangular cross-section, with beneficial effects seen in clinical use. The phase transformation from austenite to martensite led to a significant decrease in file stiffness both in bending and torsion, which was noticeable in the moment versus deformation curve. When the files were deformed under bending or torsion up to failure, a higher angle of rotation was possible before failure for the triangular section, especially in torsion and, for small pitches, in bending. A higher fatigue life can be expected in clinical use with the triangular-shaped cross-section than for the square cross-section under equivalent file deformations, especially with small pitch values. These results suggest a clinical recommendation for the use of files with triangular-shaped cross-sections and small pitch, in order to minimize ledging and maximize fatigue life.

Under the conditions of the ISO 3630 standard, the orientation of the bending plane with respect to the cross-section of the file had a significant effect on the stiffness and the strength of the file. This effect should be taken into account when designing, reporting, and interpreting similar test results.

Further works on this topic could be focused on studying the mechanical response of endodontic instruments with variable parameters (e.g., in terms of pitch and cross-section) throughout their active length. The bending fatigue life of the endodontic files in cases where the loading conditions do not represent a fully reversed fatigue phenomenon (e.g., adaptive or reciprocating motions) also deserves attention in future investigations.

Author Contributions: Conceptualization, A.P.-G. and V.R.-C.; methodology, A.P.-G. and V.R.-C.; software, V.R.-C.; investigation, A.P.-G. and V.R.-C.; resources, A.Z.-M. and V.F.-M.; writing—original draft preparation, A.P.-G.; writing—review and editing, V.R.-C.; supervision, A.Z.-M. and V.F.-M.; project administration, A.Z.-M. and V.F.-M. All authors have read and agreed to the published version of the manuscript.

Funding: This research received no external funding.

Institutional Review Board Statement: Not applicable.

Informed Consent Statement: Not applicable.

Data Availability Statement: Not applicable.

Conflicts of Interest: The authors declare no conflict of interest.

Appendix A. Post-Processing of the Finite Element Analysis Results

Appendix A.1. Assessment of the Maximum von Mises Stress and Maximum Principal Strain Values in the Endodontic File

Due to the nature of the finite element method, stress and strain singularities may appear in the vicinity of those regions of the model where boundary conditions are applied or in those areas nearby geometric stress increases. These singularities imply that unrealistically large values of stress–strain are obtained as a consequence of the numerical treatment used to derive these magnitudes from the nodal displacement results. There are many researchers who have claimed that the stress–strain results at singularity points cannot be considered when evaluating the strength of endodontic files [41,42].

Several strategies can be found in the literature to address this issue. Żmudzki [43] proposed to exclude the stress results at these points, instead extrapolating the extreme value from the stress values in the surrounding nodes. A different approach has been used by Baek [36], who determined the maximum stress level as the mean value of the top 1% von Mises equivalent stress values in the finite element model. In this work, the maximum von Mises stress σ_{max} at a given analysis frame is defined as the maximum stress level that is reached by a certain amount λ of the total volume of the file (V_{tot}). To determine this magnitude, the steps below were followed:

- Let $i \in [1, n_e]$ refer to each of the n_e tetrahedral finite elements in the model, and $j \in [1, 4]$ refer to the integration points in each tetrahedral element. The von Mises stress at a given element and integration point is denoted as σ_{ij}, and the volume associated with each integration point is denoted as $V_{ij} = V_i/4$ (where V_i is the volume of element i).

- The von Mises stress σ_{ij} and the volume V_{ij} at each integration point of the model are retrieved and stored in an array Σ with $n_i = 4 \cdot n_e$ rows. Each row m in Σ contains the von Mises stress and the volume associated with a given integration point, with the shape

$$\Sigma[m] = [\sigma_{ij}, V_{ij}]. \tag{A1}$$

- The rows in Σ are rearranged in such a way that the von Mises stresses are sorted in descending order. Then, the algorithm shown in Figure A1 is applied to determine the maximum von Mises stress in the analysis frame.

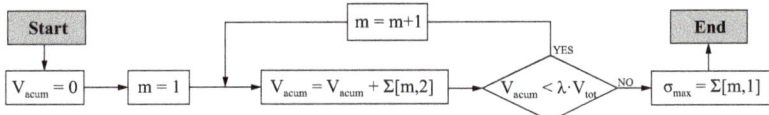

Figure A1. Algorithm to search for the maximum von Mises σ_{ij} stress in the analysis frame after the array Σ is created.

In this work, the magnitude of λ is set arbitrarily to 0.1‰, which has been shown to be a good value to avoid stress singularities while maintaining the actual stress level of the file. The same strategy was applied to determine the maximum principal strain in each analysis frame.

Appendix A.2. Determination of Bending Fatigue Life of the NiTi Endodontic Files

When the endodontic files are continuously rotated inside the root canal, they are typically subjected to a purely reversed fatigue phenomenon in which, for each rotation of the file, the bending strain alternates between nearly equal positive and negative peak values following a sinusoidal function [44]. The difference between these peak values is called the bending strain range, which is denoted by $\Delta \varepsilon$. Several studies [45–47] have demonstrated that the bending strain range and the number of cycles to failure (NCF) are correlated, and this correlation can be adequately represented by the Coffin–Manson relation:

$$\frac{\Delta \varepsilon}{2} = \varepsilon'_F \cdot N_f^c + \frac{\sigma'_F}{E} \cdot N_f^b, \tag{A2}$$

where N_f is equivalent to the NCF, ε'_F is the fatigue ductility coefficient, σ'_F is the fatigue strength coefficient, c is the fatigue ductility exponent, and b is the fatigue strength exponent.

Two issues arise when applying the Coffin–Manson relation to predict the NCF of the endodontic files from the strain results obtained from the proposed finite element model:

- On one hand, the Coffin–Manson relation is based on a uni-axial strain, but the strain results obtained from the finite element model correspond to a multi-axial strain state. Thus, a criterion to reduce the obtained multi-axial strain state to an equivalent uni-axial strain condition is required.
- On the other hand, the bending analysis conducted using the proposed finite element model does not represent the actual strain history of the endodontic file when it is rotating inside the root canal, as bending is applied in just one direction (uni-directional fatigue). Thus, a conversion method must be proposed to convert the obtained strains into a purely reversed fatigue phenomenon.

According to Roda-Casanova et al. [44], and in order to convert the multi-axial strain state into uni-axial strain, the bending strain range $\Delta \varepsilon_i$ at node i of the finite element model can be successfully approximated by:

$$\Delta\varepsilon_i = \max_{j=1\ldots n_f} (\varepsilon_{ij}^{max}) - \min_{j=1\ldots n_f} (\varepsilon_{ij}^{min}), \tag{A3}$$

where ε_{ij}^{max} and ε_{ij}^{min} are the maximum and the minimum principal strains that take place at node i at time frame j of the transient analysis, respectively. Considering that the endodontic file is continuously rotating inside the root canal, it is fair to assume that the maximum and minimum principal strains that take place at node i have the same modulus and different sign. Under this assumption, Equation (A3) can be simplified to:

$$\Delta\varepsilon_i = 2 \cdot \max_{j=1\ldots n_f} (\varepsilon_{ij}^{max}). \tag{A4}$$

Thus, by determining the maximum magnitude of the maximum principal strain in the finite element model and calculating the strain range $\Delta\varepsilon_i$ at such a node using Equation (A4), the NCF for a given specimen can be predicted through Equation (A2). The material parameters considered for the application of the Coffin–Manson relation are reflected in Table 2.

Appendix B. Literature Review

Table A1. Previous FE studies considering the effects of cross-section and pitch on rotary endodontic files.

Source	Section Type	Tip Diameter; Taper	Pitch (mm)	Material Model and Parameters	FE Code; Model Type	Boundary Conditions; Number of Nodes/Elements	Conclusions	Limitations
Xu et al., 2006 [32]	6 shapes (ProTaper, Hero642, Mtwo, ProFile, Quantec, NiTiflex)	0.4 mm, 4%	3.6	Multi-linear kinematic hardening plastic model $E_A = 34.3$ GPa, $\nu_A = 0.33$, $\sigma_L^S = 480$ MPa, $\sigma_L^E = 755$ MPa	N/A, Static	Loads: progressive 0–2.5 Nmm torsion in shank, Constraints: fixed at tip; # nodes: Not available. # elements: Not available.	(1) Sections with higher core area show lower stresses for the same torque	(1) Sections analyzed have different total areas
Kim et al., 2009 [34]	4 shapes (ProFile, HeroShaper, Mtwo, NRT)	0.3 mm; 6%	Several, N/A	$E_A = 36$ GPa, $\nu_A = 0.3$, $\sigma_L^S = 504$ MPa, $\sigma_L^E = 755$ MPa	ABAQUS; Static (cases I to IV) Dynamic (case V): Simulated shaping	Case I (or II), Load: 1 N (or 2 mm) bending in tip Constraint: shank fixed Case II (or III), Load: 2.5 Nmm (or 10°) torsion in shank Constraint: fixed at 4 mm from tip Case V, Constraint: shank rotation 240 rpm, file introduction in simulated root canal; # nodes: 7018–18,214 # elements: 5300–9440	(1) Rectangle-based sections have lower expected fatigue life than triangle-based sections	(1) Material model not clearly defined
Baek et al., 2011 [36]	4 theoretical shapes (triangle, slender rectangle, rectangle, square)	0.3 mm; 4.4%	3.2, 1.6, 1.1	$E_A = 36$ GPa, $\nu_A = 0.3$	ABAQUS; Static	Load: 20° torsion in shank Constraint: fixed at 4 mm from tip; # nodes: Not available. # elements: Not available.	(1) Rectangle-based sections, even with smaller areas, have higher torsional stiffness than triangular section; (2) Reduction in pitch increases torsional stiffness	(1) Linear material model; (2) Mesh quality not provided
Arbab-Chirani et al., 2011 [35]	5 shapes (Hero, Hero Shaper, Mtwo, ProFile, ProTaper F1)	0.2mm; 6%	Several, N/A	SMA material model, $E_A = 47$ GPa, $\nu_A = 0.3$ $\sigma_L^S = 505$ MPa	Cast3M; Static	Case 1: Load: bending at tip 3.3 mm, Constraint: shank fixed; Case 2: Load: torsion at tip 22° Constraint: shank fixed; # nodes: 66,023–73,561 # elements: 14,100–16,700	(1) ProTaper F1, Hero Shaper, and Hero are stiffer than Mtwo and ProFile; (2) Maximum stresses near the tip for both cases and similar for all the files	(1) Different pitch among files; (2) Deformations applied are low to extend martensitic transformation to a significant part of the file

Table A1. Cont.

Source	Section Type	Tip Diameter; Taper	Pitch (mm)	Material Model and Parameters	FE Code; Model Type	Boundary Conditions; Number of Nodes/Elements	Conclusions	Limitations
Versluis et al., 2012 [33]	4 theoretical shapes (triangle, slender rectangle, rectangle, square)	0.3 mm; 4%	3.2, 1.6, 1.1	SMA material model, $E_A = 36$ GPa, $\nu_A = 0.3$, $\sigma_S^L = 504$ MPa, $\sigma_L^L = 600$ MPa	MSC.Marc; Static	Load: bending at tip 5 mm (all possible orientations with respect to the cross-section). Constraint: shank axis orientation and shank end location fixed; # nodes: Not available. # elements: Not available.	(1) Flexural stiffness and stress decreases with decreasing pitch; (2) Decreasing the pitch reduces the oscillation of stress when the file rotates; (3) Flexural stiffness and stress correlates with center-core area; (4) Effect of section greater than that of pitch; (5) Maximum stress is affected by bending orientation for rectangular section	(1) Deformations applied are low to extend martensitic transformation to a significant part of the file (max. stresses below 504 MPa)
De Arruda et al., 2014 [10]	3 shapes (Mtwo, RaCe, PTU F1)	0.25 mm; 6%	Several (Not available)	Shape-memory alloy material model implemented as ABAQUS sub-routine, $E_A = 42.53$ GPa, $\nu_A = 0.33$, $\sigma_S^L = 492$ MPa, $\sigma_L^L = 630$ MPa	ABAQUS; Static	Case 1: Load: bending in shank from 0° to 45° (two perpendicular orientations). Constraint: fixed at 3 mm from tip Case 2: Load: 3 Nmm torsion in shank. Constraint: fixed at 3 mm from tip; # nodes: 84,126–91,372 # elements: 48,460–55,009	(1) Finite element analysis results agree with experimental results; (2) RaCe and Mtwo are more flexible than PTU F1 in bending and torsion; (3) Shape of the section affects the maximum stress and the variation in stress with bending orientation	(1) Only three section geometries and two orientations for bending considered; (2) Different pitch among files
Ha et al., 2015 [37]	4 theoretical shapes (triangle, slender rectangle, rectangle, square)	0.3 mm; 4.4%	3.2, 1.6, 1.1	$E_A = 26$ GPa, $\nu_A = 0.3$	ABAQUS; Not available.	Load: Prescribed rotation inside the root canal. Constraint: Contact with friction in 3 simulated root canal (15°, 30°, 45° curvature), shank axis orientation & shank end location fixed; # nodes: 10,230–18,042 # elements: 8325–15,540	(1) The square cross-section shows the highest 'screw-in' force and reaction torque; (2) 'Screw-in' force and reaction torque are higher for greater pitch and higher root canal curvature	(1) Linear material model; (2) Very low friction coefficient (0.1) considered between file and root canal; (3) Solid surface used as root canal model; (4) Only 3 root canal geometries considered
Basser-Ahamed et al., 2018 [51]	5 theoretical shapes (triangle T, convex triangle C, concave triangle U, combined CTU, combined UTC)	0.25 mm; 6%	1.6	File: $E_A = 36$ GPa, $\nu_A = 0.3$ Root canal: $E = 18.6$ GPa, $\nu_A = 0.3$	ANSYS; Not available.	Load: Torque 2 Nm. Constraint: Contact with simulated root canal (45° curvature), shank axis orientation and shank end location fixed, rotation of 180° at 240 rpm; File: # nodes: 16,750–42,785 # elements: 75,430–152,432 Root canal: # nodes: 3000 # elements: 3500	(1) A combined section CTU (C coronal third, T middle third, U apical third) presents lower stresses than constant section	(1) Geometry of the root canal not clearly defined; (2) Contact and friction conditions undefined; (3) Does not consider changes in dentin properties within the root canal; (4) Effect of pitch not analyzed

References

1. Walia, H.; Brantley, W.; Gerstein, H. An initial investigation of the bending and torsional properties of nitinol root canal files. *J. Endod.* **1988**, *14*, 346–351. [CrossRef]
2. Esposito, P.; Cunningham, C. A comparison of canal preparation with nickel-titanium and stainless steel instruments. *J. Endod.* **1995**, *21*, 173–176. [CrossRef]
3. Bergmans, L.; Van Cleynenbreugel, J.; Wevers, M.; Lambrechts, P. Mechanical root canal preparation with NiTi rotary instruments: Rationale, performance and safety. Status Report for the American Journal of Dentistry. *Am. J. Dent.* **2001**, *14*, 324–333. [PubMed]
4. Parashos, P.; Gordon, I.; Messer, H. Factors influencing defects of rotary nickel-titanium endodontic instruments after clinical use. *J. Endod.* **2004**, *30*, 722–725. [CrossRef] [PubMed]
5. Spili, P.; Parashos, P.; Messer, H. The impact of instrument fracture on outcome of endodontic treatment. *J. Endod.* **2005**, *31*, 845–850. [CrossRef]
6. Plotino, G.; Grande, N.M.; Cordaro, M.; Testarelli, L.; Gambarini, G. A Review of Cyclic Fatigue Testing of Nickel-Titanium Rotary Instruments. *J. Endod.* **2009**, *35*, 1469–1476. [CrossRef]
7. Scattina, A.; Alovisi, M.; Paolino, D.S.; Pasqualini, D.; Scotti, N.; Chiandussi, G.; Berutti, E. Prediction of cyclic fatigue life of nickel-titanium rotary files by virtual modeling and finite elements analysis. *J. Endod.* **2015**, *41*, 1867–1870. [CrossRef]
8. Peters, O.; Barbakow, F. Dynamic torque and apical forces of ProFile .04 rotary instruments during preparation of curved canals. *Int. Endod. J.* **2002**, *35*, 379–389. [CrossRef]
9. Kuhn, G.; Tavernier, B.; Jordan, L. Influence of structure on nickel-titanium endodontic instruments failure. *J. Endod.* **2001**, *27*, 516–520. [CrossRef]
10. De Arruda Santos, L.; López, J.; De Las Casas, E.; De Azevedo Bahia, M.; Buono, V. Mechanical behavior of three nickel-titanium rotary files: A comparison of numerical simulation with bending and torsion tests. *Mater. Sci. Eng. C* **2014**, *37*, 258–263. [CrossRef]
11. Pruett, J.; Clement, D.; Carnes, D., Jr. Cyclic fatigue testing of nickel-titanium endodontic instruments. *J. Endod.* **1997**, *23*, 77–85. [CrossRef]
12. Parashos, P.; Messer, H. Rotary NiTi Instrument Fracture and its Consequences. *J. Endod.* **2006**, *32*, 1031–1043. [CrossRef] [PubMed]
13. Topçuoğlu, H.; Topçuoğlu, G. Cyclic Fatigue Resistance of Reciproc Blue and Reciproc Files in an S-shaped Canal. *J. Endod.* **2017**, *43*, 1679–1682. [CrossRef] [PubMed]
14. Siqueira, J., Jr.; Rôças, I. Polymerase chain reaction-based analysis of microorganisms associated with failed endodontic treatment. *Oral Surgery Oral Med. Oral Pathol. Oral Radiol. Endod.* **2004**, *97*, 85–94. [CrossRef]
15. Strindberg, L. The Dependence of the Results of Pulp Therapy on Certain Factors: An Analytic Study Based on Radiographic and Clinical Follow-Up Examinations. *Acta Odontol. Scand.* **1956**, *14*, 1–175.
16. Yang, Q.; Shen, Y.; Huang, D.; Zhou, X.; Gao, Y.; Haapasalo, M. Evaluation of Two Trephine Techniques for Removal of Fractured Rotary Nickel-titanium Instruments from Root Canals. *J. Endod.* **2017**, *43*, 116–120. [CrossRef]
17. Fu, M.; Zhang, Z.; Hou, B. Removal of broken files from root canals by using ultrasonic techniques combined with dental microscope: A retrospective analysis of treatment outcome. *J. Endod.* **2011**, *37*, 619–622. [CrossRef]
18. Ruiz-Sánchez, C.; Faus-Llacer, V.; Faus-Matoses, I.; Zubizarreta-Macho, A.; Sauro, S.; Faus-Matoses, V. The influence of niti alloy on the cyclic fatigue resistance of endodontic files. *J. Clin. Med.* **2020**, *9*, 3755. [CrossRef]
19. Zupanc, J.; Vahdat-Pajouh, N.; Schäfer, E. New thermomechanically treated NiTi alloys—A review. *Int. Endod. J.* **2018**, *51*, 1088–1103. [CrossRef]
20. Faus-Llacer, V.; Kharrat, N.; Ruiz-Sanchez, C.; Faus-Matoses, I.; Zubizarreta-Macho, A.; Faus-Matoses, V. The effect of taper and apical diameter on the cyclic fatigue resistance of rotary endodontic files using an experimental electronic device. *Appl. Sci.* **2021**, *11*, 863. [CrossRef]
21. Turpin, Y.; Chagneau, F.; Vulcain, J. Impact of two theoretical cross-sections on torsional and bending stresses of nickel-titanium root canal instrument models. *J. Endod.* **2000**, *26*, 414–417. [CrossRef] [PubMed]
22. Sekar, V.; Kumar, R.; Nandini, S.; Ballal, S.; Velmurugan, N. Assessment of the role of cross section on fatigue resistance of rotary files when used in reciprocation. *Eur. J. Dent.* **2016**, *10*, 541–545. [CrossRef] [PubMed]
23. Kwak, S.; Ha, J.H.; Lee, C.J.; El Abed, R.; Abu-Tahun, I.; Kim, H.C. Effects of Pitch Length and Heat Treatment on the Mechanical Properties of the Glide Path Preparation Instruments. *J. Endod.* **2016**, *42*, 788–792. [CrossRef]
24. *ISO 3630-1:2008*; Dentistry—Root-Canal Instruments—Part 1: General Requirements and Test Methods. International Organization for Standardization: Geneva, Switzerland, 2008.
25. Zhang, E.; Cheung, G.; Zheng, Y. A mathematical model for describing the mechanical behaviour of root canal instruments. *Int. Endod. J.* **2011**, *44*, 72–76. [CrossRef] [PubMed]
26. Tsao, C.; Liou, J.; Wen, P.; Peng, C.; Liu, T. Study on bending behaviour of nickel-titanium rotary endodontic instruments by analytical and numerical analyses. *Int. Endod. J.* **2013**, *46*, 379–388. [CrossRef] [PubMed]
27. Lee, M.H.; Versluis, A.; Kim, B.M.; Lee, C.J.; Hur, B.; Kim, H.C. Correlation between experimental cyclic fatigue resistance and numerical stress analysis for nickel-titanium rotary files. *J. Endod.* **2011**, *37*, 1152–1157. [CrossRef] [PubMed]
28. Montalvão, D.; Shengwen, Q.; Freitas, M. A study on the influence of Ni-Ti M-Wire in the flexural fatigue life of endodontic rotary files by using Finite Element Analysis. *Mater. Sci. Eng. C* **2014**, *40*, 172–179. [CrossRef]

29. Bonessio, N.; Pereira, E.; Lomiento, G.; Arias, A.; Bahia, M.; Buono, V.; Peters, O. Validated finite element analyses of WaveOne Endodontic Instruments: A comparison between M-Wire and NiTi alloys. *Int. Endod. J.* **2015**, *48*, 441–450. [CrossRef]
30. Chien, P.Y.; Walsh, L.J.; Peters, O.A. Finite element analysis of rotary nickel-titanium endodontic instruments: A critical review of the methodology. *Eur. J. Oral Sci.* **2021**, *129*, e12802. [CrossRef]
31. Basheer Ahamed, S.; Vanajassun, P.; Rajkumar, K.; Mahalaxmi, S. Comparative Evaluation of Stress Distribution in Experimentally Designed Nickel-titanium Rotary Files with Varying Cross Sections: A Finite Element Analysis. *J. Endod.* **2018**, *44*, 654–658. [CrossRef]
32. Xu, X.; Eng, M.; Zheng, Y.; Eng, D. Comparative study of torsional and bending properties for six models of nickel-titanium root canal instruments with different cross-sections. *J. Endod.* **2006**, *32*, 372–375. [CrossRef] [PubMed]
33. Versluis, A.; Kim, H.C.; Lee, W.; Kim, B.M.; Lee, C.J. Flexural stiffness and stresses in nickel-titanium rotary files for various pitch and cross-sectional geometries. *J. Endod.* **2012**, *38*, 1399–1403. [CrossRef] [PubMed]
34. Kim, H.; Kim, H.; Lee, C.; Kim, B.; Park, J.; Versluis, A. Mechanical response of nickel-titanium instruments with different cross-sectional designs during shaping of simulated curved canals. *Int. Endod. J.* **2009**, *42*, 593–602. [CrossRef] [PubMed]
35. Arbab-Chirani, R.; Chevalier, V.; Arbab-Chirani, S.; Calloch, S. Comparative analysis of torsional and bending behavior through finite-element models of 5 Ni-Ti endodontic instruments. *Oral Surgery Oral Med. Oral Pathol. Oral Radiol. Endod.* **2011**, *111*, 115–121. [CrossRef] [PubMed]
36. Baek, S.H.; Lee, C.J.; Versluis, A.; Kim, B.M.; Lee, W.; Kim, H.C. Comparison of torsional stiffness of nickel-titanium rotary files with different geometric characteristics. *J. Endod.* **2011**, *37*, 1283–1286. [CrossRef]
37. Ha, J.H.; Cheung, G.S.; Versluis, A.; Lee, C.J.; Kwak, S.W.; Kim, H.C. 'Screw-in' tendency of rotary nickel-titanium files due to design geometry. *Int. Endod. J.* **2015**, *48*, 666–672. [CrossRef]
38. Roda-Casanova, V.; Zubizarreta-Macho, A.; Sanchez-Marin, F.; Ezpeleta, O.; Martínez, A.; Catalán, A. Computerized generation and finite element stress analysis of endodontic rotary files. *Appl. Sci.* **2021**, *11*, 4329. [CrossRef]
39. Auricchio, F.; Petrini, L. A three-dimensional model describing stress-temperature induced solid phase transformations: Solution algorithm and boundary value problems. *Int. J. Numer. Methods Eng.* **2004**, *61*, 807–836. [CrossRef]
40. El-Anwar, M.I.; Mandorah, A.O.; Yousief, S.A.; Soliman, T.A.; Abd El-Wahab, T.M. A finite element study on the mechanical behavior of reciprocating endodontic files. *Braz. J. Oral Sci.* **2015**, *14*, 52–59. [CrossRef]
41. Stolk, J.; Verdonschot, N.; Huiskes, R. Management of stress fields around singular points in a finite element analysis. *Comput. Methods Biomech. Biomed. Eng.* **2001**, *3*, 57–62.
42. Chen, G.; Pettet, G.; Pearcy, M.; McElwain, D. Comparison of two numerical approaches for bone remodelling. *Med. Eng. Phys.* **2007**, *29*, 134–139. [CrossRef] [PubMed]
43. Żmudzki, J.; Chladek, W. Stress present in bone surrounding dental implants in FEM model experiments. *J. Achiev. Mater. Manuf. Eng.* **2008**, *27*, 71–74.
44. Roda-Casanova, V.; Pérez-González, A.; Zubizarreta-Macho, Á.; Faus-Matoses, V. Fatigue Analysis of NiTi Rotary Endodontic Files through Finite Element Simulation: Effect of Root Canal Geometry on Fatigue Life. *J. Clin. Med.* **2021**, *10*, 5692. [CrossRef] [PubMed]
45. Cheung, G.S.; Darvell, B.W. Fatigue testing of a NiTi rotary instrument. Part 1: Strain-life relationship. *Int. Endod. J.* **2007**, *40*, 612–618. [CrossRef]
46. Figueiredo, A.M.; Modenesi, P.; Buono, V. Low-cycle fatigue life of superelastic NiTi wires. *Int. J. Fatigue* **2009**, *31*, 751–758. [CrossRef]
47. Maletta, C.; Sgambitterra, E.; Furgiuele, F.; Casati, R.; Tuissi, A. Fatigue properties of a pseudoelastic NiTi alloy: Strain ratcheting and hysteresis under cyclic tensile loading. *Int. J. Fatigue* **2014**, *66*, 78–85. [CrossRef]

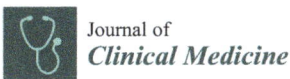

Article

Root and Root Canal Configuration Characterization Using Microcomputed Tomography: A Systematic Review

Mohmed Isaqali Karobari [1,2,*], Sohaib Arshad [3], Tahir Yusuf Noorani [1,*], Naveed Ahmed [4], Syed Nahid Basheer [5], Syed Wali Peeran [6], Anand Marya [7], Charu Mohan Marya [8], Pietro Messina [9] and Giuseppe Alessandro Scardina [9,*]

1 Conservative Dentistry Unit, School of Dental Sciences, Health Campus, Universiti Sains Malaysia, Kubang Kerian, Kota Bharu 16150, Kelantan, Malaysia
2 Department of Conservative Dentistry & Endodontics, Saveetha Dental College & Hospitals, Saveetha Institute of Medical and Technical Sciences University, Chennai 600077, Tamil Nadu, India
3 Periodontics Unit, School of Dental Sciences, Health Campus, Universiti Sains Malaysia, Kubang Kerian, Kota Bharu 16150, Kelantan, Malaysia; ehab_arshad@hotmail.com
4 Department of Medical Microbiology and Parasitology, School of Medical Sciences, Universiti Sains Malaysia, Kubang Kerian, Kota Bharu 16150, Kelantan, Malaysia; naveed.malik@student.usm.my
5 Department of Restorative Dental Sciences, College of Dentistry, Jazan University, Jazan 45142, Saudi Arabia; snbasheer@jazanu.edu.sa
6 Department of Periodontics, Armed Forces Hospital Jizan, Jazan 82722, Saudi Arabia; doctorsyedwali@yahoo.com
7 Department of Orthodontics, Saveetha Dental College & Hospitals, Saveetha Institute of Medical and Technical Sciences University, Chennai 600077, Tamil Nadu, India; amarya@puthisastra.edu.kh
8 Department of Public Health Dentistry, Sudha Rustagi College of Dental Sciences and Research, Faridabad 121002, Haryana, India; maryacm@co.uk
9 Department of Surgical, Oncological and Stomatological Disciplines, University of Palermo, 90133 Palermo, Italy; pietro.messina01@unipa.it
* Correspondence: dr.isaq@gmail.com (M.I.K.); dentaltahir@yahoo.com (T.Y.N.); alessandro.scardina@unipa.it (G.A.S.)

Abstract: This systematic review's objective was to conduct a complete analysis of the literature on the root canal morphology using advanced micro-computed tomography. The electronic web databases PubMed, Scopus, and Cochrane were examined for research papers concerning the chosen keywords, evaluating the root canal morphology using Micro-CT, published up to 2021. The articles were searched using MeSH keywords and searched digitally on four specialty journal websites. DARE2 extended (Database of Attributes of Reviews of Effects) was used to assess bias risk. The information was gathered from 18 published studies that strictly met the criteria for inclusion. In the included studies, a total of 6696 samples were studied. The studies were conducted on either maxillary (n-2222) or mandibular teeth (n-3760), permanent anteriors (n-625), and Third molars (n-89). To scan samples, a Scanco Medical machine in was used in 10 studies, Bruker Micro-CT in 34, and seven other machines were utilized in the rest. Bruker Micro-CT software from Kontich, Belgium, VG-Studio Max 2.2 software from Volume Graphics, Heidelberg, Germany, was the most commonly used software. The minimum Voxel size (resolution) adopted in the included studies was 11.6 µm. However, 60 µm was the maximum. Most studies classified the root canal morphology using Vertucci's classification system (n-16) and the four-digit system (n-6).

Keywords: dental anatomy; dental pulp; dental diagnostic imaging; endodontics; morphology; Micro-CT; root; root canal

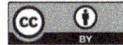

1. Introduction

Endodontic therapy aims to thoroughly clean and obturate the whole system of the root canal. However, to prevent endodontic failure and execute successful root canal therapy, specific determinants play an essential role [1,2]. Precise shaping, cleaning, and filling of all spaces previously filled by the radicular pulp tissues or pulp capping/pulpotomy to maintain healthy dental pulp is required. The morphologic uniqueness of each root necessitates a comprehensive knowledge of variations in the root canal system, which should be reflected during the diagnostic and treatment process [3]. Research upon the root canal morphology in lasting teeth has revealed that the root canal's amount and classification can differ by ethnicity, gender, and in different populations, within the same population, and uniquely in each person [4,5]. Furthermore, it is possible that a variety of morphologic root canal system configurations exist; as a result, each tooth should be evaluated separately using a proper classification system [6].

The investigation of external and internal anatomy of different teeth using many in vitro and in vivo techniques were performed in the beginning of 20th century [7]. Various in vitro techniques were used to identify root and canal morphology which includes root sectioning, staining, tooth clearing, microscopic investigation, radiographic investigations using conventional radiographs, and three-dimensional techniques such as CBCT and microcomputed tomography (MCT) [8]. The in vivo techniques include conventional radiographic examinations, retrospective evaluation of patients' data, clinical evaluation during root canal treatment, digital radiography, and advanced radiographic techniques such as CBCT [8]. An investigation showed a technique by using longitudinal sectioning to produce a sagittal view of pulp space from pulp chamber to the root apex [9]. Opaque wax was used to fill the exposed canals, but this method showed lateral canals very rarely [10]. Rosenstiel (1957) introduced a technique using a Radio opaque material to reproduce the root canals. A study demonstrated a simple in vitro technique to evaluate both endodontically treated and untreated root canal systems. The following steps were used in the technique to make teeth transparent. Firstly, teeth were decalcified using nitric acid, then dehydrated using alcohol, and finally cleared with methyl salicylate [11].

Digital radiography, magnetic resonance imaging (MRI), densitometry, ultrasound, and computed tomography (CT) are just a few of the noninvasive dental imaging technologies that have been developed in recent years. However, most of these approaches are restricted since they only provide a 2-dimensional (2-D) examination of the root canal system (RCS) and cannot be easily compared subjectively or quantitatively with other samples [12]. Furthermore, these methods do not allow for synchronized 3-dimensional (3-D) examination of teeth surface and interior anatomy [13]. In endodontic research, microcomputed tomography (Micro-CT) has acquired much interest since it displays high-resolution (10 µm) tooth morphological structures and has proven to be an essential information source for dentists, as shown in Figure 1 [14]. Microcomputed tomography is a nondestructive and reproducible ex vivo research method and is considered as the research method that offers the foremost possibility for an accurate examination of the morphology of the root canal system.

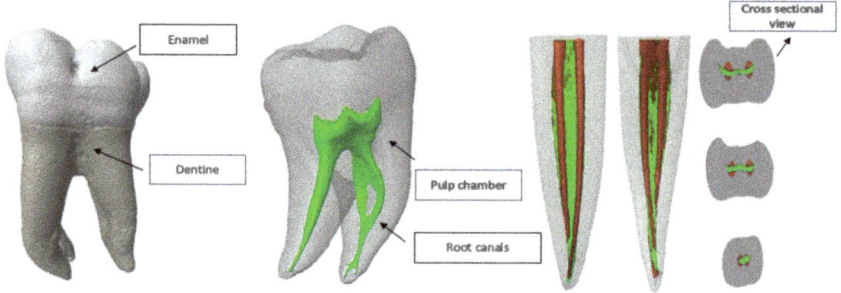

Figure 1. Micro-CT in endodontics.

The ex vivo investigation is used in Micro-CT imaging, which is widely accepted because of its accuracy, repeatability, and noninvasiveness, all of which are superior to other commonly used research methods [15]. Maxillary central incisors have one root and one main canal. Rarely, at a 6% rate, one canal of central maxillary teeth splits into two parts at the apical foramina which can be classified as Vertucci type V [16]. Apical root canal morphology should be considered because of its main effect on the success of root canal treatment. In the study of Adorno et al. [17], accessory canals in the apical 3 mm in the Japanese population were found among 46% of the specimens. Over the years, different studies have been conducted to understand the root canal morphology of premolars using different research methods [18] and different populations [19–21]. The frequency of a single canal is 54–88.5%. However, multiple canals were reported in 11.5–46% of cases [21,22]. In the study of Pan et al. [23], the prevalence of maxillary first premolar teeth with one main root canal was 67.8%, with two roots at 31.9%, and with two canals at 88.2%. In the Malaysian population, according to Vertucci's classification, the second premolar was detected as single-root type I with the rate of 58.2% [16]. In posterior teeth, mandibular first molars are recognized to exhibit various complex and distinct morphological variations of the root canal system [24,25]. This tooth usually has two roots, but sometimes it has three, with two or three canals in the mesial root and one, two, or three canals in the distal root [26,27]. When only one distal root canal is present, it is often buccolingually oval, and untreated surface areas were shown to be as high as 59–79% when rotary instruments were used for the shaping procedure [28].

Similarly, a study on the Burmese population showed that the prevalence of two canals in mesiobuccal roots of the upper first molar teeth decrease gradually towards the upper third molars. About 85.2% of the 270 roots of the maxillary teeth had one root canal at the apex, 14% had two apical canals, and 0.8% had three apical canals [25,29]. Moreover, the morphology of root canals was explored, white spot lesions on enamel were identified, and enamel demineralization with therapy were assessed using Micro-CT [30,31]. The latest evidence demonstrated the ability to scan isthmuses successfully, while another claimed to detect inorganic material within a tooth root [32,33]. The nondestructive Micro-CT imaging method allows for multiple exposures and data collection. As a result, this imaging method is beneficial for evaluating experimental endodontics [34]. The goal of this systematic review was to carry out a thorough examination of the literature on root canal physiology using sophisticated microcomputed tomography.

2. Methods

2.1. Study Protocol and Registration

The Reporting Items preferred for Meta-Analysis and systematic Review (PRISMA) procedures (http://www.prisma-statement.org, accessed on 10 April 2022) were respected in this work. The current systematic review is registered in PROSPERO with the number CRD42021278968.

2.2. Research Question

Studies about assessment of root canal morphologies through microcomputed tomography were selected based on the "PICOS" (PRISMA-P 2016) technique:

- P (population): Extracted teeth models
- I (intervention): Assessment by Micro-CT
- C (comparison): None
- O (result): Root and root canal morphologies
- S (study design): In vitro studies

2.3. Search Strategies

The electronic online databases search was conducted for research papers based on selected keywords, assessing root canal morphology using Micro-CT, published until March 2022. The number of studies obtained from each dataset is displayed in Table 1. The articles were searched using MeSH keywords and searched digitally on four specialty journal websites. The MeSH keywords were searched in PubMed and Scopus initially, as per our initial search criteria. Further, to add more scientific evidence related to the topic, the search was carried out in Cochrane. Furthermore, to include the latest articles up to the last search date published in the specialty journals as it may take some time for the articles to be included in the indexes after they are published, the search on websites of four endodontic specialty Journals were performed, including the Journal of Endodontics, the International Endodontic Journal, the Australian Endodontic Journal, and the Iranian Endodontic Journal.

Table 1. Information of sources and search strategies using MeSH keywords.

Database	Search Strategies	Results
PubMed	(((((((((((((Tooth Root[Title/Abstract]) OR (Tooth anatomy[Title/Abstract])) OR (Tooth histology[Title/Abstract])) OR (Tooth diagnosis[Title/Abstract])) OR (Tooth diagnostic imaging[Title/Abstract])) OR (Root canal morphology[Title/Abstract])) OR (Root canal configuration[Title/Abstract])) OR (Root canal system[Title/Abstract])) OR (Dental Pulp Cavity[Title/Abstract])) OR (Dental anatomy[Title/Abstract])) OR (Dental histology[Title/Abstract])) OR (Dental diagnosis[Title/Abstract])) OR (Dental diagnostic imaging[Title/Abstract]) **AND** (((((((X-ray Microtomography[Title/Abstract]) OR (X-ray methods[Title/Abstract])) OR (Micro-CT[Title/Abstract])) OR (micro computed tomography[Title/Abstract])) OR (microcomputed tomography[Title/Abstract])) OR (microcomputed tomography[Title/Abstract])) OR (Micro-CT[Title/Abstract])) OR (Micro-CT[Title/Abstract])	236
Scopus	Tooth Root OR Tooth anatomy OR Tooth histology OR Tooth diagnosis OR Tooth diagnostic imaging OR Root canal morphology OR Root canal configuration OR Root canal system OR Dental Pulp Cavity OR Dental anatomy OR Dental histology OR Dental diagnosis OR Dental diagnostic imaging **AND** X-ray Microtomography OR X-ray methods OR Micro-CT OR micro computed tomography OR microcomputed tomography OR microcomputed tomography OR Micro-CT OR Micro-CT	131
Cochrane	Tooth Root OR Tooth anatomy OR Tooth histology OR Tooth diagnosis OR Tooth diagnostic imaging OR Root canal morphology OR Root canal configuration OR Root canal system OR Dental Pulp Cavity OR Dental anatomy OR Dental histology OR Dental diagnosis OR Dental diagnostic imaging **AND** X-ray Microtomography OR X-ray methods OR Micro-CT OR micro computed tomography OR microcomputed tomography OR microcomputed tomography OR Micro-CT OR Micro-CT	483
ScienceDirect	(Root canal morphology OR Root canal configuration OR Root canal system OR Dental Pulp Cavity) AND (Micro-CT OR micro computed tomography OR microcomputed tomography OR Micro-CT OR Microtomography)	2179
	Total	3029

2.4. Data Sources

Two separate researchers (M.I.K and N.A.) performed an electronic literature search on 20 March 2022, using MeSH terms and keywords, as well as the Boolean operators "OR" and "AND" to compile relevant material using appropriate filters. The keywords used were "Tooth Root/anatomy and histology", "Tooth Root/diagnosis", "Tooth Root/diagnostic imaging", "Tooth root", "dental pulp cavity", "Micro-CT", and "X-ray Microtomography/methods". The required literature was then gathered using proper filters by combining these key terms with the Boolean operators "OR" and "AND" as shown in Table 1. Furthermore, a hand search was also conducted by two different reviewers using keywords such as "Root canal morphology," "Root canal configuration," "Root canal system," "Micro-computed tomography," "Micro-computed tomography," and "Micro-CT" from databases such as PubMed, Scopus, ScienceDirect, and Cochrane.

2.5. Eligibility Criteria

A literature search was performed to uncover studies that used Micro-CT to assess root canal morphology. Two reviewers used the PICOS approach to examine the entire texts of the remaining papers and set inclusion and exclusion criteria. The year of publication was not restricted in any way. On 20 March 2021, the final database search was accomplished. A third reviewer's decision was used to settle disagreements. Figure 2 illustrates the inclusion and exclusion criteria.

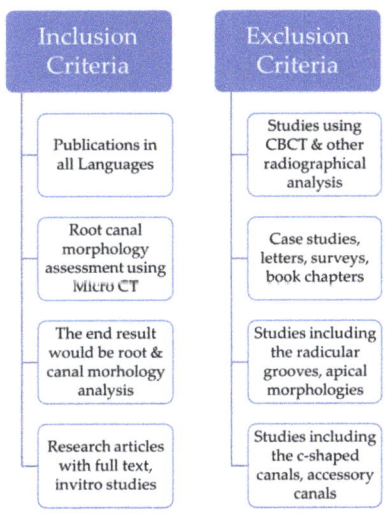

Figure 2. Inclusion and Exclusion Criteria.

2.6. Study Selection

The studies that examined the assessment of root canal morphology using the Micro-CT technique, which are published in various medical journals, were found through a random check of research papers from online sources. Two researchers evaluated relevant studies against previously defined inclusion and exclusion criteria to substantiate the search technique, as shown in Figure 2.

2.7. Data Extraction

Two reviewers (M.I.K and S.A.) assessed the titles and abstracts of the publications for the inclusion/exclusion criteria mentioned above, and "relevant" articles were chosen for a full-text reading. This procedure was carried out independently, with the help of a third researcher (NA), in the event of any questions or conflicts. A manual hand search was also carried out using different keywords, and studies were included based on selected criteria.

2.8. Quality Assessment and Risk of Bias of Research Articles

The papers were selected for inclusion and exclusion based on their titles, abstracts, and inclusion and exclusion criteria. Following the screening process, full-text articles were reviewed one by one, and the material's quality was evaluated. The articles were rated for allotment biases, preference biases, involvement integrity, allocation concealment, withdrawals and dropouts, confusion, data collection methods, and statistical analysis using internal and external validity guidelines. A total of 60 papers were screened for quality, with nine being rejected due to a lack of information about the processes, teeth, research nature, and outcomes.

The Joanna Briggs Institute (JBI) critical assessment checklist was used to appraise the quality of the included studies [35]. This checklist assessed nine items: (i) appropriate sampling frame, (ii) proper sampling technique, (iii) adequate sample size, (iv) study subject and setting description, (v) sufficient data analysis, (vi) use of valid methods for the identified conditions, (vii) valid measurement for all the participants, (viii) use of appropriate statistical analysis, and (ix) adequate response rate. Answers such as yes, no, unclear, or not applicable are assigned to each item. The 'yes' response received a 1 score, whereas the 'no' and 'unclear' responses received ratings of 0. Finally, the average score for each item was computed. The quality of studies with scores below and above the mean was then classified as good or poor quality, respectively. The study was included or excluded based on the methodological quality assessment. (Supplementary Table S1).

Two researchers (M.I.K. and N.A.) oversaw scoring, and they used the JBI criteria to base their scores. After comparing the results of their individual questions, they resolved any discrepancies to arrive at an 'agreed score'. All of the 51 included studies individually had a total score of $\geq$70%. Hence, both the researchers (M.I.K and N.A.) showed agreement for most of the included studies and were given >70% scores, thus limiting the bias.

3. Results

3.1. Study Selection Results

PubMed yielded a total of 236 research papers using MeSH keywords, 483 from Cochrane using MeSH keywords, 131 from Scopus using MeSH keywords, and 2179 from ScienceDirect. Following the removal of duplicate articles (98), a total of 2931 studies were recognized for further consideration. After reading the titles of the articles, another 2519 were eliminated. In addition, 352 additional articles were eliminated after reading the abstracts. By reading the full texts of the residual 60 articles, they were evaluated for further selection; nine more articles were eliminated. The data were extracted from the 51 studies that strictly met the eligibility criteria. Figure 3 depicts the selection criteria as it follows the PRISMA guidelines. These 51 articles were examined for the current study based on the quality of the research studies.

3.2. Study Features

The studies' basic features included in the systematic review are summarized in Table 2. The studies were performed in various countries, lasted varying amounts of time, and were published in various journals. Each included study was published in a good, reputed journal indexed in Web of Science/PubMed/Scopus. The technical characteristics, such as sample size, type of teeth, instrument used, resolution, software, classification system, methods, outcomes, and conclusion, were omitted from the systematic review. Most of the reports comprised were issued in the Journal of Endodontics (n-13). In contrast, six were published in the International Endodontic Journal, four in the Clinical Oral Investigations, two in the Scientific reports, two in the Journal of Conservative Dentistry, two in Oral Surgery, Oral Medicine, Oral Pathology, Oral Radiology, and Endodontology, two in the Archives of Oral Biology, two in the Journal of Applied Oral Sciences, two in Clinical Oral Investigations, two in Clinical Anatomy, one in the Australian Endodontic Journal, one in the International Journal of Oral Sciences, one in the Swiss Dental Journal, one in the European Endodontic Journal, one in Acta Odontologica Latinoamericana, one in the Journal of Dental Sciences, one in the Nigerian Journal of Clinical Practice, one in the International Medical Journal of Experimental and Clinical Research, one in the British Journal of Oral and Maxillofacial Surgery, one in The Saudi Dental Journal, one in Imaging Science in Dentistry, one in Medical Principles and Practice, one in The Bulletin of Tokyo Dental College, and one in Annals of Anatomy. All the included studies were published between 2008–2022. The research included was carried out in a variety of nations, including Brazil (n-16), China (n-7), Egypt (n-5), Germany (n-5), Poland (n-3), the United States (n-2), Korea (n-2), Turkey (n-2), New Zealand (n-1), Chile (n-1), France (n-1), Myanmar (n-1), Saudi Arabia (n-1), Italy (n-1), Japan (n-1), and the United Arab Emirates (n-1).

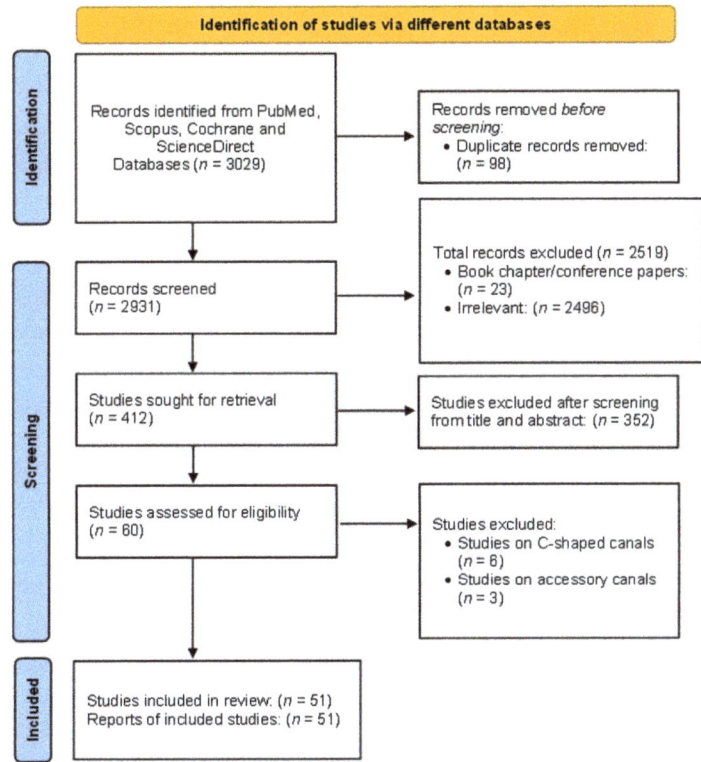

Figure 3. PRISMA flowchart showing the selection process of articles retrieved from different web sources.

Table 2. Studies included in the systematic review.

No.	Study Reference	Journal	Population	Year of Publication
1	[36]	Journal of Endodontics	Egyptians	2015
2	[37]	Journal of Endodontics	Germans	2019
3	[3]	Journal of Endodontics	Swiss Germans	2020
4	[38]	Journal of Applied Oral Sciences	Brazilians	2019
5	[39]	Journal of Endodontics	Americans	2013
6	[40]	International Endodontic Journal	Brazilians	2015
7	[41]	Clinical Oral Investigations	Koreans	2012
8	[42]	Australian Endodontic Journal	Brazilians	2018
9	[43]	Journal of Endodontics	Brazilians	2014
10	[44]	Journal of Endodontics	Brazilians	2015
11	[45]	Journal of Endodontics	Brazilians	2016
12	[46]	International Endodontic Journal	New Zealanders	2011
13	[47]	Journal of Endodontics	Brazilians	2013

Table 2. Cont.

No.	Study Reference	Journal	Population	Year of Publication
14	[48]	International Endodontic Journal	Brazilians	2017
15	[49]	Journal of Endodontics	Egyptians	2016
16	[50]	International Journal of Oral science	Egyptians	2017
17	[51]	Journal of Endodontics	Swiss Germans	2020
18	[52]	Archives of Oral Biology	Chinese	2018
19	[53]	Journal of Conservative Dentistry	Brazilians	2018
20	[54]	Scientific Reports	Chilean	2021
21	[55]	Journal of Conservative Dentistry	Brazilians	2018
22	[56]	Swiss Dental Journal	Egyptians	2017
23	[57]	Journal of Endodontics	Americans	2019
24	[58]	European Endodontic Journal	Brazilians	2020
25	[59]	Clinical Anatomy	Polandians	2018
26	[60]	Acta Odontológica Latinoamericana	Brazilians	2020
27	[61]	Journal of Dental Sciences	Chinese	2022
28	[62]	Oral Surgery, Oral Medicine, Oral Pathology, Oral Radiology, and Endodontology	Italians	2008
29	[63]	Journal of Endodontics	Brazilians	2013
30	[64]	Clinical Oral Investigations	Chinese	2021
31	[65]	Scientific Reports	Chinese	2017
32	[66]	Nigerian Journal of Clinical Practice	Egyptians	2020
33	[67]	International Medical Journal of Experimental and Clinical Research	Chinese	2021
34	[68]	British Journal of Oral and Maxillofacial Surgery	France	2005
35	[1]	International Endodontic Journal	Brazilians	2013
36	[69]	Clinical Oral Investigations	Chinese	2021
37	[70]	International Journal of Dentistry	Myanmar	2021
38	[71]	The Saudi Dental Journal	Saudis	2016
39	[72]	International Endodontic Journal	Brazilians	2012
40	[73]	Scientific Reports	Swiss Germans	2021
41	[74]	Clinical Oral Investigations	Chinese	2013
42	[75]	Journal of Applied Oral Science	Brazilians	2016
43	[76]	Journal of Endodontics	Swiss Germans	2020
44	[77]	Imaging Science in Dentistry	Turkish	2021
45	[78]	International Endodontic Journal	Italians	2009
46	[79]	Clinical Anatomy	Polish	2018
47	[22]	Medical Principles and Practice	Emiratis	2017
48	[80]	The Bulletin of Tokyo Dental College	Japanese	2011
49	[81]	Oral Surgery, Oral Medicine, Oral Pathology, Oral Radiology, and Endodontology	Koreans	2009
50	[12]	Annals of Anatomy	Polish	2018
51	[82]	Archives of Oral Biology	Turkish	2020

In the studies included, a total of 6696 samples were studied. The studies were conducted on either maxillary (n-2222) or mandibular teeth (n-3760), permanent anteriors (n-625), and third molars (n-89). Of the total maxillary and mandibular teeth, 970 were maxillary first molars, 262 were maxillary second molars, 659 were both maxillary first and second molars, 331 were maxillary premolars, 789 were mandibular first molars, 158 were mandibular second molars, 529 were mandibular first premolars, 1254 were mandibular incisors, 281 were mandibular canines, and the remaining 1463 were mixed. The authors used different reagents to store the samples (70% Alcohol, 0.5% sodium azide solution, or 10% formalin). To scan samples, a Scanco Medical machine was used in 10 studies, a Bruker Micro-CT machine in 34 studies, Micro-CT Inveon, Siemens Medical Solutions, Knoxville in two studies, VGStudio Max 2.2 in one study, Nikon Metrology Inc, Brighton in one study, Nanotom S, General Electric in one study, Kodak, Rochester, New York, USA in one study, and HMX 225-ACTIS 4, Tesco, Inc in one study.

Bruker Micro-CT software from Kontich, Belgium (n-27), software VG-Studio Max 2.2 from Volume Graphics, Germany Heidelberg (n-10), NRecon software (n-5), CTAn v.1.12 software Mimics 17.01, Materialize, Leuven, Belgium (n-4), MICs 10.01 software Materialise, Leuven, Belgium (n-1), Image processing language (n-1), On-Demand 3D software from Cybermed, Seoul, Republic of Korea (n-2), Cobra software Siemens Medical Solutions, Knoxville (n 1), and MeVisLab v3.2 software (MeVis Medical Solutions AG, Bremen, Germany) (n-1) was used in the studies to interpret the data about root canal morphologies. The minimum Voxel size (resolution) adopted in included studies was 11.6 μm. However, 60 μm was the maximum resolution adopted in included studies. Most studies classified the root canal morphology using Vertucci's classification system (n-16) and the four-digit system (n-6). Furthermore, Weine's classification system (n-3), Pucci & Reig (1944), a new classification system by Ahmed et al., Pomeranz 's classification and the American Association of Endodontics system for classification were also used. The technical characteristics of the studies are shown in Table 3.

Table 3. Characteristics of the included studies.

Study Reference	Sample Size	Sample Type	Micro-CT Machine	Voxel Size (Resolution)	Software Used	Classification System	Technique	Results	Conclusion
[x]	179	Maxillary first molars *	Scanco Medical, Bruttisellen, Switzerland	20 μm	Heidelberg, Germany Volume Graphics VG-Studio Max 2.2;	fourfour-digit system	Endodontic access cavity was prepared with a high-speed and round bur, pulp stones were removed by ultrasonic scaler if needed, and at the end, the pulp chamber was rinsed with sodium hypochlorite following suction for drying and assessment of Micro-CT morphology of the root canal.	In mesiobuccal roots, the most prevalent root canal configurations were 1-1-1/1 (45.8%), 1-1-2/2 (25.1%), and 1-2-2/2 (10.1%), while in distobuccal roots, the most prevalent root canal configurations were 1-1-1/1 (97.2%) and 1-1-1/1 palatal (10.1%) (98.9 percent).	Maxillary first molars have a wide range of root canal configurations. According to this study, the mesiobuccal root has only one main foramen and one root canal entrance.
[x]	125	Permanent Anteriors	Scanco Medical, Bruttisellen, Switzerland	20 μm	Heidelberg, Germany Volume Graphics VG-Studio Max 2.2;	four-digit system	Rendering software was used to visualize the various tooth structures generated from the Micro-CT scans. Red was used to color the pulp chamber and RCS, white for the enamel/crown area, and transparent grey for the root/dentin area. The root canal configuration was determined when the roots were split into three.	The most prominent root canal configurations were 1-1-1/1 (56%), 1-2-1/1 (17.6%), and 1-1-1/2 (10.4%); however, 19 teeth had a total of nine root canal combinations (15.2 percent).	The study discovered variations in the morphology of root canal of anterior teeth in the German population, the most prevalent root canal configuration being 1-1-1/1.
[ ]	109	Mandibular first premolar *	Scanco Medical, Bruttisellen, Switzerland	16 μm	Heidelberg, Germany Volume Graphics VG-Studio Max 2.2;	four-digit system	The pulp chamber and root canals were red, the enamel was white, and the dentin was a translucent grey tint to distinguish tooth features. The root canal configuration was determined by dividing the roots into thirds and using the RCC method to generate a four-digit code system. The first three digits of the code system indicate the number of root canals at the coronal boundary of the coronal, middle, and apical thirds of a root; the fourth digit, divided by a slash, represents the number of physiological foramina.	The most common root canal configurations were 1-1-1/1 (70.6%), 1-1-2/2 (7.3%), and 1-2-1/1 (7.3%).	The researchers discovered differences in the morphology of root canal of maxillary first premolars in the German-Swiss population, with 1-1-1/1 root canal configurations being the most prevalent (70.6 percent).

Table 3. Cont.

Study Reference	Sample Size	Sample Type	Micro-CT Machine	Voxel Size (Resolution)	Software Used	Classification System	Technique	Results	Conclusion
[38]	500	Maxillary and mandibular: Anteriors, premolars, and molars	Bruker Micro-CT, Kontich, Belgium	26 μm	Bruker Micro-CT, Kontich, Belgium	Pucci & Reig (PR) (1944) and American Association of Endodontics	CT scanning for root canal morphology.	According to the PR, significant canals were found in 100% of the teeth studied, with the exception of the second mesiobuccal canal in the maxillary first and second molars, which had a frequency of 87 and 75 percent, respectively. In terms of the major canal, the AAE classification revealed the same results as the PR classification.	The variation of the RCS was accurately described by Micro-CT, which was proved by the PR and AAE classifications, with some discrepancies observed for upper molars.
[39]	18	human hemi-maxilla	Scanco Medical, Bruttisellen, Switzerland	20 μm	Image processing language (version 5.15; Scanco Medical)	—	The hemi-maxillae were taken from cadavers used in medical research and teaching (with prior agreement). Teeth from the human hemi-maxillae were extracted, washed with 3% NaOCl, and imaged using a CT scanner.	Thirteen first molars and fourteen second molars from eighteen cadavers were studied. Two canals were found in 100% of maxillary first molar MB roots (100 percent). Two canals were found in 57 percent of maxillary second molar MB roots.	Micro-CT canal numbers were considerably different from digital periapical radiograph counts in cadaver maxillary teeth, but not from 3-D CBCT counts.
[40]	32	Mesial roots of mandibular first molars	Bruker Micro-CT, Kontich, Belgium	19.6 μm	Bruker Micro-CT, Kontich, Belgium	Vertucci's classification	Group 1 and Group 2 (n = 10), Group 3 (n = 12). Based on Micro-CT scans and presenting several canal configurations, were evaluated followed by a clearing technique.	Type I root canals were found in a considerably limited number of cleaned teeth, but type II root canals were found in all cases.	The evaluation technique and anatomy type significantly affected the accuracy of detecting mesial root canal shape among the tooth population examined.
[41]	154	Extracted human maxillary first molar mesiobuccal roots **	SkyScan, Aartselaar, Belgium	15.9 μm	On-Demand 3D software (Cybermed, Seoul, Republic of Korea).	Vertucci's classification	The mesiobuccal roots of maxillary first molars with more than two canals were examined using 154 Micro-CT scans. Weine and Vertucci's classifications were used to classify the root canal configurations of multiple-canalled MB roots.	73.4 percent of the MB roots had multiple canals. The most common canal type was Weine type III. In 29.2 percent and 17.7 percent of MB roots, respectively, nonclassifiable configuration types were found.	The current study indicates that configuration classifications may need to be modified to reflect MB root morphology better.

Table 3. Cont.

Study Reference	Sample Size	Sample Type	Micro-CT Machine	Voxel Size (Resolution)	Software Used	Classification System	Technique	Results	Conclusion
[42]	104	Extracted human mandibular first molars	Bruker Micro-CT, Kontich, Belgium	12.1 μm	Bruker Micro-CT, Kontich, Belgium	Vertucci's classification	The mesial RCS were modelled in 3-D and assessed.	The morphology of mandibular molars' mesial root canals was highly variable. The most common root canal configuration was Vertucci type IV (46.2 percent).	The morphology of the mesial root canals of mandibular molars was discovered to be very diverse in a Brazilian community. Clinicians must have a thorough understanding of the mandibular first molar mesial root canal architecture.
[43]	100	Extracted single-rooted human mandibular incisors	Bruker Micro-CT, Kontich, Belgium	12.1 μm	Bruker Micro-CT, Kontich, Belgium	Vertucci's classification	A Micro-CT system was used to scan the specimen. At five different levels in the apical third, the software was used to assess the length of the teeth and the number of canal orifices.	The mandibular central and lateral incisors had average lengths of 20.71 and 21.56 mm, respectively. One, two, or three canal orifices were discovered during a cross-section examination of the apical third. According to qualitative assessments of 3-D models of the RCS of the central and lateral incisor teeth, Vertucci's type I (50 and 62 percent) the most common configuration.	The most common canal configurations in mandibular incisors were Vertucci's types I and III.
[44]	100	Extracted mandibular first molars	Bruker Micro-CT, Kontich, Belgium	19.6 μm	Bruker Micro-CT, Kontich, Belgium	Vertucci's classification	The teeth were scanned in a Micro-CT device after being mounted on a custom attachment.	In 76 percent of the distal roots, a single root canal was discovered. In 13%, 8%, and 3% of the sample, respectively, two, three, and four canals were discovered. In 13 cases, the RCS configuration did not fit into Vertucci's classification.	Single root canals were seen in a significant percentage of the mandibular first molars' distal roots. Canal configurations not included in Vertucci's configuration scheme were discovered in 13% of the samples.
[45]	169	Extracted Maxillary first molars	Bruker Micro-CT, Kontich, Belgium	60 μm	Bruker Micro-CT, Kontich, Belgium	Vertucci's classification	By sectioning the molar at the cementoenamel junction, the palatal root was obtained. Micro-CT was used to scan the roots.	Vertucci type I was used for classifying all canals. Sixty-six percent of the canals had oval cross-sections. In 95 percent of the samples, the major foramen did not line up with the root apex. Straight canals accounted for just 8% of the canals.	Type I was discovered in the palatal roots. However, when treating these roots, several variables must be addressed, such as the frequent occurrence of moderate/severe curvatures, cross-sections, oval-shaped, and the presence of many roots.

Table 3. *Cont.*

Study Reference	Sample Size	Sample Type	Micro-CT Machine	Voxel Size (Resolution)	Software Used	Classification System	Technique	Results	Conclusion
[46]	20	Extracted maxillary first molars ***	SkyScan Micro-CT scanner (SkyScan 1172 X-ray Microtomography, Antwerp, Belgium), twelve-bit digital cooled CCD camera with fiber optics	11.6 μm	T Converter (Amira 4.1; Mercury Computer System Inc. Chelmsford, MA, USA) (ECAD-2-12210 PMC; Mercury Computer System Inc.)	Weine and Vertucci's classification	The mesiobuccal root of the maxillary first molar was placed in a 7 mm plastic container. To remove the adhering from hard and soft tissues, the roots were cleansed, and the mesiobuccal root was removed at the furcation level.	The root canal systems of a large percentage of the roots examined were complex, with 90 percent having a second mesiobuccal canal. Only 60% of root canals could be classified using the Weine classification system, while 70% could be classified using the Vertucci system.	Micro-CT enables a more thorough analysis of root canal anatomy, revealing that the morphology of the mesiobuccal root of maxillary first molar teeth is complicated, and that existing morphological categories are insufficient to capture this complexity.
[47]	340	Extracted Mandibular incisors	Skyscan 1174 (Bruker Micro-CT, Kontich, Belgium)	19 μm	NRecon software, CTAn v.1.12 software (SkyScan, Belgium)	Vertucci classification	The numbers of canals were categorized using the Vertucci classification system, and the apical third was measured in 3-D. For each anatomic categorization, the data was reported as a median and range.	A single root canal was found in all of the specimens (N = 257). Vertucci type III (N = 56) was the second most common morphology. This anatomical group accounts for 92 percent of the total sample. At the 1 mm apical level, oval canals were found 16.7% of the time for Vertucci type I and 37.5 percent of the time for Vertucci type II. At the 3 mm apical level, oval canals increased to 32.4 percent and 76.2 percent for Vertucci type I and III, respectively.	Type I and III forms were found in 92 percent of the mandibular incisors examined. In these morphological configurations, oval-shaped canals in the apical third were common, and they were more common in type III.

49

Table 3. Cont.

Study Reference	Sample Size	Sample Type	Micro-CT Machine	Voxel Size (Resolution)	Software Used	Classification System	Technique	Results	Conclusion
[43]	100	Extracted fused-rooted maxillary second molar	Skyscan 1174 (Bruker Micro-CT, Kontich, Belgium)	19.6 μm	(NRecon. 1.6.3; Bruker Micro-CT), CTAn v. 1.16 (Bruker Micro-CT), and CTVolv. 2.3 software (Bruker Micro-CT).	Vertucci classification	At 1, 2, and 3 mm from the anatomical apex of the fused roots, the morphology of the RCS was assessed using the Vertucci classification.	Type 3, Distobuccal root fused with Palatal root (27 percent), Type 4, Mesiobuccal root fused with Distobuccal root, and Palatal root fused with MB or DB roots were the most common root canal fusions (32 percent).	In the root canal system of maxillary second molars with fused roots, merging canals were common.
[49]	118	Mandibular first molars *	Scanco Medical, Bruttisellen, Switzerland	20 μm	Heidelberg, Germany Volume Graphics, VG Studio Max 2.2;	Four-digit system	The pulpal access cavity was prepared with a diamond bur at a high speed, pulp stones were eliminated with an ultrasonic scaler if necessary, and the pulp chamber was rinsed with sodium hypochlorite at the end.	The most common root canal configurations in the mesial root were 2-2-2/2 (31.4%), 2-2-1/1 (15.3%), and 2-2-2/3 (11.9%); there were also 24 additional root canal configurations in this root. In the distal root, 1-1-1/1 (58.5%), 1-1-1/2 (10.2%), and 16 different root canal configurations were found.	The root canal configurations of mandibular first molars vary greatly. Many morphologic differences were found in both the mesial and distal roots.
[50]	123	Maxillary second molar *	Scanco Medical, Bruttisellen, Switzerland	20 μm	Heidelberg, Germany Volume Graphics VG Studio Max 2.2,	Four-digit system	Endodontic access cavities were generated under a microscope for further investigation of the tooth's internal morphology; making sure not to affect the root canal system morphology or the pulp chamber floor.	The most common root canal configurations in the mesiobuccal root were 2-2-2/2 (19.5%), 2-2-1/1 (14.6%), and 2-1-1/1 (13.0 percent). A total of 93.5 percent of distobuccal roots and 96.7 percent of palatal roots had a 1-1-1/1 arrangement, respectively.	The most common root canal configurations in the mesiobuccal root were 1-1-1/1 (26%).
[51]	116	Maxillary second premolar *	Scanco Medical, Bruttisellen, Switzerland	16 μm	Heidelberg, Germany Volume Graphics VG Studio Max 2.2,	Four-digit system	The maxillary first premolars were scanned with a Micro-CT scanner. The pulp chamber and Root canal configuration (RCC) were depicted in red to identify tooth anatomy, the enamel in white, and the dentin in a transparent grey tint.	The most seen (RCCs) in Maxillary second premolar (Mx2s) were 1-1-1/1 (35.3%), 1-1-1/2 (21.6%), and 2-1-1/1 (14.7 percent). A total of 11 less common RCCs were discovered. There was just one root in all Mx2Ps.	Within the study's limits, maxillary second premolars had a significant RCC.

Table 3. Cont.

Study Reference	Sample Size	Sample Type	Micro-CT Machine	Voxel Size (Resolution)	Software Used	Classification System	Technique	Results	Conclusion
[52]	260	130 Maxillary and 130 Mandibular molars ***	(Bruker micro- CT, Kontich, Belgium) Skyscan 1174	43.3 μm	(Materialize, Leuven, Belgium) Mimics 17.01	Weine's classification	A semiautomated segmentation method was used to recreate the interior and exterior tooth anatomy. The basic tooth model and the pulp cavity model were combined using a Boolean formula to create a new tooth model. The cavities in this tooth model were filled in. After that, the teeth models were evaluated qualitatively and quantitatively.	A single fused root (51.5 percent) and a single root canal system (49.2 percent) were the most common root/canal types for maxillary molars; typical three-rooted molars were only found in 25.4 percent, and secondary MB canals were only seen in 2 percent. 25% The type 1-1 canal was the most common configuration for mesial and distal root canal systems. A total of 47.7% of mandibular molars were single-rooted, while 32.3 percent had a single root canal system; 20 single-rooted and 60 double-rooted molars had separate mesial and distal root canal systems (61.5%).	The root canal system of the third molars can be physically different in several ways. The degree of canal variation was small in most cases, and the canal form was clear.
[53]	80	Mandibular canines	SkyScan 1173 v2 Micro-CT (Bruker Micro-CT, Kontich, Belgium)	12.1 μm	NRecon software (v1.6.1); Bruker, Kontich, Belgium), (CTAn v. 1.14.4, Bruker Micro-CT Kontich, Belgium), and (CTVol v. 2.2.1, Bruker Micro-CT, Kontich, Belgium)	Vertucci's classification	The number of canals, root canal configurations according to Vertucci's classification, root length and number and location of lateral canals, the presence of apical delta, perimeter, roundness, and minor and major diameters at cervical, medium, and apical thirds and 1 mm from the foramen were evaluated.	All canals were classified as Vertucci Type 1. Lateral canals were verified in 42.4% of the roots, in apical third. The cross-sections at the cementoenamel junction and 1 mm from the apex were oval in 38.3% and 79.4% of the canals, respectively.	The root canal of single-rooted canines evaluated in the present study was classified as Vertucci type I.

Table 3. Cont.

Study Reference	Sample Size	Sample Type	Micro-CT Machine	Voxel Size (Resolution)	Software Used	Classification System	Technique	Results	Conclusion
[3]	186	Mandibular first premolar	SkyScan 1278, Bruker, Kontich, Belgium	50 μm	CTAn v.1.12 software (Bruker Micro-CT), Kontich, Belgium	Vertucci's and Ahmed's classification	All the samples were emerged in 5% sodium hypochlorite for 30 min and reserved in 10% neutral buffered formalin. Dental calculus was removed by using an ultrasonic scaler and stored in a moisturizing solution at room temperature. All teeth were scanned using a high- resolution Micro-CT device.	Radicular grooves were observed in 39.25% of teeth. The ASUDAS scores for radicular grooves were 60.75%, 13.98%, 12.36%, 10.22%, 2.15%, and 0.54%, from grade 0 to grade 5, respectively.	Mandibular first premolars showed a wide range of anatomical variations. Ahmed's criteria allowed for the classification of the internal anatomy of the root canal in a more precise and practical way than Vertucci's criteria. Teeth with multiple root canals had a higher incidence of radicular grooves and a more complex morphology compared with teeth with a single root canal.
[5]	520	Mandibular incisors	SkyScan 1176, Bruker Micro-CT, Kontich, Belgium	17.42 μm	CTAn (V1.11.8; SkyScan, Belgium) software, NRecon (V1.6.4.7; SkyScan, Belgium) software, and Data Viewer (V1.5.1.2; SkyScan, Belgium) software	–	All the samples were evaluated 9 mm from the apex using digital radiographs in buccolingual (BL) and mesiodistal (MD) directions. Root canal diameters obtained in measurements were 3, 6, and 9 mm from the apex.	Between all the incisors, 121 (23.3%) were flattened; 215 (41.3%) oval; 142 (27.3%) rounded; 23 (4.5%) round; and 19 (3.6%) with BL flatness 9 mm from the apex.	Oval root canals are predominant in mandibular incisors with a single canal at 9 mm from apex.
[6]	93	Mandibular second molar	Microcomp- uted tomography (VGStudio Max 2.2; Volume-graphics, Heidelberg, Germany)	20 μm	VGStudio Max 2.2; Volume- graphics, Heidelberg, Germany software	–	Teeth were cleaned and access cavities were prepared. The pulp chamber root was carefully removed by cutting along the pulp chamber walls. When required, ultrasonic tips were used to re- move pulp stones.	The most frequently observed root canal configurations in the mesial root were 2-2-1/1 (32.3%), 2-2-2/2 (28.0%), 1-1-1/1 (6.5%), and 2-1-1/1 (6.5%); an additional twelve different root canal configurations were also found here. In the distal root, the RCC 1-1-1/1 was observed in 81.7%; another ten different root canal configurations with a frequency of less than 5% were also observed in this root.	The root canal configuration of mandibular second molars showed a great variety. When compared with the first mandibular molar in a historical control from the same sample, the mandibular second molar presented less morphological diversifications.

Table 3. *Cont.*

Study Reference	Sample Size	Sample Type	Micro-CT Machine	Voxel Size (Resolution)	Software Used	Classification System	Technique	Results	Conclusion
[7]	47	Maxillary first and second molar	Nikon Metrology Inc. Brighton, MI, USA	-	VG Studio MAX 2.1 software (Volume Graphics GmbH, Heidelberg, Germany)	-	Teeth were mounted on a cylindrical specimen holder and scanned by mCT.	The palatal root of maxillary first molars was found to have statistically significantly thinner dentin than second molars on the palatal aspect of the root 8–11 mm from the apex, correlating to the coronal and middle thirds of the root. First molar palatal roots also had a statistically significantly wider canal mesiodistally than second molars at 13–15 mm from the apex.	The absence of an apical constriction in 76.6% of the specimens highlights the importance of creating an apical seat through instrumentation to maintain obturation materials.
[8]	96	Maxillary first molar mesiobuccal root	Micro-CT system (Skyscan 1173; Bruker Co., Kontich, Belgium)	21.39 μm	NRecon soft-ware v1.6.9.4 (Bruker Co., Kontich, Belgium), InstaRecon® v.1.3.9.2 (IR-CBR Server, University of Illinois Research Park, Illinois, EUA), CTAn v.1.14.4.1, Dataviewer, and CTVox software (Bruker Co., Kontich, Belgium)	Weine's and Vertucci's classification	Three-Dimensional images of mesiobuccal root were analyzed regarding the number of pulp chamber orifices, the number and classification of the canals, the presence of accessory canals in different thirds of the root, and the number and type of apical foramina.	A single entrance orifice was found in 53.0% of the samples, two in 43.9%, and only 3.1% had three orifices. The second mesiobuccal root canal (MB2) was present at some portion of the root in 87.5% of the specimens. A single apical foramen was present in 16.7%, two in 22.9%, and three or more foramina in 60.4% of the roots. Only 55.3% and 76.1% of the root canals could be arranged by Weine's and Vertucci's classifications, respectively.	The most commonly found type in this study was Weine type IV/Vertucci type V, and accessory canals were more detected at the apical third, followed by the middle and cervical thirds of the root, respectively.

Table 3. Cont.

Study Reference	Sample Size	Sample Type	Micro-CT Machine	Voxel Size (Resolution)	Software Used	Classification System	Technique	Results	Conclusion
[=]	374	Mandibular first, second and third molar	Micro-CT scanner (Nanotom S, General Electric)	13.68 μm	CTVox, CTAnalyser and CTVol (SkyScan®)	Vertucci's classification	All the molars were scanned with a Micro-CT scanner (Nanotom S, General Electric)	In the mesial roots of mandibular molars, the most frequent Vertucci type of canal configuration was type IV, except for the mandibular third molar where type I was most common. Type I was most common in the distal root.	Knowledge of the complex anatomy of the mandibular molars can make root canal therapy more likely to succeed.
[6]	89	Mandibular incisor	SkyScan 1173 microtomograph (Bruker Micro-CT, Kontich, Belgium)	12.11 μm	NRecon v1.6.6.0 software (Bruker Micro-CT, Kontich, Belgium)	Vertucci's classification	All the lower incisors were scanned with a micro-CT and reconstructed with NRecon software. Two-Dimensional parameters (perimeter, root length, circularity, and canal diameter) and 3D parameters (volume, surface area, and structure model index) were evaluated with CTAn and CTVol software.	It was found that 89.9% of the canals had a single main root canal (type I), followed by type II (6.7%) and III (3.4%), while 5.6% of the specimens presented lateral canals and 1.1% had an apical delta. Mean volume and surface area were 31.80 mm^3 and 90.58 mm^2, respectively. The most prevalent shape of the root canal at CEJ level was circular (41.6%) and 1 mm from the apex, and 73% of the samples were classified as oval.	Incisors have a single root with a relatively simple anatomy, and internal anatomical variations may offer a high degree of technical complexity.
[6]	136	Mandibular first molar	Micro-CT system (mCT-50; Scanco Medical, Bassersdorf, Switzerland)	30 μm	Mimics 18.0 software (Materialise, Leuven, Belgium)	–	All the teeth were scanned with Mimics 18.0 software (Materialise, Leuven, Belgium). The 3-dimensional models of the teeth with root canal systems were constructed and made transparent by adjusting the transparency. The tooth axes based on the shape of the tooth was calculated automatically based on principal component analysis.	The measurements of the maximum curvature of coronal root canals in the axial direction were: in three-canals two-rooted teeth, the average angles of curvatures were 23, 25, and 11 for MB, ML, and DB canals; in four-canals two-rooted teeth were 23, 25, 12, and 16 for MB, ML, DB, and DL canals, respectively; in four-canals three-rooted teeth were 25, 27, 17, and 39 for MB, ML, DB, and DL canals, respectively.	The results of this study are similar to those previously obtained using CBCT and can help us design endodontic approaches.

Table 3. Cont.

Study Reference	Sample Size	Sample Type	Micro-CT Machine	Voxel Size (Resolution)	Software Used	Classification System	Technique	Results	Conclusion
[62]	30	Premolar	X-Ray microfocus CT scanner (SkyScan 1072; SkyScan, Aart- selaar, Belgium)	19.1 μm	software (NRecon V1.4.0; SkyScan), CT-analyzer V1.6; SkyScan	—	All the radiographs were made in the buccolingual (BL) and mesiodistal (MD) direction to evaluate the root canal anatomy and to identify the radiographic apex using X-ray microfocus CT scanner (SkyScan 1072, SkyScan, Aart-selaar, Belgium).	At all levels of analysis, the BL diameter was greater than the MD diameter for both the canal and the root. Generally, canal and root increased coronally. Buccal and lingual wall thicknesses were greater than mesial and distal at all levels. Canal diameters were at 1 mm from the apex.	Oval canals are frequently present, including in the last few apical millimeters of the root canals.
[63]	105	Mandibular premolar	Micro-CT system (SkyScan 1174v2; Bruker Micro-CT, Kontich, Belgium)	18 μm	NRecon v.1.6.3; Bruker Micro-CT	—	The samples were mounted on a custom attachment and scanned in a Micro-CT system (SkyScan 1174v2; Bruker Micro-CT, Kontich, Belgium)	Overall, specimens had one root with a main canal that divided into mesiobuccal, distobuccal, and lingual canals at the furcation level. Mean length of the teeth was 22.9 and 2.06 mm, and the configuration of the pulp chamber was mostly triangle-shaped. Mean distances from the furcation to the apex and cementoenamel junction were 9.14, 2.07, 5.59, and 2.19 mm.	Type IX configuration of the root canal system was found in 16 of 105 (15.2%) extracted mandibular premolars with radicular grooves.
[64]	72	Maxillary first molar	Micro-CT scanning (SkyScan 1174; Bruker Micro-CT, Kontich, Belgium)	22.4 μm	Mimics 15.01 (Materialise, Leuven, Belgium) software	Vertucci's classification	Each specimen was scanned along the tooth axis with a voxel size of 22.4 μm using Micro-CT scanning (SkyScan 1174; Bruker Micro-CT, Kontich, Belgium). The root canal configuration in the MB roots was examined and described by Vertucci's classification.	MB2 canals were detected in 76.4% (55/72) of the total sample teeth. The incidence of accessory canals was 56.9% (41/72). The mean ratio of D/d was generally "greatest to least".	The occurrence of finding MB2 in maxillary second molar is high.

Table 3. *Cont.*

Study Reference	Sample Size	Sample Type	Micro-CT Machine	Voxel Size (Resolution)	Software Used	Classification System	Technique	Results	Conclusion
[65]	178	Mandibular first premolar	Micro-CT scanner (Micro-CT Inveon; Siemens Medical Solutions, Knoxville, TN, USA)	15 μm	Cobra software (Siemens Medical Solutions, Knoxville, TN)	Vertucci's classification	All samples were scanned using a Micro-CT scanner (Micro-CT Inveon; Siemens Medical Solutions, Knoxville, TN) with voxel sizes of 15 μm × 15 μm × 15 μm. The in-built Cobra software (Siemens Medical Solutions, Knoxville, TN) was used for the 3-D reconstruction and analysis.	Almost all the samples were single-rooted (99.4%). In total, 64.04% of teeth possessed type I canal systems, while 34.27% had two canals, and 1.69% had three canals. According to ASUDAS, the scores of radicular grooves were 56.74%, 16.85%, 12.36%, 10.11%, 3.37%, and 0.56%, respectively, from grade 0 to grade 5. The roots with radicular grooves (grade 3 or 4) were defined as Tome's anomalous root and these roots have a high incidence of C-shape configurations (66.67%) and multiple-canal systems (100%).	There is obvious variation of the root anatomy and root canal morphology of mandibular first premolar among the southwestern Chinese population, which is very complex and requires careful assessment for endodontic treatment.
[66]	240	Mandibular molar	Micro-CT scanner (SkyScan 1174, SkyScan, Bruker, Belgium)	32.17 μm	software (SkyScan 1174, SkyScan, Bruker, Belgium)	Pomeranz's classification	All the samples were scanned with a Micro-CT scanner (SkyScan 1174, SkyScan, Bruker, Belgium).	The evaluation of three-dimensional (3-D) images of this study showed that no significant difference was found between the percentage of MM (27.5%) and MD canals (22.5%) ($p = 0.2064$); however, there was a significant difference between the percentage of teeth having both extra canals (10%) and teeth having only one of these canals ($p < 0.05$). The confluent configuration (71%) was significantly higher than the other configurations ($p < 0.05$).	The presence of MM canals was higher than that of MD canals; however, the difference was nonsignificant. The occurrence of both extra canals in the same tooth was less significant than the occurrence of only one of either MM or MD canals. The extra canals detected had a higher percentage of the confluent configuration rather than the fin or the independent configurations.

Table 3. *Cont.*

Study Reference	Sample Size	Sample Type	Micro-CT Machine	Voxel Size (Resolution)	Software Used	Classification System	Technique	Results	Conclusion
[?]	274	Maxillary premolars and molar	Micro CT inveon; Siemens Medical Solutions, Knoxville, TN)	15 μm	MICs 10.01 software (Materialise, Leuven, Belgium)	Vertucci's classification	After access cavity pulp chamber was cleaned and an 15 k file was inserted in the canal, X-rays were taken from the mesiodistal and buccolingual direction.	The root canals of the maxillary posterior teeth showed more significant curvature in the mesiodistal direction than in the buccolingual direction ($p < 0.05$). The MB2 root canal of maxillary molars showed severe bending in the mesiodistal direction: 25.16 ± 6.6 degrees and 28.05 ± 8.65 degrees in first and second molars, respectively. The detection rate of MB2 was 48% in maxillary first molars and 32% in maxillary second molars.	The maxillary posterior teeth showed obvious root canal bending variation and root canal configuration differences. Mostly, the root canals of maxillary premolars showed moderate curvature, while the root canals of maxillary molars showed moderate to severe bending.
[?]	11	Third molar	The Skyscan 1072 X-ray computed microtomograph (Skyscan, Aartselaar, Belgium)	19.74 μm	ANT software (release 2.05, Skyscan, Aartselaar, Belgium)	—	The enamel crown was sealed onto poly (methylmethacrylate) blocks with commercial cyanoacrylic glue. Poly (methylmethacrylate) is a radiolucent polymer and these blocks allowed the teeth to be handled easily inside the Micro-CT system. The Skyscan 1072 X-ray computed microtomograph (Skyscan, Aartselaar, Belgium) was used for scanning.	Most roots had a single canal that tapered to the apex. Several canals seemed to have a thin, ribbon-like appearance with focal areas of contact between the walls of the dentine.	Microcomputed tomography seems to be a promising way of studying dental anatomy.
[1]	100	Mandibular canine	ICT scanner (Skyscan 1174v2; Bruker Micro-CT, Kontich, Belgium)	19.6 μm	NRecon v. 1.6.3; Bruker Micro-CT and CTAn v. 1.12 software (Bruker Micro-CT).	—	After being washed in running water for 24 h, each tooth was dried, mounted on a custom attachment, and scanned in an ICT scanner (Skyscan 1174v2; Bruker Micro-CT, Kontich, Belgium).	The length of the roots ranged from 12.53 to 18.08 mm. Thirty-one specimens had no accessory canals. The location of the apical foramen varied considerably. The mean distance from the root apex to the major apical foramen was 0.27 and 0.25 mm, and the major diameter of the major apical foramen ranged from 0.16 to 0.72 mm. Mean major and minor diameters of the canal 1 mm short of the foramen were 0.43 and 0.31 mm.	The anatomy and morphology of the root canal of single-rooted canine varied widely in different levels of the root.

Table 3. Cont.

Study Reference	Sample Size	Sample Type	Micro-CT Machine	Voxel Size (Resolution)	Software Used	Classification System	Technique	Results	Conclusion
[69]	208	Mandibular incisors	Micro-CT scanner (μCT-50; Scanco Medical, Bassersdorf, Switzerland)	30 μm	MeVisLab v3.2 software (MeVis Medical Solutions AG, Bremen, Germany)	Vertucci's classification	All the samples were scanned with a Micro-CT scanner (μCT-50; Scanco Medical).	Three canal categories, labeled as Single (77.88%), Merged (15.87%), and Separated (6.25%), were summarized. The most frequent constriction type in main foramina was single constriction (42.53%). Wide and narrow diameters are in a single main foramen. During the virtual root-end resection, 97.12% of roots underwent successful resection at the 2 mm level.	This study provides detailed information about the root canal morphology and thickness of the crown and root of mandibular incisors in a Chinese population. The most frequent canal configuration was the Single type (77.88%), and more than half (55.2%) of the specimens demonstrated the presence of a constriction.
[70]	101	Maxillary first molar	SkyScan 1272 scanner (Bruker Micro-CT, Belgium)	10 μm	NRecon software (Bruker Micro-CT), CTAn software (Bruker Micro-CT) and CTVol software (Bruker Micro-CT)	Vertucci's classification	All the samples were scanned with a SkyScan 1272 scanner (Bruker Micro-CT, Belgium).	Eighty-three (82.18%) mesiobuccal roots had multiple canals. The most common canal type is type IV (45.5%), followed by type II (17.8%) and I (17.8%) canals. Type III, V, VI, VII, and VIII canals are less than 10% in total. Seven additional canal types were seen for 10% in total. Fourteen (13.86%) distobuccal roots had multiple canals, and the predominant canal type is type I (86.1%), followed by type II (5.9%) and V (4%) canals. Three additional canal types were observed for 4% in total. All palatal roots possessed the simplest type I canal.	The results of this study reiterate that the root canal configuration of Burmese MFMs is quite complex, especially the mesiobuccal root possessing the highest incidence of additional canals, lateral canals, and apical delta, and isthmuses among three roots.
[71]	100	Maxillary second premolar	SkyScan 1172 X-ray Micro-CT scanner (Bruker Corp., Antwerp, Belgium)	27.4 μm	SkyScan CT-Volume v2.2 software (Bruker Corp., Antwerp, Belgium)	Vertucci classification	All the samples were scanned by SkyScan 1172 X-ray Micro-CT scanner (Bruker Corp., Antwerp, Belgium).	Number of roots were: one root (67%), two roots (30%), three roots (3%), and root canal classifications were IV and V (both found in 23% of teeth), followed by type I (17%), type III (9%), type II (7%), and type VII (2%).	The root canal morphology of maxillary second premolars in the Saudi Arabian subpopulation is complex and requires cautious evaluation prior to endodontic treatment.

Table 3. Cont.

Study Reference	Sample Size	Sample Type	Micro-CT Machine	Voxel Size (Resolution)	Software Used	Classification System	Technique	Results	Conclusion
[2]	25	Maxillary second molar	Micro-CT scanner (SkyScan 1174v2; SkyScan N.V., Kontich, Belgium)	22.6 μm	NRecon v1.6.4; SkyScan	–	A Micro-CT scanner 1174v2; SkyScan N.V., Kontich, Belgium) was used for scanning all teeth.	The specimens were classified as types I ($n = 16$), II ($n = 7$), and III ($n = 2$). The size of the roots was similar ($p > 0.05$), and most of them presented straight with one canal, except the mesio/buccal that showed two canals in 24% of the samples.	Considering the evaluation of the external and internal anatomy of four-rooted maxillary second molars, it can be concluded that most of the samples were classified as type I.
[3]	101	Mandibular canine	Bruker SkyScan	10.0 μm	Bruker Micro-CT, Control software version 1.1.19, Kontich, Belgium	–	Bruker SkyScan was used for scanning for samples.	The root canal configurations were 1-1-1/1 (74.5%) and 1-1-1/2 (14.3%). Physiological foramen was observed in 80.0% of the MaCas, two in 16.3%, three in 1.0%, and four in 2.0%.	Single-rooted mandibular canines (MaCas) were the most frequently observed (97.0%) ones.
[4]	115	Mandibular first premolar	Siemens Inveon CT, Munich, Germany	14.97 μm	Mimics 10.01 software (Materialise, Leuven, Belgium)	Vertucci classification	Mimics 10.01 software (Materialise, Leuven, Belgium) was used for 3-D imaging.	Canal configuration types I (65.2%), III (2.6%), V (22.6%), and VII were identified (0.9%).	The data obtained in this study revealed complex root morphology with a high prevalence of multiple canals, more than half of which exhibited type I canal patterns.
[5]	55	Mandibular first molar	Micro-CT system (SkyScan 1174v2; Bruker-Micro-CT, Kontich, Belgium)	19.6 μm	NRecon v1.6.3; Bruker Micro-CT, Kontich, Belgium	–	Three-Dimensional models were reconstructed after binarization of the source images, exported by Micro-CT, Kontich, Belgium).	Mesial roots showed a complex distribution of the root canal system in comparison to the distal roots. Almost all distal roots had one root canal and one apical foramen with few accessory canals.	Distolingual roots generally have a short length, severe curvature, and a single root canal with a low apical diameter.

Table 3. Cont.

Study Reference	Sample Size	Sample Type	Micro-CT Machine	Voxel Size (Resolution)	Software Used	Classification System	Technique	Results	Conclusion
[76]	115	Maxillar first premolar	Micro-CT unit (mCT 40; Scanco Medical, Bruttisellen, Switzerland)	16 μm	VGStudio Max 2.2; Volume Graphics, Heidelberg, Germany	—	A Micro-CT unit (mCT 40; Scanco Medical, Bruttisellen, Switzerland) was used for scanning all the samples.	Root canal configurations were in 30 single-rooted teeth, 2-2-2/2 (30.0%), 1-2-2/2 (13.3%), 1-2-1/2 (10%), and 2-2-1/2 (10.0%), and in two-rooted maxillary roots 1-1-1/1 (56.8%), 1-1-1/2 (29.6%), and 1-1-2/2 (8.6%) in the buccal root, and 1-1-1/1 (92.6%) and 1-1-1/2 (6.2%) in the palatal root's root canal configuration appeared most frequently.	The results of this study provide detailed morphologic root canal configuration information. Single-rooted teeth showed more morphologic diversifications more frequently than two- or three-rooted premolars. Within two-rooted premolars, the buccal root had higher root canal configuration variety, accessory canals, and foramina numbers than the palatal root.
[77]	40	Mandibular first molar	micro- CT scanner (SkyScan 1172 X-ray Micro-CT; SkyScan, Ant- werp, Belgium)	—	SkyScan Micro-CT software for 3-D analysis on sagittal, coronal, and axial slices	Vertucci classification	Forty mandibular first molars were cleaned and stored. Micro-CT scanner (SkyScan 1172 X-ray Micro-CT; SkyScan, Ant- werp, Belgium) were used to scane all the teeth.	The mesial roots of mandibular first molars had canal configurations of type I (15%), type II (7.5%), type III (25%), type IV (10%), type V (2.5%), type VI (7.5%), and type VII (7.5%).	Frequent variations were detected in mesial roots of mandibular first molars. Clinicians should take into consideration the complex structure of the root canal morphology before commencing root canal treatment.
[78]	30	Maxillary first molar	SkyScan 1072, SkyScan b.v.b.a, Aartselaar, Belgium	19.1 μm	NRecon V1.4.0; SkyScan b.v.b.a	Vertucci classification	Maxillary first molar teeth having three separate roots were randomly selected for microtomographic analysis.	The MB2 canal was present in 80% of specimens and was independent in 42% of these cases. When present, the MB2 canal merged with the MB1 canal in 58% of cases.	The MB root canal anatomy was complex: a high incidence of MB2 root canals, isthmuses, accessory canals, apical deltas, and loops was found.
[79]	208	Maxillary first and second molar	CTVox, CTAnalyser and CTVol (SkyScan®)	13.68 μm	CTVox, CTAnalyser and CTVol (SkyScan®)	Vertucci classification	After cleaning all the maxillary molars, they were scanned by CTVox, CTAnalyser and CTVol (SkyScan®).	The mesiobuccal root was the most variable with respect to canal configuration, with type I being the most common configuration followed by type II and type IV. Type I was the most common canal configuration in the distobuccal and palatal root.	It is important to know the morphology of the root canal system in order to perform endodontic treatment correctly.

Table 3. Cont.

Study Reference	Sample Size	Sample Type	Micro-CT Machine	Voxel Size (Resolution)	Software Used	Classification System	Technique	Results	Conclusion
[12]	50	Mandibular first premolar	Micro-CT scanner (Sky-Scan 1172 X-ray micro-tomograph; SkyScan, Antwerp, Belgium)	11.94 μm	NRecon/InstaRecon reconstruction en- gine; SkyScan	Vertucci's classification	A Micro-CT scanner (Sky-Scan 1172 X-ray micro-tomography; SkyScan, Antwerp, Belgium) was used to scan all the mandibular first premolar.	Variable root canal configurations were types I, III, IV, V, and VII. The examined teeth exhibited the following two additional root canal configurations, which did not fit the classification: types 1–2–3 and types 1–3.	A complex morphology of mandibular first premolars were observed with a high prevalence of multiroot canal systems.
[50]	90	Maxilary first molar	HMX 225-ACTIS 4, Tesco, Inc	50 μm	VGStudio Max 2.2; Volume- graphics, Heidelberg, Germany software	Weine's classification	Before measuring, the 3-D reconstruction was prepared using volumetric analysis.	Single root canal was observed in 44%.	The authors concluded that the images were classified based on numeric criteria obtained by Micro-CT.
[51]	46	Maxilary first molar	Micro-CT (SkyScan 1072; SkyScan, Aartselaar, Bel- gium)	19.5 μm	V-Works 4.0, Cybermed, Seoul, Korea	–	Mesiobuccal root of maxillary first molar were scanned using Micro-CT (SkyScan 1072; SkyScan, Aartselaar, Belgium).	In these MB roots, 65.2% had two canals, 28.3% had only one canal, and 6.5% had three canals. The most common root canal configuration was two distinct canals (type III: 37.0%), followed by one single canal (type I: 28.3%), two canals that joined together (type II: 17.4%), one canal that split into two (type IV: 10.9%), and three canals (type V: 6.5%).	Micro-CT provided an in-depth analysis of canal configurations, as well as length, curvature, and location of calcified segments.
[12]	78	Maxilary third molar	Micro-CTscanner (SkyScan® 1172, Aartselaar, Belgium)	13.68 μm	NRecon software (SkyScan®)	–	All the maxillary third molars were scanned by Micro-CTscanner(SkyScan® 1172, Aartselaar, Belgium).	Maxillary third molars possessed one or three roots, which principally curved buccally/palatally (75.9%), had one to four root canals, and typically no apical constriction (84.4%). The average external root length was 11.89 ± 1.53 mm, while root canal length was 10.18 ± 0.35 mm.	In some cases, the anatomy of maxillary third molars may not be as complicated as previously documented. During root canal treatment, the frequent deviation of the apical foramen from the radiographic apex should be considered, as should the absence of an apical constriction in the majority of cases.

Table 3. *Cont.*

Study Reference	Sample Size	Sample Type	Micro-CT Machine	Voxel Size (Resolution)	Software Used	Classification System	Technique	Results	Conclusion
[82]	30	Mandibular first molar	SkyScan 1172; Bruker-Micro-CT, Kontich, Belgium	-	CTVol v. 2.3.2.0 software (Bruker- Micro-CT)	-	All the roots were scanned by SkyScan 1172; Bruker-Micro-CT, Kontich, Belgium.	Mesiobuccal (MB) and mesiolingual (ML) canals were positioned within 2.5 mm from the anatomic apex, and the origin and exit of accessory canals were observed mostly between 1.0 and 2.0 mm from the apex in the group.	The presence of bifid apex in the mesial root of mandibular first molars might be a predictive factor for a complex canal anatomy at the apical third with an increasing number of accessory canals.

* Stored in 70% Alcohol. ** Stored in 0.5% sodium azide solution at 4 °C. *** Stored in 10% formalin.

4. Discussion

Micro-CT analysis has proven useful in a wide variety of applications in dental research. It can provide high-resolution images, as well as qualitative and quantitative analysis of teeth [83,84]. To achieve long-term treatment success, endodontic anatomical knowledge is required. As a result, a detailed description of the apical region is required [85]. Until now, there was a scarcity of detailed information on the anatomy of the RCS; therefore, 3-D, high-resolution techniques dominated. Compact commercial systems are now available and are quickly becoming vital in many academic and corporate research laboratories. It is possible to study a wide range of specimens using Micro-CT to examine mineralized tissue, teeth, bone, and materials such as ceramics, polymers, and biomaterial scaffolds [86–89]. Micro-CT provides a repeatable, nondestructive, and noninvasive technique for nonclinical ex vivo evaluation with this goal in mind, enabling measured values of the structures investigated and providing critical info regarding minimal structures such as the end part of the apical portion of teeth [49,50,90,91].

Even though data is challenging to come by, it appears that a large group of researchers agree that Micro-CT gives more objective information than traditional 2-D optical techniques [92], the clearing procedure, or scanning microscopy [44]. As a result, in the present study, a substantial number of sufficiently recognized teeth were evaluated using Micro-CT, allowing for a thorough statistical analysis of the sample. Compared with other investigating techniques, the advantages of Micro-CT produce extraordinary resolution 3-D and 2-D figures, with possibilities of rescanning the sample and volumetric analysis of external and internal structures. The Micro-CT system using a microfocal spot X-ray source and a high-resolution detector is projected in several directions to obtain a three-dimensional reconstructed image of the sample. Since the imaging process is nondestructive, the unique properties of the same sample can be tested multiple times, and the sample can still be used after scanning for further biological and mechanical testing [89]. Some of the recent applications of Micro-CT in dental research includes enamel thickness and tooth measurement [93], analysis of root canal morphology and evaluation of root canal preparation [94], craniofacial skeletal development and structure [95], biomechanics, tissue engineering, determination of mineral concentrations of teeth [96], and the measurement of implant stability and osseointegration [97]. The main disadvantage of Micro-CT is that it cannot be utilized in medical practices due to elevated radiation heights, the operating cost, time taken to process data, cost-effectiveness, and safety [98,99].

The current study provides an overview of the Micro-CT studies for root canal morphology. The data included in this systematic review are secondary information collected from various past research studies. Secondary data are prone to flaws or biases present in the original data, which might eventually appear in the study's findings. For example, it may appear in the analysis technique, or the smallest number of teeth examined in the research. However, the goal was to give the dentistry and endodontic communities a Micro-CT-based analysis of the massive data on the root canal morphology.

Endodontic therapy, both nonsurgical and surgical, needs a thorough understanding of tooth anatomy and morphology [100,101]. Because it is used to instrument and fill root canals to a considerable extent, the morphological interpretation of the apical region should be accurate. Understanding the apical region and the configuration of the root canals is an essential and challenging condition that the clinician must have to make judgments about during endodontic therapy [102].

Despite the fact that the permanent anterior maxillary and mandibular teeth are typically single-rooted, studies suggest that an auxiliary root might be present [103]. Earlier studies in other ethnicities, comprising Turkish, American, Brazilian, and Indian communities, found that all maxillary incisor teeth were single-rooted [104–106]. This suggests that the number of roots in maxillary incisors does not differ structurally throughout all populations. Nevertheless, it is important to note that the presence of a double-rooted maxillary anterior has only been confirmed in a few case studies [103]. However, studies revealed a double-rooted mandibular anterior [4]. Numerous root canal morphology differences in mandibular incisors were documented [37,43,47]. The current review showed that the most common type of root canal morphology classified using the four-digit system was 1-1-1, Type I using Vertucci's classification system, and Type 1-1 using Weine's classification. According to previous research, Vertucci type I in mandibular incisors can range between 55% and 87% [107]. In two earlier investigations of Turkish populations, type I in the mandibular incisors was lower [108,109]. The most common type of root canal configuration identified in this study was type I (75 percent), similar to Vertucci's results [16]. Both mandibular incisors had 88% of type 1 configuration, according to Madeira and Hetem [110]. Furthermore, De Almeida, MM et al. revealed that the most common was type III from the Vertucci classification (16%) [47].

The mandibular first molar is not only the most treated endodontically, but it also presents several anatomic difficulties. The diversity includes isthmuses, several canals, apical ramifications, and lateral canals [3]. Additionally, the distal surface of the mesial root has a thin patch of dentin referred to as a danger zone because there is a higher chance of perforation of dentin in this region during mechanical instrumentation. Hence, orthograde and retrograde endodontic treatment in this tooth may be difficult because of its unusual form [40,102]. The anatomy of the mandibular second molar has been widely investigated, notably using the cleaning procedure [102]. According to previous research, the frequency of C-shaped canals is between 31 and 45% (mostly of Asian people) [52,111–113]. Various classifications of the tridimensional distributions of RCS and the transverse sections have also been published subsequently [114,115].

The canal shape of posterior maxillary teeth varies significantly between races and geographical locations. As per Mohara et al., Brazilians have a 64.2 percent frequency of MB2 in the foremost permanent molar and a 33.5 percent incidence in the subsequent permanent maxillary molar, respectively [116]. In South Africa, type IV root canals are widespread in maxillary primary molar and type I root canals are the most familiar in a maxillary second molar, according to the Vertucci classification of the root canal [117]. According to Li et al., the most common maxillary first premolar anatomy in the Chinese population is one root with two canals (58.0 percent), and the most common canal morphology is type IV (42.7 percent) [118]. Guo et al., on the other hand, examined the maxillary first molars' morphology amongst the North American population and discovered that Asians had a higher occurrence of type I (35.0 percent) and type IV (45.0 percent) configurations than whites (type IV: 36.3 percent, type I: 23.4 percent) [119]. As a result, root canal shape varies depending on where you live. Relevant studies in native communities can help dentists better analyze and understand root canal therapy while also adding to the body of information about root and canal morphology in humans.

The current work uses Micro-CT imaging of many samples to provide a detailed assessment of root canal morphology of the mandibular and maxillary teeth. This knowledge will help practitioners comprehend and anticipate the challenges of 3-D endodontic therapy, particularly during root canal shaping and cleaning. This study revealed that the maxillary first molar and mandibular first premolars had a higher incidence of morphological endodontic variables than the other maxillary and mandibular molars and incisors, indicating that they are more complicated.

5. Study Limitations

We searched data from a small number of significant websites for our systematic review. Articles that have appeared in other publications not indexed in the indices searched may have been ignored. We have also only included items published in English; as a result, publications in other languages may have been overlooked. A limited number of studies have been performed using Micro-CT.

6. Conclusions

This review used Micro-CT studies to provide detailed information atop the anatomy of the root and canal morphology in permanent dentition of various populations. Further, it revealed wide disparities concerning root and canal morphology in permanent dentition, which could perhaps derive from the geographical area studied. In Micro-CT findings, the mandibular incisors followed by maxillary molars were the most studied teeth. The use of multiple categorization systems and Micro-CT allowed for a more precise description of the root canal system and its ramifications, with some inconsistencies noted for molars. This Micro-CT study adds to the existing categorization methods by providing a detailed description of the diversity among root canals and their ramifications and clinically relevant data on the presence and location of lateral canals in all human tooth groups.

Supplementary Materials: The following supporting information can be downloaded at: https://www.mdpi.com/article/10.3390/jcm11092287/s1, Table S1: Quality of included studies by JBI critical appraisal checklist for included studies.

Author Contributions: Conceptualization, M.I.K. and T.Y.N.; methodology, M.I.K., S.A., N.A., S.N.B. and T.Y.N.; software, S.N.B. and S.W.P.; validation, A.M. and C.M.M.; formal analysis, A.M. and C.M.M.; investigation, M.I.K., S.A. and N.A.; resources, S.N.B. and S.W.P.; data curation, M.I.K., S.A. and N.A.; writing—original draft preparation, M.I.K., S.A. and A.M.; writing—review and editing, T.Y.N., P.M. and G.A.S.; visualization, N.A.; supervision, T.Y.N. and G.A.S.; project administration, M.I.K.; funding acquisition, P.M. All authors have read and agreed to the published version of the manuscript.

Funding: This systematic review received no outside funding.

Institutional Review Board Statement: Not applicable.

Informed Consent Statement: Not applicable.

Data Availability Statement: The data used in the current study will be made available at a reasonable request.

Conflicts of Interest: The authors declared no conflict of interest.

References

1. Versiani, M.A.; Pécora, J.D.; de Sousa-Neto, M.D. Root and Root Canal Morphology of Four-rooted Maxillary Second Molars: A Micro–Computed Tomography Study. *J. Endod.* **2012**, *38*, 977–982. [CrossRef] [PubMed]
2. Bernardi, S.; Bianchi, S.; Fantozzi, G.; Leuter, C.; Continenza, M.A.; Macchiarelli, G. Morphometric study on single-root premolars in a European population sample: An update on lengths and diameters. *Eur. J. Anat.* **2019**, *23*, 17–25.
3. Wolf, T.G.; Kim, P.; Campus, G.; Stiebritz, M.; Siegrist, M.; Briseño-Marroquín, B. 3-Dimensional Analysis and Systematic Review of Root Canal Morphology and Physiological Foramen Geometry of 109 Mandibular First Premolars by Micro–computed Tomography in a Mixed Swiss-German Population. *J. Endod.* **2020**, *46*, 801–809. [CrossRef] [PubMed]
4. Karobari, M.I.; Noorani, T.Y.; Halim, M.S.; Ahmed, H.M.A. Root and canal morphology of the anterior permanent dentition in Malaysian population using two classification systems: A CBCT clinical study. *Aust. Endod. J.* **2020**, *47*, 202–216. [CrossRef] [PubMed]
5. Karobari, M.I.; Noorani, T.Y.; Halim, M.S.; Dummer, P.M.H.; Ahmed, H.M.A. Should inter-canal communications be included in the classification of root canal systems? *Int. Endod. J.* **2019**, *52*, 917–919. [CrossRef] [PubMed]
6. Karobari, M.I.; Parveen, A.; Mirza, M.B.; Makandar, S.D.; Nik Abdul Ghani, N.R.; Noorani, T.Y.; Marya, A. Root and Root Canal Morphology Classification Systems. *Int. J. Dent.* **2021**, *2021*, 6682189. [CrossRef] [PubMed]
7. Ahmed, N.; Arshad, S.; Basheer, S.N.; Karobari, M.I.; Marya, A.; Marya, C.M.; Taneja, P.; Messina, P.; Yean, C.Y.; Scardina, G.A. Smoking a Dangerous Addiction: A Systematic Review on an Underrated Risk Factor for Oral Diseases. *Int. J. Environ. Res. Public Health* **2021**, *18*, 11003. [CrossRef]
8. Ahmad, I.A. Root and root canal morphology of Saudi Arabian permanent dentition. *Saudi Endod. J.* **2015**, *5*, 99–106. [CrossRef]
9. Sommer, L.H. 0-F. Bennett, PG Campbell and DR Weyenberg. *J. Am. Chem. Soc.* **1957**, *79*, 3295. [CrossRef]
10. Gupta, B.; Tiwari, B.; Raj, V.; Kashyap, B.; Chandra, S.; Dwivedi, N. Transparent tooth model: A study of root canal morphology using different reagents. *Eur. J. Gen. Dent.* **2014**, *3*, 66–70. [CrossRef]
11. Robertson, D.; Leeb, I.J.; Mckee, M.; Brewer, E. A clearing technique for the study of root canal systems. *J. Endod.* **1980**, *6*, 421–424. [CrossRef]
12. Tomaszewska, I.M.; Leszczyński, B.; Wróbel, A.; Gładysz, T.; Duncan, H.F. A micro-computed tomographic (Micro-CT) analysis of the root canal morphology of maxillary third molar teeth. *Ann. Anat.-Anat. Anz.* **2018**, *215*, 83–92. [CrossRef] [PubMed]
13. Grande, N.M.; Plotino, G.; Gambarini, G.; Testarelli, L.; D'Ambrosio, F.; Pecci, R.; Bedini, R. Present and future in the use of Micro-CT scanner 3D analysis for the study of dental and root canal morphology. *Annali dell'Istituto Superiore di Sanita* **2012**, *48*, 26–34. [PubMed]

14. Acar, B.; Kamburoğlu, K.; Tatar, İ.; Arıkan, V.; Çelik, H.H.; Yüksel, S.; Özen, T. Comparison of micro-computerized tomography and cone-beam computerized tomography in the detection of accessory canals in primary molars. *Imaging Sci. Dent.* **2015**, *45*, 205. [CrossRef] [PubMed]
15. Solomonov, M.; Paqué, F.; Fan, B.; Eilat, Y.; Berman, L.H. The Challenge of C-shaped Canal Systems: A Comparative Study of the Self-Adjusting File and ProTaper. *J. Endod.* **2012**, *38*, 209–214. [CrossRef] [PubMed]
16. Vertucci, F.J. Root canal anatomy of the human permanent teeth. *Oral Surg. Oral Med. Oral Pathol.* **1984**, *58*, 589–599. [CrossRef]
17. Adorno, C.; Yoshioka, T.; Suda, H. Incidence of accessory canals in Japanese anterior maxillary teeth following root canal filling ex vivo. *Int. Endod. J.* **2010**, *43*, 370–376. [CrossRef]
18. Zillich, R.; Dowson, J. Root canal morphology of mandibular first and second premolars. *Oral Surg. Oral Med. Oral Pathol.* **1973**, *36*, 738–744. [CrossRef]
19. Khedmat, S.; Assadian, H.; Saravani, A.A. Root canal morphology of the mandibular first premolars in an Iranian population using cross-sections and radiography. *J. Endod.* **2010**, *36*, 214–217. [CrossRef]
20. Awawdeh, L.; Abdullah, H.; Al-Qudah, A. Root form and canal morphology of Jordanian maxillary first premolars. *J. Endod.* **2008**, *34*, 956–961. [CrossRef]
21. Celikten, B.; Orhan, K.; Aksoy, U.; Tufenkci, P.; Kalender, A.; Basmaci, F.; Dabaj, P. Cone-beam CT evaluation of root canal morphology of maxillary and mandibular premolars in a Turkish Cypriot population. *BDJ Open* **2016**, *2*, 15006. [CrossRef] [PubMed]
22. Alkaabi, W.; AlShwaimi, E.; Farooq, I.; Goodis, H.E.; Chogle, S.M. A micro-computed tomography study of the root canal morphology of mandibular first premolars in an Emirati population. *Med. Princ. Pract.* **2017**, *26*, 118–124. [CrossRef] [PubMed]
23. Pan, J.Y.Y.; Parolia, A.; Chuah, S.R.; Bhatia, S.; Mutalik, S.; Pau, A. Root canal morphology of permanent teeth in a Malaysian subpopulation using cone-beam computed tomography. *BMC Oral Health* **2019**, *19*, 14. [CrossRef] [PubMed]
24. Villas-Bôas, M.H.; Bernardineli, N.; Cavenago, B.C.; Marciano, M.; del Carpio-Perochena, A.; de Moraes, I.G.; Duarte, M.H.; Bramante, C.M.; Ordinola-Zapata, R. Micro–Computed Tomography Study of the Internal Anatomy of Mesial Root Canals of Mandibular Molars. *J. Endod.* **2011**, *37*, 1682–1686. [CrossRef] [PubMed]
25. Gulabivala, K.; Aung, T.; Alavi, A.; Ng, Y.L. Root and canal morphology of Burmese mandibular molars. *Int. Endod. J.* **2001**, *34*, 359–370. [CrossRef]
26. Gulabivala, K.; Opasanon, A.; Ng, Y.L.; Alavi, A. Root and canal morphology of Thai mandibular molars. *Int. Endod. J.* **2002**, *35*, 56–62. [CrossRef]
27. Gu, Y.; Lu, Q.; Wang, H.; Ding, Y.; Wang, P.; Ni, L. Root Canal Morphology of Permanent Three-rooted Mandibular First Molars—Part I: Pulp Floor and Root Canal System. *J. Endod.* **2010**, *36*, 990–994. [CrossRef]
28. Paqué, F.; Balmer, M.; Attin, T.; Peters, O.A. Preparation of Oval-shaped Root Canals in Mandibular Molars Using Nickel-Titanium Rotary Instruments: A Micro-computed Tomography Study. *J. Endod.* **2010**, *36*, 703–707. [CrossRef]
29. Guven, E.P. Root Canal Morphology and Anatomy. In *Human Teeth-Key Skills and Clinical Illustrations*; IntechOpen: London, UK, 2019.
30. Hamba, H.; Nikaido, T.; Inoue, G.; Sadr, A.; Tagami, J. Effects of CPP-ACP with sodium fluoride on inhibition of bovine enamel demineralization: A quantitative assessment using micro-computed tomography. *J. Dent.* **2011**, *39*, 405–413. [CrossRef]
31. Huang, T.T.; Jones, A.S.; He, L.H.; Darendeliler, M.A.; Swain, M.V. Characterisation of enamel white spot lesions using X-ray micro-tomography. *J. Dent.* **2007**, *35*, 737–743. [CrossRef]
32. Fan, B.; Pan, Y.; Gao, Y.; Fang, F.; Wu, Q.; Gutmann, J.L. Three-dimensional Morphologic Analysis of Isthmuses in the Mesial Roots of Mandibular Molars. *J. Endod.* **2010**, *36*, 1866–1869. [CrossRef] [PubMed]
33. Robinson, J.P.; Lumley, P.J.; Claridge, E.; Cooper, P.R.; Grover, L.M.; Williams, R.L.; Walmsley, A.D. An analytical Micro CT methodology for quantifying inorganic dentine debris following internal tooth preparation. *J. Dent.* **2012**, *40*, 999–1005. [CrossRef] [PubMed]
34. Rossi-Fedele, G.; Ahmed, H.M.A. Assessment of root canal filling removal effectiveness using micro–computed tomography: A systematic review. *J. Endod.* **2017**, *43*, 520–526. [CrossRef] [PubMed]
35. Joanna Briggs Institute (JBI). *Checklist for Prevalence Studies*; Joanna Briggs Institute: Adelaide, Australia, 2017.
36. Briseño-Marroquín, B.; Paqué, F.; Maier, K.; Willershausen, B.; Wolf, T.G. Root canal morphology and configuration of 179 maxillary first molars by means of micro–computed tomography: An ex vivo study. *J. Endod.* **2015**, *41*, 2008–2013. [CrossRef]
37. Wolf, T.G.; Stiebritz, M.; Boemke, N.; Elsayed, I.; Paqué, F.; Wierichs, R.J.; Briseño-Marroquín, B. 3-dimensional Analysis and Literature Review of the Root Canal Morphology and Physiological Foramen Geometry of 125 Mandibular Incisors by Means of Micro–Computed Tomography in a German Population. *J. Endod.* **2020**, *46*, 184–191. [CrossRef]
38. Mazzi-Chaves, J.F.; Silva-Sousa, Y.T.C.; Leoni, G.B.; Silva-Sousa, A.C.; Estrela, L.; Estrela, C.; Jacobs, R.; Sousa-Neto, M.D.d. Micro-computed tomographic assessment of the variability and morphological features of root canal system and their ramifications. *J. Appl. Oral Sci.* **2020**, *28*, e20190393. [CrossRef]
39. Domark, J.D.; Hatton, J.F.; Benison, R.P.; Hildebolt, C.F. An ex vivo comparison of digital radiography and cone-beam and micro computed tomography in the detection of the number of canals in the mesiobuccal roots of maxillary molars. *J. Endod.* **2013**, *39*, 901–905. [CrossRef]

40. Ordinola-Zapata, R.; Bramante, C.; Versiani, M.; Moldauer, B.; Topham, G.; Gutmann, J.; Nuñez, A.; Duarte, M.H.; Abella, F. Comparative accuracy of the Clearing Technique, CBCT and Micro-CT methods in studying the mesial root canal configuration of mandibular first molars. *Int. Endod. J.* **2017**, *50*, 90–96. [CrossRef]
41. Kim, Y.; Chang, S.-W.; Lee, J.-K.; Chen, I.-P.; Kaufman, B.; Jiang, J.; Cha, B.Y.; Zhu, Q.; Safavi, K.E.; Kum, K.-Y. A micro-computed tomography study of canal configuration of multiple-canalled mesiobuccal root of maxillary first molar. *Clin. Oral Investig.* **2013**, *17*, 1541–1546. [CrossRef]
42. Marceliano-Alves, M.F.; Lima, C.O.; Bastos, L.G.d.P.M.N.; Bruno, A.M.V.; Vidaurre, F.; Coutinho, T.M.; Fidel, S.R.; Lopes, R.T. Mandibular mesial root canal morphology using micro-computed tomography in a Brazilian population. *Aust. Endod. J.* **2019**, *45*, 51–56. [CrossRef]
43. Leoni, G.B.; Versiani, M.A.; Pécora, J.D.; de Sousa-Neto, M.D. Micro-computed tomographic analysis of the root canal morphology of mandibular incisors. *J. Endod.* **2014**, *40*, 710–716. [CrossRef] [PubMed]
44. Filpo-Perez, C.; Bramante, C.M.; Villas-Boas, M.H.; Duarte, M.A.H.; Versiani, M.A.; Ordinola-Zapata, R. Micro-computed tomographic analysis of the root canal morphology of the distal root of mandibular first molar. *J. Endod.* **2015**, *41*, 231–236. [CrossRef] [PubMed]
45. Marceliano-Alves, M.; Alves, F.R.F.; de Melo Mendes, D.; Provenzano, J.C. Micro-computed tomography analysis of the root canal morphology of palatal roots of maxillary first molars. *J. Endod.* **2016**, *42*, 280–283. [CrossRef] [PubMed]
46. Verma, P.; Love, R. A Micro CT study of the mesiobuccal root canal morphology of the maxillary first molar tooth. *Int. Endod. J.* **2011**, *44*, 210–217. [CrossRef]
47. De Almeida, M.M.; Bernardineli, N.; Ordinola-Zapata, R.; Villas-Bôas, M.H.; Amoroso-Silva, P.A.; Brandao, C.G.; Guimaraes, B.M.; De Moraes, I.G.; Húngaro-Duarte, M.A. Micro-computed tomography analysis of the root canal anatomy and prevalence of oval canals in mandibular incisors. *J. Endod.* **2013**, *39*, 1529–1533. [CrossRef]
48. Ordinola-Zapata, R.; Martins, J.; Bramante, C.; Villas-Boas, M.; Duarte, M.; Versiani, M. Morphological evaluation of maxillary second molars with fused roots: A Micro-CT study. *Int. Endod. J.* **2017**, *50*, 1192–1200. [CrossRef]
49. Wolf, T.G.; Paqué, F.; Zeller, M.; Willershausen, B.; Briseño-Marroquín, B. Root canal morphology and configuration of 118 mandibular first molars by means of micro-computed tomography: An ex vivo study. *J. Endod.* **2016**, *42*, 610–614. [CrossRef]
50. Wolf, T.G.; Paqué, F.; Woop, A.-C.; Willershausen, B.; Briseño-Marroquín, B. Root canal morphology and configuration of 123 maxillary second molars by means of Micro-CT. *Int. J. Oral Sci.* **2017**, *9*, 33–37. [CrossRef]
51. Wolf, T.G.; Kozaczek, C.; Campus, G.; Paqué, F.; Wierichs, R.J. Root Canal Morphology of 116 Maxillary Second Premolars by Micro-Computed Tomography in a Mixed Swiss-German Population with Systematic Review. *J. Endod.* **2020**, *46*, 1639–1647. [CrossRef]
52. Zhang, W.; Tang, Y.; Liu, C.; Shen, Y.; Feng, X.; Gu, Y. Root and root canal variations of the human maxillary and mandibular third molars in a Chinese population: A micro-computed tomographic study. *Arch. Oral Biol.* **2018**, *95*, 134–140. [CrossRef]
53. Marceliano-Alves, M.F.; de Lima, C.O.; Augusto, C.M.; Almeida Barbosa, A.F.; Vieira Bruno, A.M.; Rosa, A.M.; Lopes, R.T. The internal root canal morphology of single-rooted mandibular canines revealed by micro-computed tomography. *J. Conserv. Dent. JCD* **2018**, *21*, 588–591. [CrossRef] [PubMed]
54. Sierra-Cristancho, A.; González-Osuna, L.; Poblete, D.; Cafferata, E.A.; Carvajal, P.; Lozano, C.P.; Vernal, R. Micro-tomographic characterization of the root and canal system morphology of mandibular first premolars in a Chilean population. *Sci. Rep.* **2021**, *11*, 93. [CrossRef]
55. Espir, C.G.; Nascimento, C.A.; Guerreiro-Tanomaru, J.M.; Bonetti-Filho, I.; Tanomaru-Filho, M. Radiographic and micro-computed tomography classification of root canal morphology and dentin thickness of mandibular incisors. *J. Conserv. Dent. JCD* **2018**, *21*, 57–62. [CrossRef]
56. Wolf, T.G.; Paqué, F.; Betz, P.; Willershausen, B.; Briseño-Marroquín, B. Micro-CT assessment of internal morphology and root canal configuration of non C-shaped mandibular second molars. *Swiss Dent. J.* **2017**, *127*, 513–519.
57. Divine, K.A.; McClanahan, S.B.; Fok, A. Anatomic Analysis of Palatal Roots of Maxillary Molars Using Micro-computed Tomography. *J. Endod.* **2019**, *45*, 724–728. [CrossRef] [PubMed]
58. Camargo Dos Santos, B.; Pedano, M.S.; Giraldi, C.K.; De Oliveira, J.C.M.; Lima, I.C.B.; Lambrechts, P. Mesiobuccal Root Canal Morphology of Maxillary First Molars in a Brazilian Sub-Population—A Micro-CT Study. *Eur. Endod. J.* **2020**, *5*, 105–111. [CrossRef]
59. Tomaszewska, I.M.; Skinningsrud, B.; Jarzębska, A.; Pękala, J.R.; Tarasiuk, J.; Iwanaga, J. Internal and external morphology of mandibular molars: An original Micro-CT study and meta-analysis with review of implications for endodontic therapy. *Clin. Anat.* **2018**, *31*, 797–811. [CrossRef] [PubMed]
60. Lima, C.O.; Magalhães, L.T.; Marceliano-Alves, M.F.; de Oliveira, P.Y.; Lacerda, M.F. Internal Lower Incisor Morphology revealed by Computerized Microtomography. *Acta Odontol. Latinoam. AOL* **2020**, *33*, 33–37. [CrossRef]
61. Fu, Y.; Gao, Y.; Gao, Y.; Tan, X.; Zhang, L.; Huang, D. Three-dimensional analysis of coronal root canal morphology of 136 permanent mandibular first molars by micro-computed tomography. *J. Dent. Sci.* **2022**, *17*, 482–489. [CrossRef] [PubMed]
62. Grande, N.M.; Plotino, G.; Pecci, R.; Bedini, R.; Pameijer, C.H.; Somma, F. Micro-computerized tomographic analysis of radicular and canal morphology of premolars with long oval canals. *Oral Surg. Oral Med. Oral Pathol. Oral Radiol. Endod.* **2008**, *106*, e70–e76. [CrossRef]

63. Ordinola-Zapata, R.; Bramante, C.M.; Villas-Boas, M.H.; Cavenago, B.C.; Duarte, M.H.; Versiani, M.A. Morphologic micro-computed tomography analysis of mandibular premolars with three root canals. *J. Endod.* **2013**, *39*, 1130–1135. [CrossRef] [PubMed]
64. Shen, Y.; Gu, Y. Assessment of the presence of a second mesiobuccal canal in maxillary first molars according to the location of the main mesiobuccal canal-a micro-computed tomographic study. *Clin. Oral Investig.* **2021**, *25*, 3937–3944. [CrossRef] [PubMed]
65. Dou, L.; Li, D.; Xu, T.; Tang, Y.; Yang, D. Root anatomy and canal morphology of mandibular first premolars in a Chinese population. *Sci. Rep.* **2017**, *7*, 750. [CrossRef]
66. Alashiry, M.K.; Zeitoun, R.; Elashiry, M.M. Prevalence of middle mesial and middle distal canals in mandibular molars in an Egyptian subpopulation using micro-computed tomography. *Niger. J. Clin. Pr.* **2020**, *23*, 534–538. [CrossRef]
67. Qiao, X.; Xu, T.; Chen, L.; Yang, D. Analysis of Root Canal Curvature and Root Canal Morphology of Maxillary Posterior Teeth in Guizhou, China. *Med. Sci. Monit. Int. Med. J. Exp. Clin. Res.* **2021**, *27*, e928758. [CrossRef] [PubMed]
68. Guillaume, B.; Lacoste, J.P.; Gaborit, N.; Brossard, G.; Cruard, A.; Baslé, M.F.; Chappard, D. Microcomputed tomography used in the analysis of the morphology of root canals in extracted wisdom teeth. *Br. J. Oral Maxillofac. Surg.* **2006**, *44*, 240–244. [CrossRef]
69. Chen, M.; Wang, H.; Tsauo, C.; Huang, D.; Zhou, X.; He, J.; Gao, Y. Micro-computed tomography analysis of root canal morphology and thickness of crown and root of mandibular incisors in Chinese population. *Clin. Oral Investig.* **2022**, *26*, 901–910. [CrossRef] [PubMed]
70. Kyaw Moe, M.M.; Jo, H.J.; Ha, J.H.; Kim, S.K. Root Canal Configuration of Burmese (Myanmar) Maxillary First Molar: A Micro-Computed Tomography Study. *Int. J. Dent.* **2021**, *2021*, 3433343. [CrossRef]
71. Elnour, M.; Khabeer, A.; AlShwaimi, E. Evaluation of root canal morphology of maxillary second premolars in a Saudi Arabian sub-population: An in vitro microcomputed tomography study. *Saudi Dent. J.* **2016**, *28*, 162–168. [CrossRef]
72. Versiani, M.A.; Pécora, J.D.; Sousa-Neto, M.D. Microcomputed tomography analysis of the root canal morphology of single-rooted mandibular canines. *Int. Endod. J.* **2013**, *46*, 800–807. [CrossRef]
73. Wolf, T.G.; Anderegg, A.L.; Haberthür, D.; Khoma, O.Z.; Schumann, S.; Boemke, N.; Wierichs, R.J.; Hlushchuk, R. Internal morphology of 101 mandibular canines of a Swiss-German population by means of Micro-CT: An ex vivo study. *Sci. Rep.* **2021**, *11*, 21281. [CrossRef] [PubMed]
74. Liu, N.; Li, X.; Liu, N.; Ye, L.; An, J.; Nie, X.; Liu, L.; Deng, M. A micro-computed tomography study of the root canal morphology of the mandibular first premolar in a population from southwestern China. *Clin. Oral Investig.* **2013**, *17*, 999–1007. [CrossRef] [PubMed]
75. Rodrigues, C.T.; de Oliveira-Santos, C.; Bernardineli, N.; Duarte, M.A.H.; Bramante, C.M.; Minotti-Bonfante, P.G.; Ordinola-Zapata, R. Prevalence and morphometric analysis of three-rooted mandibular first molars in a Brazilian subpopulation. *J. Appl. Oral Sci.* **2016**, *24*, 535–542. [CrossRef] [PubMed]
76. Wolf, T.G.; Kozaczek, C.; Siegrist, M.; Betthäuser, M.; Paqué, F.; Briseño-Marroquín, B. An Ex Vivo Study of Root Canal System Configuration and Morphology of 115 Maxillary First Premolars. *J. Endod.* **2020**, *46*, 794–800. [CrossRef]
77. Şallı, G.A.; Egil, E. Evaluation of mesial root canal configuration of mandibular first molars using micro-computed tomography. *Imaging Sci. Dent.* **2021**, *51*, 383–388. [CrossRef]
78. Somma, F.; Leoni, D.; Plotino, G.; Grande, N.M.; Plasschaert, A. Root canal morphology of the mesiobuccal root of maxillary first molars: A micro-computed tomographic analysis. *Int. Endod. J.* **2009**, *42*, 165–174. [CrossRef]
79. Tomaszewska, I.M.; Jarzębska, A.; Skinningsrud, B.; Pękala, P.A.; Wroński, S.; Iwanaga, J. An original Micro-CT study and meta-analysis of the internal and external anatomy of maxillary molars-implications for endodontic treatment. *Clin. Anat.* **2018**, *31*, 838–853. [CrossRef]
80. Yamada, M.; Ide, Y.; Matsunaga, S.; Kato, H.; Nakagawa, K. Three-dimensional analysis of mesiobuccal root canal of Japanese maxillary first molar using Micro-CT. *Bull. Tokyo Dent. Coll.* **2011**, *52*, 77–84. [CrossRef]
81. Park, J.W.; Lee, J.K.; Ha, B.H.; Choi, J.H.; Perinpanayagam, H. Three-dimensional analysis of maxillary first molar mesiobuccal root canal configuration and curvature using micro-computed tomography. *Oral Surg. Oral Med. Oral Pathol. Oral Radiol. Endod.* **2009**, *108*, 437–442. [CrossRef]
82. Keleş, A.; Keskin, C.; Alqawasmi, R.; Versiani, M.A. Micro-computed tomographic analysis of the mesial root of mandibular first molars with bifid apex. *Arch. Oral Biol.* **2020**, *117*, 104792. [CrossRef]
83. Versiani, M.A.; Keleş, A. Applications of Micro-CT technology in endodontics. In *Micro-Computed Tomography (Micro-CT) in Medicine and Engineering*; Springer: Berlin/Heidelberg, Germany, 2020; pp. 183–211.
84. Peters, O.A.; Laib, A.; Rüegsegger, P.; Barbakow, F. Three-dimensional analysis of root canal geometry by high-resolution computed tomography. *J. Dent. Res.* **2000**, *79*, 1405–1409. [CrossRef] [PubMed]
85. Ayranci, L.B.; Yeter, K.Y.; Arslan, H.; Kseoğlu, M. Morphology of apical foramen in permanent molars and premolars in a Turkish population. *Acta Odontol. Scand* **2013**, *71*, 1043–1049. [CrossRef] [PubMed]
86. Guldberg, R.E.; Lin, A.S.; Coleman, R.; Robertson, G.; Duvall, C. Microcomputed tomography imaging of skeletal development and growth. *Birth Defects Res. Part C Embryo Today Rev.* **2004**, *72*, 250–259. [CrossRef] [PubMed]
87. Zhang, C.; Chen, Z.; Liu, J.; Wu, M.; Yang, J.; Zhu, Y.; Lu, W.W.; Ruan, C. 3D-printed pre-tapped-hole scaffolds facilitate one-step surgery of predictable alveolar bone augmentation and simultaneous dental implantation. *Compos. Part B Eng.* **2022**, *229*, 109461. [CrossRef]

88. Fang, H.; Zhu, D.; Yang, Q.; Chen, Y.; Zhang, C.; Gao, J.; Gao, Y. Emerging zero-dimensional to four-dimensional biomaterials for bone regeneration. *J. Nanobiotech.* **2022**, *20*, 26. [CrossRef] [PubMed]
89. Swain, M.V.; Xue, J. State of the art of Micro-CT applications in dental research. *Int. J. Oral Sci.* **2009**, *1*, 177–188. [CrossRef] [PubMed]
90. Plotino, G.; Grande, N.M.; Pecci, R.; Bedini, R.; Pameijer, C.H.; Somma, F. Three-dimensional imaging using microcomputed tomography for studying tooth macromorphology. *J. Am. Dent. Assoc.* **2006**, *137*, 1555–1561. [CrossRef]
91. Rhodes, J.; Ford, T.P.; Lynch, J.; Liepins, P.; Curtis, R. Micro-computed tomography: A new tool for experimental endodontology. *Int. Endod. J.* **1999**, *32*, 165–170. [CrossRef]
92. Marroquín, B.B.; El-Sayed, M.A.; Willershausen-Zönnchen, B. Morphology of the physiological foramen: I. Maxillary and mandibular molars. *J. Endod.* **2004**, *30*, 321–328. [CrossRef]
93. Smith, T.M.; Harvati, K.; Olejniczak, A.J.; Reid, D.J.; Hublin, J.J.; Panagopoulou, E. Brief communication: Dental development and enamel thickness in the Lakonis Neanderthal molar. *Am. J. Phys. Anthropol.* **2009**, *138*, 112–118. [CrossRef]
94. Cheung, L.H.; Cheung, G.S. Evaluation of a rotary instrumentation method for C-shaped canals with micro-computed tomography. *J. Endod.* **2008**, *34*, 1233–1238. [CrossRef] [PubMed]
95. Luan, Q.; Desta, T.; Chehab, L.; Sanders, V.; Plattner, J.; Graves, D. Inhibition of experimental periodontitis by a topical boron-based antimicrobial. *J. Dent. Res.* **2008**, *87*, 148–152. [CrossRef] [PubMed]
96. Zhang, X.; Rahemtulla, F.; Zhang, P.; Beck, P.; Thomas, H.F. Different enamel and dentin mineralization observed in VDR deficient mouse model. *Arch. Oral Biol.* **2009**, *54*, 299–305. [CrossRef]
97. Freilich, M.; Shafer, D.; Wei, M.; Kompalli, R.; Adams, D.; Kuhn, L. Implant system for guiding a new layer of bone. Computed microtomography and histomorphometric analysis in the rabbit mandible. *Clin. Oral Implant. Res.* **2009**, *20*, 201–207. [CrossRef] [PubMed]
98. Anderson, P.; Yong, R.; Surman, T.; Rajion, Z.; Ranjitkar, S. Application of three-dimensional computed tomography in craniofacial clinical practice and research. *Aust. Dent. J.* **2014**, *59*, 174–185. [CrossRef]
99. Loch, C.; Schwass, D.R.; Kieser, J.A.; Fordyce, R.E. Use of micro-computed tomography for dental studies in modern and fossil odontocetes: Potential applications and limitations. *NAMMCO Sci. Publ.* **2018**, *10*, 1–24. [CrossRef]
100. Peters, O.A.; Boessler, C.; Paqué, F. Root canal preparation with a novel nickel-titanium instrument evaluated with micro-computed tomography: Canal surface preparation over time. *J. Endod.* **2010**, *36*, 1068–1072. [CrossRef]
101. Xu, T.; Tay, F.R.; Gutmann, J.L.; Fan, B.; Fan, W.; Huang, Z.; Sun, Q. Micro–computed tomography assessment of apical accessory canal morphologies. *J. Endod.* **2016**, *42*, 798–802. [CrossRef]
102. Baratto Filho, F.; Zaitter, S.; Haragushiku, G.A.; de Campos, E.A.; Abuabara, A.; Correr, G.M. Analysis of the Internal Anatomy of Maxillary First Molars by Using Different Methods. *J. Endod.* **2009**, *35*, 337–342. [CrossRef]
103. Ahmed, H.; Hashem, A. Accessory roots and root canals in human anterior teeth: A review and clinical considerations. *Int. Endod. J.* **2016**, *49*, 724–736. [CrossRef]
104. Altunsoy, M.; Ok, E.; Nur, B.G.; Aglarci, O.S.; Gungor, E.; Colak, M. A cone-beam computed tomography study of the root canal morphology of anterior teeth in a Turkish population. *Eur. J. Dent.* **2014**, *8*, 302–306. [CrossRef] [PubMed]
105. Amardeep, N.S.; Raghu, S.; Natanasabapathy, V. Root canal morphology of permanent maxillary and mandibular canines in Indian population using cone beam computed tomography. *Anat. Res. Int.* **2014**, *2014*, 731859.
106. Nogueira Leal da Silva, E.J.; Queiroz de Castro, R.W.; Nejaim, Y.; Vespasiano Silva, A.I.; Haiter-Neto, F.; Silberman, A.; Cohenca, N. Evaluation of root canal configuration of maxillary and mandibular anterior teeth using cone beam computed tomography: An in-vivo study. *Quintessence Int.* **2016**, *47*, 19–24.
107. Miyashita, M.; Kasahara, E.; Yasuda, E.; Yamamoto, A.; Sekizawa, T. Root canal system of the mandibular incisor. *J. Endod.* **1997**, *23*, 479–484. [CrossRef]
108. Kartal, N.; Yanıkoğlu, F.Ç. Root canal morphology of mandibular incisors. *J. Endod.* **1992**, *18*, 562–564. [CrossRef]
109. Sert, S.; Bayirli, G.S. Evaluation of the root canal configurations of the mandibular and maxillary permanent teeth by gender in the Turkish population. *J. Endod.* **2004**, *30*, 391–398. [CrossRef]
110. Madeira, M.C.; Hetem, S. Incidence of bifurcations in mandibular incisors. *Oral Surg. Oral Med. Oral Pathol.* **1973**, *36*, 589–591. [CrossRef]
111. Seo, M.; Park, D. C-shaped root canals of mandibular second molars in a Korean population: Clinical observation and in vitro analysis. *Int. Endod. J.* **2004**, *37*, 139–144. [CrossRef]
112. Wang, Y.; Guo, J.; Yang, H.-B.; Han, X.; Yu, Y. Incidence of C-shaped root canal systems in mandibular second molars in the native Chinese population by analysis of clinical methods. *Int. J. Oral Sci.* **2012**, *4*, 161–165. [CrossRef]
113. Zheng, Q.; Zhang, L.; Zhou, X.; Wang, Q.; Wang, Y.; Tang, L.; Song, F.; Huang, D. C-shaped root canal system in mandibular second molars in a Chinese population evaluated by cone-beam computed tomography. *Int. Endod. J.* **2011**, *44*, 857–862. [CrossRef]
114. Fan, B.; Cheung, G.S.; Fan, M.; Gutmann, J.L.; Bian, Z. C-shaped canal system in mandibular second molars: Part I—anatomical features. *J. Endod.* **2004**, *30*, 899–903. [CrossRef]
115. Min, Y.; Fan, B.; Cheung, G.S.; Gutmann, J.L.; Fan, M. C-shaped canal system in mandibular second molars Part III: The morphology of the pulp chamber floor. *J. Endod.* **2006**, *32*, 1155–1159. [CrossRef] [PubMed]

116. Mohara, N.T.; Coelho, M.S.; de Queiroz, N.V.; Borreau, M.L.S.; Nishioka, M.M.; de Jesus Soares, A.; Frozoni, M. Root anatomy and canal configuration of maxillary molars in a Brazilian subpopulation: A 125-µm cone-beam computed tomographic study. *Eur. J. Dent.* **2019**, *13*, 082–087. [CrossRef] [PubMed]
117. Buchanan, G.D.; Gamieldien, M.Y.; Tredoux, S.; Vally, Z.I. Root and canal configurations of maxillary premolars in a South African subpopulation using cone beam computed tomography and two classification systems. *J. Oral Sci.* **2020**, *62*, 93–97. [CrossRef] [PubMed]
118. Li, Y.-h.; Bao, S.-j.; Yang, X.-w.; Tian, X.-m.; Wei, B.; Zheng, Y.-l. Symmetry of root anatomy and root canal morphology in maxillary premolars analyzed using cone-beam computed tomography. *Arch. Oral Biol.* **2018**, *94*, 84–92. [CrossRef]
119. Guo, J.; Vahidnia, A.; Sedghizadeh, P.; Enciso, R. Evaluation of root and canal morphology of maxillary permanent first molars in a North American population by cone-beam computed tomography. *J. Endod.* **2014**, *40*, 635–639. [CrossRef]

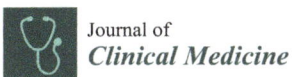

Article

Confocal Laser Scanner Evaluation of Bactericidal Effect of Chitosan Nanodroplets Loaded with Benzalkonium Chloride

Mario Alovisi [1,*], Damiano Pasqualini [1], Narcisa Mandras [2], Janira Roana [2], Pietro Costamagna [1], Allegra Comba [1], Roberta Cavalli [3], Anna Luganini [4], Alfredo Iandolo [5], Lorenza Cavallo [2], Nicola Scotti [1] and Elio Berutti [1]

[1] Department of Surgical Sciences, Dental School, University of Turin, 10126 Turin, Italy; damiano.pasqualini@unito.it (D.P.); costamagna@hotmail.it (P.C.); allegra.comba@unito.it (A.C.); nicola.scotti@unito.it (N.S.); elio.berutti@unito.it (E.B.)
[2] Department of Public Health and Pediatrics, University of Turin, 10126 Turin, Italy; narcisa.mandras@unito.it (N.M.); janira.roana@unito.it (J.R.); lorenza.cavallo@unito.it (L.C.)
[3] Department of Drug Science and Technology, University of Turin, 10126 Turin, Italy; roberta.cavalli@unito.it
[4] Department of Life Sciences and Systems Biology, University of Turin, 10126 Turin, Italy; anna.luganini@unito.it
[5] Department of Medicine, Surgery and Dentistry, Salerno Medical School, University of Salerno, 84084 Salerno, Italy; iandoloalfredo@unisa.it
* Correspondence: mario.alovisi@unito.it

Abstract: The aim was to evaluate the antibacterial efficacy and penetration depth into dentinal tubules of a solution of chitosan nanodroplets (NDs) loaded with Benzalkonium Chloride (BAK). Seventy-two human single-root teeth with fully formed apex were used. Cylindrical root dentin blocks were longitudinally sectioned and enlarged to a size of a Gates Glidden drill #4. After sterilization, root canals were infected with *Enterococcus faecalis* ATCC 29212 and further incubated for three weeks. Specimens were assigned to three experimental groups ($n = 20$), plus positive ($n = 6$) and negative ($n = 6$) controls. In the first group, irrigation was achieved with 2 mL of NDs solution loaded with BAK (NDs-BAK), in the second with 2 mL of 5% sodium hypochlorite (NaOCl) and in the last with 2 mL of 2% chlorhexidine (CHX). Specimens were rinsed and vertically fractured. Confocal laser scanning microscopy (CLSM) and viability staining were used to analyze the proportions of dead and live bacteria quantitatively. The volume ratio of red fluorescence (dead) was calculated in 3D reconstructions. Data were analyzed by one-way ANOVA and post hoc Bonferroni tests ($p < 0.05$). The ratio of red fluorescence over the whole green/red fluorescence resulted in a significant comparison of NDs-BAK with NaOCl ($p < 0.01$) and NaOCl with CHX ($p < 0.01$). No differences were found between NDs-BAK and CHX ($p > 0.05$). The mean depth of efficacy was, respectively: NDs-BAK 325.25 µm, NaOCl 273.36 µm and CHX 246.78 µm with no statistical differences between groups. The NaOCl solution showed the highest antimicrobial efficacy, but nanodroplets with BAK seemed to have the same effect as CHX with a high depth of efficacy.

Keywords: nanodroplets; confocal laser microscope; benzalkonium chloride; chlorhexidine; sodium hypochlorite; viability staining

---

Citation: Alovisi, M.; Pasqualini, D.; Mandras, N.; Roana, J.; Costamagna, P.; Comba, A.; Cavalli, R.; Luganini, A.; Iandolo, A.; Cavallo, L.; et al. Confocal Laser Scanner Evaluation of Bactericidal Effect of Chitosan Nanodroplets Loaded with Benzalkonium Chloride. *J. Clin. Med.* **2022**, *11*, 1650. https://doi.org/10.3390/jcm11061650

Academic Editors: Edgar Schäfer and Lorenzo Drago

Received: 18 January 2022
Accepted: 14 March 2022
Published: 16 March 2022

Publisher's Note: MDPI stays neutral with regard to jurisdictional claims in published maps and institutional affiliations.

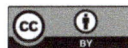

Copyright: © 2022 by the authors. Licensee MDPI, Basel, Switzerland. This article is an open access article distributed under the terms and conditions of the Creative Commons Attribution (CC BY) license (https://creativecommons.org/licenses/by/4.0/).

1. Introduction

The prevalence of apical periodontitis among adult populations is more than 35–40% and increases with age [1,2]. Although epidemiological studies reported an elevated endodontic treatment success rate, many apical periodontal lesions seem to affect previously root-filled teeth [2,3].

To achieve long-term success, removing the pulp tissue remnants, bacteria and microbial toxins from the root canal system is essential. However, nickel–titanium (NiTi) rotary instrumentation only acts on the central root canal volume, leaving lateral canals and isthmuses untouched after preparation [4,5]. Therefore, microorganisms remaining in the root canal system after treatment or re-colonizing the filled canal system are considered an important cause of endodontic failure [6].

Recent microcomputed tomography (micro-CT) studies have demonstrated that large areas of the root canal walls remain untouched, emphasizing the importance of chemical irrigation [5,7,8]. Nevertheless, irrigation is an essential part of root canal debridement because it allows for cleaning beyond what might be achieved by root canal instrumentation alone [9,10].

The remarkable reduction in preparation size and taper and treatment time for even simpler and minimally invasive shaping protocols encourages the development of more efficient irrigation systems [11]. Sodium hypochlorite (NaOCl) is the most used irrigant during root canal preparation due to its high capacity for tissue dissolution and a well-known antimicrobial activity [12]. Surfactants are associated with NaOCl to improve its properties, such as dissolution of organic tissues, antimicrobial activity and penetration into the root canal system [13].

Many other antimicrobial agents have been proposed for root canal irrigation, such as chlorhexidine (CHX) and benzalkonium chloride (BAK) [14,15]. The latter is a cationic detergent composed of quaternary ammonium. BAK causes structural disorganization, loss of cytoplasmic membrane integrity and other destructive effects against bacteria [16]. Moreover, in concentrations up to 5%, it is claimed to provide antibacterial properties and long-lasting effects due to its ability to inhibit proteases [17].

The effectiveness of BAK administration deep into the root canal and tissues, coronal through the dentinal microtubules, could be augmented using nanodroplets (NDs) [18]. Experimental NDs with chitosan shells have been recently proposed [19]. Chitosan (CS) is a nontoxic biopolymer derived by the deacetylation of chitin and, due to its catatonic nature, it has broad antimicrobial activity against bacteria, with a high killing rate through interaction with the bacterial cell wall [20]. This interaction between chitosan and the bacterial cell depends on the hydrophilicity of the cell wall, which could explain the lower toxicity of chitosan to mammalian cells [18–20]. Therefore, NDs with chitosan shells offer different advantages such as a broad spectrum of antibacterial activity, biocompatibility and the ability of a long-lasting release of antimicrobial substances [21,22]. However, no studies are available about the potential in vitro efficacy of a solution of NDs loaded with BAK for the improvement of the endodontic disinfection.

Recent studies have visualized bacteria in dentinal tubules by confocal laser scanning microscopy (CLSM), which has been reported to be an appropriate way, not just to visualize bacteria, but also to identify live and dead bacteria in the infected dentin [23,24].

This study evaluated the antibacterial efficacy and depth of penetration into dentinal tubules of a solution of NDs loaded with BAK through CLSM images compared with NaOCl and CHX.

2. Materials and Methods

2.1. Manufacturing of NDs and Characterization

A decafluoropentane nano-emulsion was obtained and stabilized with dipalmitoyl phosphatidylcholine and palmitic acid (1% w/v). Afterward, a chitosan solution (2.7% w/v) at pH = 5.5 was added dropwise under stirring. The NDs formulation was sterilized through ultraviolet (UV)-C ray exposure for 20 min. To evaluate sterilization efficacy, UV-C-treated NDs were incubated with cell culture Gibco Dulbecco's Modified Eagle Medium (DMEM) in a humidified CO_2/air incubator at 37 °C, up to 72 h. No microbial contamination was observed when NDs and FITC-labeled NDs were checked by optical microscopy. Physic-chemical characterization of chitosan-shelled/decafluoropentane-cored NDs formulation with BAK was performed in vitro to evaluate the size, morphology and surface charge [19].

2.2. Antimicrobial Activity of Benzalkonium Chloride against E. faecalis

The antibacterial activity of NDs loaded with BAK was evaluated comparatively with the free BAK by quantitative analyses. *Enterococcus faecalis* ATCC 29212 was used as the model organism. The broth microdilution assay for quantitative analysis was carried out in accordance with the CLSI M100-S27 to determine the lowest concentration (minimal inhibitory concentration, MIC) and the minimum bactericidal concentration (MBC) of NDs loaded with BAK and free BAK, which inhibit the growth of bacteria.

Seventy-two human single-root teeth with fully formed apex were extracted for periodontal reasons and stored in 4% thymol solution. All samples were collected with informed consent and the Ethical Committee of the University of Turin approved the study protocol (Approval code: DS_00052_2021; Approval date: 20 June 2021). A root dentin block of 4 mm was horizontally sectioned from 1 mm below the cementoenamel junction by a 0.5 mm-thick diamond saw (Isomet 5000; Buehler Ltd., Lake Bluff, IL, USA) at 1000 rpm under water cooling. A Gates Glidden drill #4 (1.1 mm in diameter) (Tulsa Dentsply, Tulsa, OK, USA) at 300 rpm under water cooling was used to enlarge root canals. The smear layer was removed using EDTA 10% for 5 min. Specimens were then packaged and sterilized.

2.3. Irrigation Protocol

Sixty-six of 72 sterilized specimens were placed in multi-well support under a laminar flow biohazard cabinet (CLANLAF-VFR 1206, Racine, WI, USA). Six negative controls (C−) (without bacteria) were used to ensure the efficacy of the sterilization procedures. The root canals of 66 remaining specimens were infected, with an overnight culture of *E. faecalis* ATCC 29212, to match the turbidity of 3×10^8 colony-forming units/mL (CFU/mL) as confirmed by colony counts in triplicate, in Brain Heart Infusion (BHI; Oxoid, Milan, Italy) broth. They were further incubated aerobically with 5% CO_2 at 37 °C for three weeks to allow penetration of *E. faecalis* into dentin tubules. The fresh broth was replaced every fourth day. The purity of the cultures was checked regularly. After three weeks of infection, a control group with six untreated samples was set up as positive control (C+), and the remaining specimens were randomly subdivided into three groups to compare the antimicrobial efficacy of nanodroplets charged with BAK to different types of disinfectants. In the group NDs-BAK ($n = 20$), irrigation was performed for 3 min with 2 mL of NDs solution loaded with BAK; in the group NaOCl ($n = 20$), irrigation was performed for 3 min with 2 mL of 5% NaOCl; and in the group CHX ($n = 20$), irrigation was performed for 3 min with 2 mL of 2% chlorhexidine (CHX).

Each cylindrical dentin block was fractured into two semi-cylindrical halves by making a thin groove in the middle of the specimen, using a low-speed handpiece with a small round bur (Tulsa Dentsply). The size of the fine specimen was about $4 \times 4 \times 2$ mm, and the corresponding irrigant in each group was applied on the internal surface [25].

2.4. Confocal Laser Scanning Microscopy Analysis

Specimens' root canals were accurately rinsed with sterile saline solution, and then Live/Dead Backlight (L/D) viability testing was used to detect viable and dead bacteria: Syto 9 (20/1) and PI (120/1) with a 1:1 ratio (20,000:20,000 µL). Specimens were immersed in the L/D viability test solution, agitated and stocked in a dark container for 30 min; the excess of L/D was then removed with repeated saline solution rinses. Specimens were stocked in a microscopy chamber after having positioned 100 µL of saline solution in the multi-well, and then stocked in a dark room until the CLSM examination. The specimens were then washed in sterile water for 1 min and vertically fractured through the root canal into two flat halves to expose a fresh surface of longitudinally visible dentin canals for CLSM examination [25]. CLSM analysis microscopy imaging was performed using a confocal Olympus IX70 (Olympus optical co. GMBH. Hamburg, Germany) Fluorescence Microscope with illumination by a Krypton/Argon laser (488 nm). Two detection channels captured Syto9 and PI. Emission wavelengths of 505–550 nm (green, Syto9) and 650–750 nm (red, PI) were collected to visualize Syto 9 and PI, respectively. Six additional uninfected samples were stained under the same protocol and used as negative controls to set channel thresholds and ensure standardization [25]. Images were taken using an HCX PL APO CS 20×/0.7 NA oil immersion objective with a different zoom of 2. The software ImageJ (NIH, Bethesda, MD, USA) acquired confocal laser scanning microscopic images at a 1024 × 1024 pixel scan area. For the tested samples, each group's mean depth of action was calculated from ten separate measurements for every single image, adjusted for the red color channel. The mean ratio of red fluorescence over the whole red/green fluorescence (red fluorescence ratio), indicating the proportion of dead cells for each group, was calculated from merged images and three-dimensional reconstructions. This measurement was considered a surrogate marker of bactericidal efficacy.

2.5. Statistical Analyses

Mean depths of action were recorded, and differences were analyzed with one-way ANOVA and post hoc Bonferroni testing ($p < 0.05$). The Kolmogorov–Smirnov test for normality was used to analyze the data distribution of the antibacterial effect. The data were collected, and the differences among groups were analyzed by Kruskal–Wallis and Dunn's post hoc test ($p < 0.05$).

3. Results

The results for MIC and MBC for *E. faecalis* ATCC 29212 showed that BAK (0.023 µg/mL and 0.046 µg/mL, respectively), and NDs-BAK (0.046 µg/mL and 0.186 µg/mL, respectively), were strongly antibacterial. MIC and MBC of CHX were determined as 0.0037 µg/mL and 0.0015 µg/mL, respectively, which resulted in complete inhibition of bacterial growth.

The penetration of *E. faecalis* from the root canal side into the dentinal tubules was verified with CLSM. The negative control group showed no bacterial contamination. The mean depth of action and the mean proportion of dead cells volume (red fluorescence ratio) for each group are reported in Figure 1 and Tables 1 and 2. The three groups exhibited similar mean depths of action: NDs-BAK 325.25 µm, NaOCl 273.36 µm and CHX 246.78 µm, respectively. It was slightly higher in NDs-BAK, but the differences were not statistically significant ($p > 0.05$).

Table 1. Mean depth of action and antimicrobial activity (Red Fluorescence Ratio) of NDs-BAK (nanodroplets with Benzalkonium Chloride), CHX (chlorhexidine), NaOCl (sodium hypochlorite), C+ (positive controls) and C− (negative controls). Nd: data not determined.

	NDs-BAK	NaOCl	CHX	C+	C−
Mean Depth of Action (µm)	325.25 ± 134.52	273.36 ± 181.49	246.78 ± 75.88	0.52 ± 0	Nd
Red Fluorescence Ratio (%)	68.78 ± 0.0956	91.23 ± 0.1066	65.14 ± 0.1362	0.01 ± 0	Nd

Table 2. Comparison among groups of the tested parameters depth of action and antimicrobial effect. NDs-BAK (nanodroplets with Benzalkonium Chloride), CHX (chlorhexidine) and NaOCl (sodium hypochlorite). Level of statistical significance ($p < 0.05$).

	Mean Difference (Mean Depth of Action)	*p*-Value	Mean Difference (Red Fluorescence Ratio)	*p*-Value
NDs-BAK vs. NaOCl	11,493	$p > 0.05$	−20,131	$p < 0.01$
NDs-BAK vs. CHX	15,092	$p > 0.05$	2596	$p > 0.05$
NaOCl vs. CHX	3599	$p > 0.05$	22,727	$p < 0.001$

The mean red fluorescence ratio(s) was higher in NaOCl (91.23%), whereas it was similar between the NDs-BAK and CHX groups (68.78% and 65.14%, respectively) (Table 1). The NaOCl solution showed higher antimicrobial efficacy, whereas nanodroplets with BAK seemed to have the same effect as CHX. There was a statistical difference comparing NDs-BAK with NaOCl ($p < 0.01$) and NaOCl with CHX ($p < 0.001$) related to the antimicrobial activity (Table 2). No differences were found between NDs-BAK and CHX ($p > 0.05$). The positive controls showed a lower mean fluorescence ratio and negative controls were also analyzed (Figure 1, Table 1).

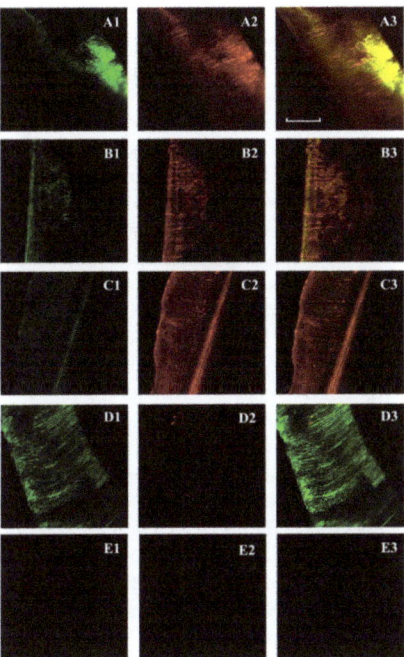

Figure 1. Confocal laser scanning microscopy of *Enterococcus faecalis*-infected dentinal tubules after different irrigation protocols and viability staining. Two-dimensional images of the green channel (**A1–D1**); two-dimensional images of the red channel (**A2–D2**); two-dimensional images of the composite reconstruction (**A3–D3**). NDs-BAK group (nanodroplets with Benzalkonium Chloride) (**A1–A3**). CHX group (chlorhexidine) (**B1–B3**). NaOCl group (sodium hypochlorite) (**C1–C3**). Positive controls (**D1–D3**) and negative controls (**E1–E3**). The pulpal side is represented on the left side for each image and the scale length is 300 μm.

4. Discussion

The experimental data reported that the innovative solution consisting of NDs loaded with BAK displayed a high depth of action inside dentinal tubules and an antibacterial efficacy comparable to CHX.

It has been shown that the success of endodontic treatment depends on two factors: the eradication of bacteria from the root canal system and the absence of reinfection [26,27]. During endodontic treatment, a central role is played by the irrigants that are used to clean the root canal and to eliminate the bacterial biofilm [28]. The most common way to eradicate this infection is to clean the root canal with a dilute solution of sodium hypochlorite [9,10]. Usually, its activity is time-dependent, and several agitation techniques have been proposed to activate irrigants and optimize root canal disinfection with modern low-tapered and time-sparing shaping techniques [9–11,29,30]. However, there is not a single irrigating solution that alone sufficiently covers all the functions required for an ideal root canal cleaning [9,10].

BAK is often referred to as a synthetic antimicrobial agent with a broad-spectrum antimicrobial function, and its activity could be increased by a delayed release deep inside dentinal tubules [15,16,18]. Therefore, this in vitro study evaluated the antibacterial efficacy and depth of action of an innovative solution of chitosan NDs loaded with BAK proposed for endodontic irrigation and with supposed long-lasting antimicrobial activity.

Previous studies reported a high antibacterial activity of BAK against Gram-positive and Gram-negative bacteria, the latter being slightly less sensitive [16,31]. *E. faecalis* is physically and ecologically strong, and it is often present in persistent endodontic infections. Therefore, it is widely used to test the effectiveness of the endodontic disinfecting agents [31]. Finally, Enterococcus' shape is quite round, and they have a relatively small cell diameter, which makes it easier to force them into dentinal tubules [24,32].

After exposure to the antibacterial solutions, the infected dentin specimens were fractured to obtain a fresh dentin surface for CLSM analysis. The border of the fractured root dentin surface was first localized with the microscope to ensure a reproducible scanning field [25]. The bacterial presence could not be determined until the images were processed, ensuring a blindfold evaluation [25,33]. Moreover, representative data from all randomly selected areas with an excellent signal-to-noise fluorescence ratio were obtained due to the presence of bacteria in the dentinal tubules [25]. However, background fluorescence was occasionally observed within the canal lumen and the root canal samples showed auto-fluorescent materials not to be confused with bacteria [23–25]. Nevertheless, the background fluorescence intensity was minimal within the tubules and there was no inference with the signal generated from bacteria [33].

Confocal-laser scanning microscope visualized the presence of microorganisms in the root canal dentinal tubules due to its ability to penetrate below the surface of the specimen and to include the dentin canals that are not open on the surface [2,25,32,33].

Microorganism selection depends on the focus of the study and an endodontic biofilm consists mostly of Enterococcus faecalis. Usually, the common analyzed variables are counts of colony-forming units or the percentage of dead bacteria determined by confocal laser scanning microscopy after applying a differentiating stain. These models are helpful to evaluate new antimicrobial treatment options, even if a new therapy has yet to be proven in randomized controlled clinical trials [34].

In the present study, the CLSM analysis showed no statistical difference among groups concerning the depth of action, even if the NDs-BAK solution seemed to penetrate deeper on the limit of statistical significance. Previous studies showed lower BAK dentin tubular penetration, but the use of a NDs carrier could be beneficial for a deeper irrigant penetration [35,36]. The overall efficacy of the tested NDs-BAK solution was similar to CHX. These results seem in accordance with the available literature, despite the differences in methodology [17]. In conclusion, within the limitation of this in vitro study based on CLSM analysis, nanodroplets charged with BAK, although they failed to show the same antibacterial efficacy of NaOCl, proved as effective as the CHX solution, with deep penetration ability inside tubules [21,22].

Author Contributions: Conceptualization: M.A., N.M., P.C., E.B. and D.P.; Methodology: N.M., J.R., P.C., M.A., L.C., A.L., A.C., N.S. and R.C.; Software: A.L., P.C., M.A. and N.S.; Data Analysis: A.I., D.P., N.M., J.R., A.L., L.C. and N.S.; Visualization: A.I., E.B., A.C. and N.S.; Supervision and Project Administration: M.A., E.B., A.I., D.P. and R.C.; Writing: M.A., N.M., J.R., P.C., A.C. and L.C.; Reviewing and Editing: E.B., R.C., N.S. and A.I. All authors have read and agreed to the published version of the manuscript.

Funding: For the development of this study no funds have been received.

Institutional Review Board Statement: Seventy-two human single-root teeth with fully formed apex were stored in 4% thymol solution after extraction. The teeth were extracted for periodontal reasons and all samples were collected with informed consent. The Ethical Committee of the University of Turin approved the study protocol (Approval code: DS_00052_2021; Approval date: 20 June 2021).

Informed Consent Statement: Not applicable.

Acknowledgments: The authors declare no competing conflict of interest with the materials discussed in this manuscript.

Conflicts of Interest: The authors affirm that any conflict of interest is disclosed.

References

1. Eriksen, H.M.; Kirkevang, L.; Petersson, K. Endodontic epidemiology and treatment outcome: General considerations. *Endod. Top.* **2002**, *2*, 1–9. [CrossRef]
2. Tibúrcio-Machado, C.S.; Michelon, C.; Zanatta, F.B.; Gomes, M.S.; Marin, J.A.; Bier, C.A. The global prevalence of apical periodontitis: A systematic review and meta-analysis. *Int. Endod. J.* **2021**, *54*, 712–735. [CrossRef] [PubMed]
3. Pak, J.G.; Fayazi, S.; White, S.N. Prevalence of periapical radiolucency and root canal treatment: A systematic review of cross-sectional studies. *J. Endod.* **2012**, *38*, 1170–1176. [CrossRef] [PubMed]
4. Peters, O.A. Current challenges and concepts in the preparation of root canal systems: A review. *J. Endod.* **2004**, *30*, 559–567. [CrossRef] [PubMed]
5. Alovisi, M.; Pasqualini, D.; Scotti, N.; Carpegna, G.; Comba, A.; Bernardi, M.; Tutino, F.; Dioguardi, M.; Berutti, E. Micro-CT evaluation of rotary and reciprocating glide path and shaping systems outcomes in maxillary molar curved canals. *Odontology* **2021**, *110*, 54–61. [CrossRef]
6. Hulsmann, M.; Peters, O.A.; Dummer, P.M.H. Mechanical preparation of root canals: Shaping goals, techniques and means. *Endod. Top.* **2005**, *10*, 30–76. [CrossRef]
7. Zhao, D.; Shen, Y.; Peng, B.; Haapasalo, M. Root Canal Preparation of Mandibular Molars with 3 Nickel-Titanium Rotary Instruments: A Micro-Computed Tomographic Study. *J. Endod.* **2014**, *40*, 1860–1864. [CrossRef] [PubMed]
8. Alovisi, M.; Cemenasco, A.; Mancini, L.; Paolino, D.; Scotti, N.; Bianchi, C.C.; Pasqualini, D. Micro-CT evaluation of several glide path techniques and ProTaper Next shaping outcomes in maxillary first molar curved canals. *Int. Endod. J.* **2017**, *50*, 387–397. [CrossRef]
9. Zehnder, M. Root canal irrigants. *J. Endod.* **2006**, *32*, 5. [CrossRef]
10. Haapasalo, M.; Shen, Y.; Qian, W.; Gao, Y. Irrigation in endodontics. *Dent. Clin. N. Am.* **2010**, *54*, 291–312. [CrossRef]
11. Gu, L.; Kim, J.R.; Ling, J.; Choi, K.K.; Pashley, D.H.; Tay, F.R. Review of contemporary irrigant agitation techniques and devices. *J. Endod.* **2009**, *35*, 791–804. [CrossRef] [PubMed]
12. Fedorowicz, Z.; Nasser, M.; Sequeira-Byron, P.; de Souza, R.F.; Carter, B.; Heft, M. Irrigants for non-surgical root canal treatment in mature permanent teeth. *Cochrane Database Syst. Rev.* **2012**, *12*, 9–17. [CrossRef] [PubMed]
13. Guerreiro, M.Y.; Belladonna, F.G.; Monteiro, L.P.; Lima, C.O.; Silva, E.J.; Brandão, J.M. The influence of the addition of surfactants to sodium hypochlorite on the removal of hard tissue debris. *Int. Endod. J.* **2020**, *53*, 1131–1139. [CrossRef] [PubMed]
14. Mohammadi, Z.; Abbott, P.V. The properties and applications of chlorhexidine in endodontics. *Int. Endod. J.* **2009**, *42*, 288–302. [CrossRef] [PubMed]
15. Bukiet, F.; Couderc, G.; Camps, J.; Tassery, H.; Cuisinier, F.; About, I.; Charrier, A.; Candoni, N. Wetting properties and critical micellar concentration of benzalkonium chloride mixed in sodium hypochlorite. *J. Endod.* **2012**, *38*, 1525–1529. [CrossRef] [PubMed]
16. Jaramillo, D.E.; Arriola, A.; Safavi, K.; de Paz, L.E. Decreased bacterial adherence and biofilm growth on surfaces coated with a solution of benzalkonium chloride. *J. Endod.* **2012**, *38*, 821–825. [CrossRef] [PubMed]
17. Arias-Moliz, M.T.; Ruiz-Linares, M.; Cassar, G.; Ferrer-Luque, C.M.; Baca, P.; Ordinola-Zapata, R.; Camilleri, J. The effect of benzalkonium chloride additions to AH Plus sealer. Antimicrobial, physical and chemical properties. *J. Dent.* **2015**, *43*, 846–854. [CrossRef]
18. Shrestha, A.; Kishen, A. Antibacterial nanoparticles in endodontics: A review. *J. Endod.* **2016**, *42*, 1417–1426. [CrossRef]
19. Khadjavi, A.; Stura, I.; Prato, M.; Minero, V.G.; Panariti, A.; Rivolta, I.; Gulino, G.R.; Bessone, F.; Giribaldi, G.; Quaglino, E.; et al. 'In Vitro', 'In Vivo' and 'In Silico' investigation of the anticancer effectiveness of oxygen-loaded chitosan-shelled nanodroplets as potential drug vector. *Pharm. Res.* **2018**, *35*, 75–81. [CrossRef]
20. Shrestha, A.; Kishen, A. The effect of tissue inhibitors on the antibacterial activity of chitosan nanoparticles and photodynamic therapy. *J. Endod.* **2012**, *38*, 1275–1278. [CrossRef]
21. Banche, G.; Prato, M.; Magnetto, C.; Allizond, V.; Giribaldi, G.; Argenziano, M.; Khadjavi, A.; Gulino, G.R.; Finesso, N.; Mandras, N.; et al. Antimicrobial chitosan nanodroplets: New insights for ultrasound-mediated adjuvant treatment of skin infection. *Future Microbiol.* **2015**, *10*, 929–939. [CrossRef] [PubMed]
22. Argenziano, M.; Bressan, B.; Luganini, A.; Finesso, N.; Genova, T.; Troia, A.; Giribaldi, G.; Banche, G.; Mandras, N.; Cuffini, A.M.; et al. Comparative evaluation of different chitosan species and derivatives as candidate biomaterials for oxygen-loaded nanodroplet formulations to treat chronic wounds. *Mar. Drugs* **2021**, *19*, 112. [CrossRef] [PubMed]
23. Zapata, R.O.; Bramante, C.M.; de Moraes, I.G.; Bernardineli, N.; Gasparoto, T.H.; Graeff, M.S.; Campanelli, A.P.; Garcia, R.B. Confocal laser scanning microscopy is appropriate to detect viability of Enterococcus faecalis in infected dentin. *J. Endod.* **2008**, *34*, 1198–1201. [CrossRef] [PubMed]
24. Parmar, D.; Hauman, C.H.; Leichter, J.W.; McNaughton, A.; Tompkins, G.R. Bacterial localization and viability assessment in human ex vivo dentinal tubules by fluorescence confocal laser scanning microscopy. *Int. Endod. J.* **2011**, *44*, 644–651. [CrossRef] [PubMed]
25. Ma, J.; Wang, Z.; Shen, Y.; Haapasalo, M. A new noninvasive model to study the effectiveness of dentin disinfection by using confocal laser scanning microscopy. *J. Endod.* **2011**, *37*, 1380–1385. [CrossRef] [PubMed]
26. Haapasalo, M.; Endal, U.; Zandi, H.; Coil, J.M. Eradication of endodontic infection by instrumentation and irrigation solutions. *Endod. Top.* **2005**, *10*, 77–102. [CrossRef]

27. Mandras, N.; Pasqualini, D.; Roana, J.; Tullio, V.; Banche, G.; Gianello, E.; Bonino, F.; Cuffini, A.M.; Berutti, E.; Alovisi, M. Influence of Photon-Induced Photoacoustic Streaming (PIPS) on root canal disinfection and post-operative pain: A randomized clinical trial. *J. Clin. Med.* **2020**, *9*, 3915. [CrossRef]
28. Siqueira, J.F. Endodontic infections: Concepts, paradigms, and perspectives. *Oral Surg. Oral Med. Oral Pathol. Oral Radiol. Endodontol.* **2002**, *94*, 281–293. [CrossRef]
29. Del Carpio-Perochena, A.E.; Bramante, C.M.; Duarte, M.A.; Cavenago, B.C.; Villas-Boas, M.H.; Graeff, M.S.; Bernardineli, N.; de Andrade, F.B.; Ordinola-Zapata, R. Biofilm dissolution and cleaning ability of different irrigant solutions on intraorally infected dentin. *J. Endod.* **2011**, *37*, 1134–1138. [CrossRef]
30. Iandolo, A.; Dagna, A.; Poggio, C.; Capar, I.; Amato, A.; Abdellatif, D. Evaluation of the actual chlorine concentration and the required time for pulp dissolution using different sodium hypochlorite irrigating solutions. *J. Conserv. Dent.* **2019**, *22*, 108–113. [CrossRef]
31. Gjorgievska, E.; Apostolska, S.; Dimkov, A.; Nicholson, J.W.; Kaftandzieva, A. Incorporation of antimicrobial agents can be used to enhance the antibacterial effect of endodontic sealers. *Dent. Mater.* **2013**, *29*, e29–e34. [CrossRef] [PubMed]
32. Komiyama, E.Y.; Lepesqueur, L.S.; Yassuda, C.G.; Samaranayake, L.P.; Parahitiyawa, N.B.; Balducci, I.; Koga-Ito, C.Y. Enterococcus species in the oral cavity: Prevalence, virulence factors and antimicrobial susceptibility. *PLoS ONE* **2016**, *11*, e016300. [CrossRef] [PubMed]
33. Mandras, N.; Alovisi, M.; Roana, J.; Crosasso, P.; Luganini, A.; Pasqualini, D.; Genta, E.; Arpicco, S.; Banche, G.; Cuffini, A.; et al. Evaluation of the bactericidal activity of a hyaluronic acid-vehicled clarithromycin antibiotic mixture by confocal laser scanning microscopy. *Appl. Sci.* **2020**, *10*, 761. [CrossRef]
34. Eick, S. Biofilm Models for the Evaluation of Dental Treatment. *Monogr. Oral Sci.* **2021**, *29*, 38–52. [PubMed]
35. Baron, A.; Lindsey, K.; Sidow, S.J.; Dickinson, D.; Chuang, A.; McPherson, J.C., 3rd. Effect of a Benzalkonium Chloride Surfactant-Sodium Hypochlorite Combination on Elimination of Enterococcus faecalis. *J. Endod.* **2016**, *42*, 145–149. [CrossRef] [PubMed]
36. Wang, Z.; Shen, Y.; Haapasalo, M. Effectiveness of endodontic disinfecting solutions against young and old Enterococcus faecalis biofilms in dentin canals. *J. Endod.* **2012**, *38*, 1376–1379. [CrossRef]

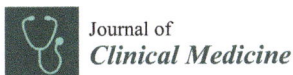

Article

Influence of Static Navigation Technique on the Accuracy of Autotransplanted Teeth in Surgically Created Sockets

Elena Riad Deglow [1], Nayra Zurima Lazo Torres [1], David Gutiérrez Muñoz [1], María Bufalá Pérez [1], Agustín Galparsoro Catalán [1], Álvaro Zubizarreta-Macho [1,2,*], Francesc Abella Sans [3] and Sofía Hernández Montero [1]

[1] Department of Implant Surgery, Faculty of Health Sciences, Alfonso X el Sabio University, 28691 Madrid, Spain; eriaddeg@uax.es (E.R.D.); nlazotor@myuax.com (N.Z.L.T.); dgutierr@uax.es (D.G.M.); mperebuf@uax.es (M.B.P.); agalpcat@uax.es (A.G.C.); shernmon@uax.es (S.H.M.)
[2] Department of Orthodontics, Faculty of Medicine and Dentistry, University of Salamanca, 37008 Salamanca, Spain
[3] Department of Endodontics, Universitat Internacional de Catalunya, 08195 Barcelona, Spain; franabella@uic.es
* Correspondence: amacho@uax.es

Citation: Riad Deglow, E.; Lazo Torres, N.Z.; Gutiérrez Muñoz, D.; Bufalá Pérez, M.; Galparsoro Catalán, A.; Zubizarreta-Macho, Á.; Abella Sans, F.; Hernández Montero, S. Influence of Static Navigation Technique on the Accuracy of Autotransplanted Teeth in Surgically Created Sockets. *J. Clin. Med.* **2022**, *11*, 1012. https://doi.org/10.3390/jcm11041012

Academic Editor: Massimo Amato

Received: 30 December 2021
Accepted: 13 February 2022
Published: 15 February 2022

Publisher's Note: MDPI stays neutral with regard to jurisdictional claims in published maps and institutional affiliations.

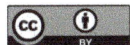

Copyright: © 2022 by the authors. Licensee MDPI, Basel, Switzerland. This article is an open access article distributed under the terms and conditions of the Creative Commons Attribution (CC BY) license (https://creativecommons.org/licenses/by/4.0/).

Abstract: The aim of this study was to analyse and compare the position of single-rooted autotransplanted teeth using computer-aided SNT drilling and conventional freehand (FT) drilling, by comparing the planned and performed position at the coronal, apical and angular level. Materials and methods: Forty single-root upper teeth were selected and distributed into the following study groups: A. Autotransplanted tooth using the computer-aided static navigation technique (SNT) ($n = 20$) and B. Autotransplanted tooth using the conventional free-hand technique (FT) ($n = 20$). Afterwards, the teeth were embedded into two experimental models and 10 single-root upper teeth were randomly autotransplanted in each experimental model. The experimental models were submitted to a preoperative cone-beam computed tomography (CBCT) scan and a digital impression by a 3D intraoral scan, in addition to a postoperative CBCT scan, after the autotransplantation. Datasets from postoperative CBCT scans of the two study groups were uploaded to the 3D implant planning software, aligned with the autotransplantation planning, and the coronal, apical and angular deviations were measured. The results were analysed using Student's *t*-test and Mann–Whitney non-parametric statistical analysis. Results: Coronal ($p = 0.079$) and angular ($p = 0.208$) statistical comparisons did not present statistically significant differences; however, statistically significant differences between the apical deviation of the SNT and FT study groups ($p = 0.038$) were also observed. Conclusions: The computer-aided static navigation technique does not provide higher accuracy in the positioning of single-root autotransplanted teeth compared to the conventional free-hand technique.

Keywords: accuracy; computed-assisted template; computer-aided static navigation; cone-beam computed tomography scan; digital impression; tooth autotransplantation

1. Introduction

Autotransplantation entails transplanting embedded, impacted or erupted teeth from one extraction site to a fresh extraction socket or surgically prepared socket [1]. The advantages of an autotransplanted tooth over a fixed osseointegrated implant include improved resistance to occlusal loading, preservation of the periodontal ligament (PDL) and surrounding bone, continuous bone growth and potentially enhanced aesthetics [2–5]. Among the indications for tooth autotransplantation are impacted or ectopic teeth, premature and/or traumatic tooth loss, tooth loss resulting from tumours or for iatrogenic reasons, congenitally missing teeth in one arch together with arch length discrepancy, or clinical signs of tooth crowding in the opposing arch, replacement of hopeless teeth and/or developmental dental anomalies [3,6,7].

The challenges of prognosticating root development and dental root resorption post transplantation meant that the 50% success rate of autologous tooth transplantation in the 1950s was relatively low [8,9]. Many studies performed since the 1990s on periodontal tissue and periodontal membrane healing and root resorption have led to a rapid increase in transplant success [3,10,11]. The immature tooth with an open apex is characterized by having an adequate blood supply and stem cells stimulating pulp revascularization post autotransplantation [12]. This revascularization promotes continuous root development and tooth vitality and, at the same time, induces normal alveolar bone growth, which is unfeasible in fixed prostheses. Hence, autotransplantation has a high success rate in immature teeth and is the most conservative and physiologic tooth replacement option [13–17], especially in young patients [6,18].

Some authors have recently determined that there is no significant difference in the success rate of autotransplantation between mature and immature teeth [19–21]. In their systematic review, Chung et al. observed that the estimated 1- and 5-year survival rates of autotransplanted teeth with completely formed roots were 98.0% and 90.5%, respectively [6].

The biological responses and wound healing behave similarly to those of avulsed teeth post replantation. Mechanical damage during extraction or continuous traumatic press-fit placement in the recipient socket could harm PDL, giving rise to gradual root resorption. These complications are overcome thanks to improvements in diagnostic and surgical techniques, particularly computer-aided rapid prototyping (CARP) models (tooth replicas) and three-dimensional (3D) printed guiding templates [22–25]. These digital techniques not only allow clinicians to select the most suitable donor tooth, according to tooth morphology, but also show them the ideal 3D position and the required dimensions of the recipient socket during surgery. Moreover, the use of tooth replicas can reduce extra oral time and possible donor tooth injury during the procedure [22,23].

However, depending on when the tooth was lost, the recipient site conditions may change. In cases of autotransplantation to a fresh extraction socket immediately after extraction of a hopeless tooth, there is usually sufficient bone [10,11,26]. However, for patients with conditions such as congenitally missing teeth or early tooth loss, the recipient site calls for surgical creation [21]. At present, 3D radiologic data are also being used for model-based surgical guides to avoid free-hand preparation of the recipient site [3,16,21–23].

Anssari Moin et al. used 10 partially edentulous human mandibular cadavers to assess the accuracy of computer-assisted template-guided autotransplantation with custom 3D designed/printed surgical tools. Their comparison of the superimposed images of the preoperatively planned donor teeth positions and the postoperative donor teeth positions revealed a mean angular deflection (alpha) of 5.6 ± 5.4°. When comparing the bodily 3D positions (a), the authors found a mean deviation of 3.15 ± 1.16 mm, resulting in a mean apical deviation of 2.61 ± 0.78 mm [24]. A comparison of superimposed images of the preoperative planning and the final donor tooth position yielded results similar to those obtained by implant-guided surgery [27]. However, there appears to be no studies comparing precision between free-hand preparation and a static navigation technique (SNT) using an implant drilling sequence.

The aim of the present study was to analyse and compare the position of single-rooted autotransplanted teeth using computer-aided SNT drilling and conventional freehand (FT) drilling, by comparing the planned and performed position at the coronal, apical and angular levels. The null hypothesis (H0) was that there is no difference between computer-aided SNT and conventional FT concerning the accuracy of single-rooted autotransplanted teeth.

2. Materials and Methods

2.1. Study Design

Forty single-rooted maxillary anterior teeth (incisors and canines), extracted for periodontal or orthodontic reasons, were selected for this study conducted at the Dental Centre of Innovation and Advanced Specialties at Alfonso X El Sabio University (Madrid, Spain) between March and April 2021. The sample size was selected according to a previous study with a power effect of 88.4 (it is considered acceptable from 80) [28]. The manuscript of this laboratory study has been written according to 2021 Preferred Reporting Items for Laboratory studies in Endodontology (PRILE) guidelines (Figure 1) [29,30]. In addition, the study was conducted in accordance with the principles defined in the German Ethics Committee's statement for the use of organic tissues in medical research (Zentrale Ethikkommission, 2003) and was authorized by the Ethical Committee of the Faculty of Health Sciences, University Alfonso X el Sabio (Madrid, Spain), in October 2020 (Process No. 05/2020). All the patients signed an informed consent form to donate the teeth for the present study.

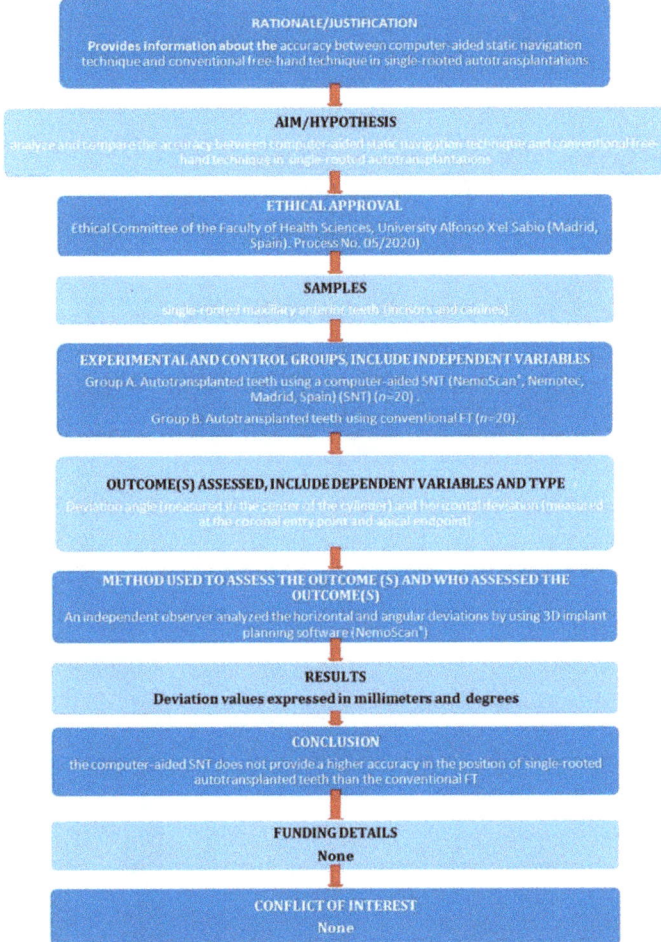

Figure 1. Preferred reporting items for laboratory studies in endodontology flowchart.

2.2. Experimental Procedure

The single-rooted teeth were embedded into two experimental epoxy resin models (Ref. 20-8130-128, EpoxiCure®, Buehler, IL, USA), each with 20 teeth. Ten teeth (for autotransplantation) were placed in the internal part of the model, and 10 teeth (used as a reference), in the external part. The teeth were randomly (Epidat 4.1, Galicia, Spain) assigned to two study groups: Group A, autotransplanted teeth using a computer-aided static navigation technique (NemoScan®, Nemotec, Madrid, Spain) (SNT) (n = 20), and Group B, autotransplanted teeth using conventional free-hand technique (FT) (n = 20).

The two experimental models were submitted to a preoperative cone-beam computed tomography (CBCT) scan (WhiteFox, Acteón Médico-Dental Ibérica S.A.U.-Satelec, Merignac, France) with the following exposure parameters: 105.0 kilovolt peak, 8.0 milliamperes, 7.20 s, and a field of view of 15 × 13 mm (Figure 2A). Subsequently, a digital impression was made using a 3D intraoral scan (True Definition, 3M ESPE™, Saint Paul, MN, USA) by means of 3D in-motion video imaging technology to generate a standard tessellation language (STL) digital file (Figure 2B). The 3D intraoral scan (True Definition) uses a cloud of points that create a tessella network, representing 3D objects as polygons composed of equilateral triangle tessellas [31,32]. The image capture procedure was performed by scanning the palatine and occlusal surface followed by the buccal surface, according to the manufacturer's recommendations. Datasets obtained from this digital workflow were uploaded to a 3D implant planning software (NemoScan®) to plan the placement of autotransplantation in Group A (Figure 2C).

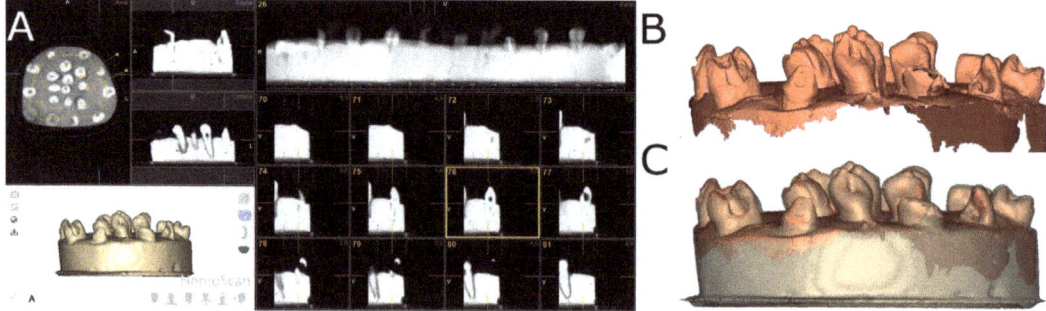

Figure 2. (**A**) CBCT scan, (**B**) STL digital files and (**C**) alignment of the digital workflow.

After matching the 3D surface scan and CBCT data (WhiteFox), each tooth in the internal part of the model was individually segmented and virtually placed between the teeth placed outside of the model (Figure 3).

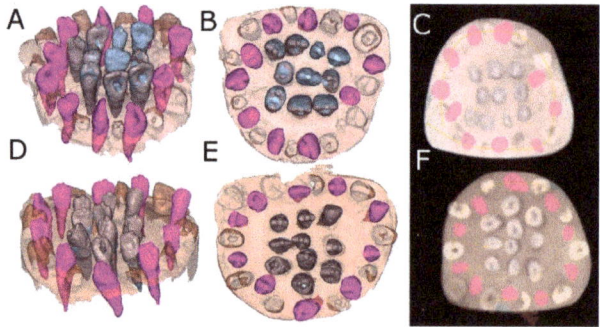

Figure 3. (**A**) Frontal, (**B**) occlusal and (**C**) apical view of the individually segmented (blue) and autotransplanted teeth (purple) between the teeth placed outside of the experimental model (pink) randomly assigned to the SNT study group. (**D**) Frontal, (**E**) occlusal and (**F**) apical view of the individually segmented (grey) and autotransplanted teeth (purple) between the teeth placed outside of the experimental model (pink) randomly assigned to the FT study group.

The surgically created sockets of the teeth were randomly assigned to the SNT study group; the drilling was performed by means of a 3D printed tooth-supported surgical template with 10 drilling sleeves of 2.5 mm in diameter (NemoScan®) (Figure 4). The dimensions of the osteotomy site preparations were designed virtually by superimposing the virtual surgical drilling burs (BioHorizons; Birmingham, AL, USA) on the roots of the autotransplanted teeth. A surgical template was then exported as an STL digital file and 3D printed for fabrication (Explora 3D Lab, Nemotec S.L, Arroyomolinos, Madrid, Spain) with medical-use resin. The osteotomy site was manually drilled with surgical burs according to each root anatomy (BioHorizons).

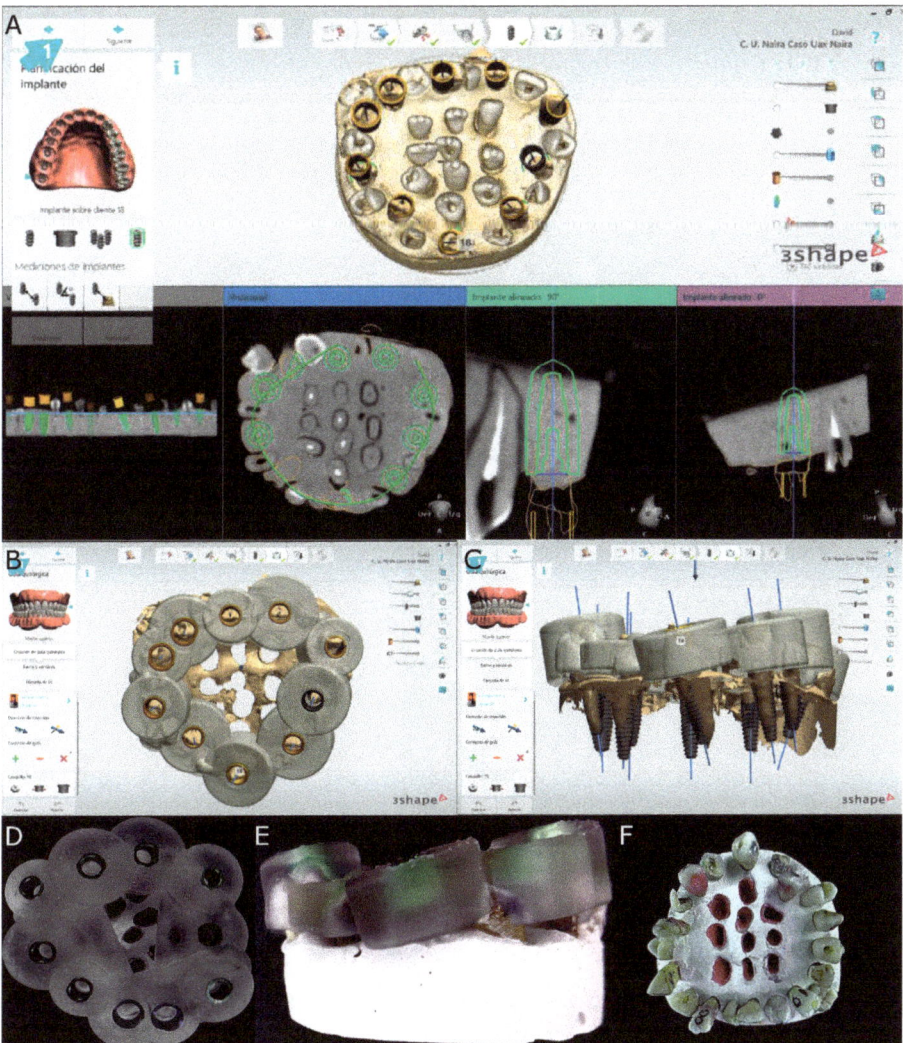

Figure 4. (**A**) Drilling site planning in the CBCT scan, (**B**) occlusal view of the surgical template design for computer-aided static navigation technique, (**C**) lateral view of the drilling bur selection according to the root dimensions, (**D**) occlusal and (**E**) lateral view of the surgical template manufactured and (**F**) occlusal view of the transplanted teeth.

On the other hand, the drilling procedure of the osteotomy site of the teeth randomly assigned to the autotransplanted tooth using conventional FT study group was performed completely manually. Subsequently, the teeth placed inside of the experimental models of epoxy resin were extracted and placed between the teeth placed outside of the experimental model until it adjusted to the previously autotransplanted planned position (Figure 4). A single operator with 10 years of surgical experience performed all autotransplanted teeth procedures.

2.3. Measurement Procedure

After performing the osteotomy site preparation and placing the autotransplanted teeth of both study groups, a postoperative CBCT scan (WhiteFox) of the experimental models were taken with the same, previously described exposure parameters. STL digital files from the planning and datasets from postoperative CBCT scans of the two study groups were uploaded to the 3D implant planning software (NemoScan®) and aligned using the 3D implant planning software (NemoScan®) to analyse the deviation angle (measured in the centre of the cylinder) and horizontal deviation (measured at the coronal entry point and apical endpoint) (Figure 5) by an independent observer.

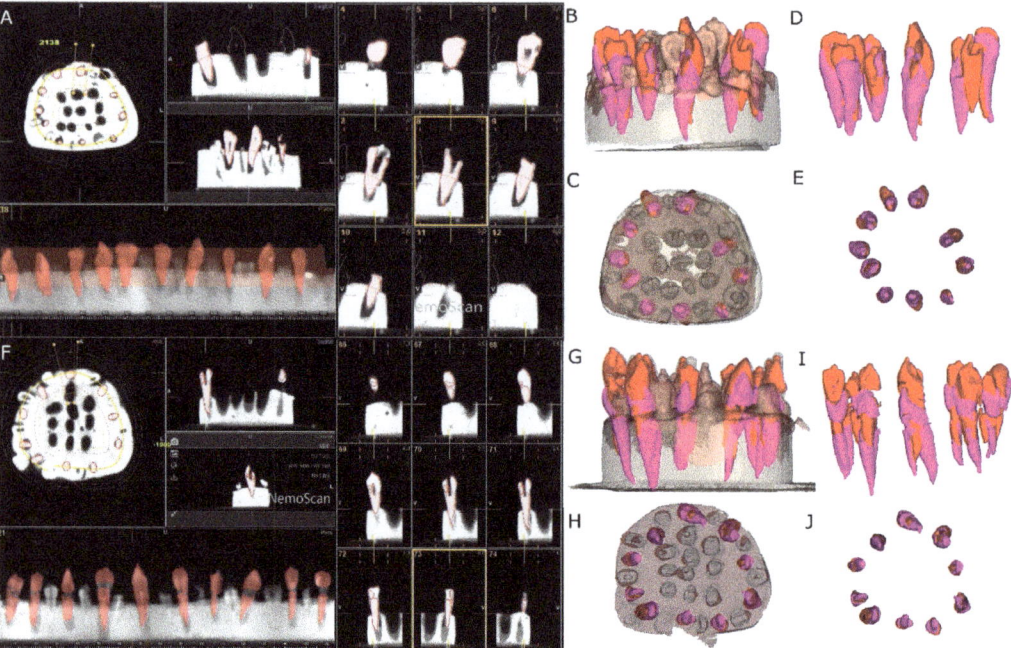

Figure 5. (**A**) Segmented teeth on the postoperative CBCT scan (red teeth), (**B**) lateral view and (**C**) apical view of the experimental models and (**D**) lateral and (**E**) apical view of the planned (pink teeth) and performed (red teeth) autotransplanted teeth without model of the conventional freehand technique study group. (**F**) Segmented teeth on the postoperative CBCT scan (red teeth), (**G**) lateral and (**H**) apical view of the experimental models and (**I**) lateral and (**J**) apical view of the planned (pink teeth) and performed (red teeth) autotransplanted teeth without model of the computer-aided static navigation technique.

2.4. Statistical Tests

All the variables of interest were recorded for statistical analysis with SAS v9.4 (SAS Institute Inc., Cary, NC, USA). Descriptive statistical analysis was expressed as means and standard deviations (SDs) for quantitative variables. Comparative analysis was performed by comparing the mean deviation between planned and performed autotransplanted tooth using Student's *t*-test, since variables had normal distribution, or Mann–Whitney non-parametric test; $p < 0.05$ was considered statistically significant.

3. Results

The means and standard deviation (SD) values for coronal, apical and angular deviation of the autotransplanted tooth using computer-aided static navigation technique and conventional freehand technique are displayed in Table 1.

Table 1. Descriptive deviation values at coronal (mm), apical (mm) and angular (°) levels of the autotransplanted tooth using computer-aided static navigation technique and conventional free-hand technique.

		n	Mean	Median	SD	Minimum	Maximum
SNT	Coronal	10	6.93	5.40 [a]	3.76	3.50	16.90
	Apical	10	6.60	5.65 [a]	2.81	3.90	13.50
	Angular	10	10.64	8.05 [a]	5.78	4.50	21.20
FT	Coronal	10	4.62	4.20 [a]	1.85	2.00	7.70
	Apical	10	4.36	3.90 [b]	1.99	2.20	8.10
	Angular	10	7.61	7.10 [a]	4.53	2.30	15.80

SNT: static navigation technique. FT: free-hand technique. [a,b] Statistically significant differences between groups ($p < 0.05$).

Mean comparison of the coronal deviation of the autotransplanted teeth randomly assigned to the SNT study group did not show a normal distribution; therefore, the comparative analysis was performed by a Mann–Whitney non-parametric test. Median comparison of the autotransplanted teeth revealed no statistically significant differences at the coronal deviation ($p = 0.079$) between the SNT (5.40 ± 3.76 mm) and FT (4.20 ± 1.85 mm) study groups (Figure 6).

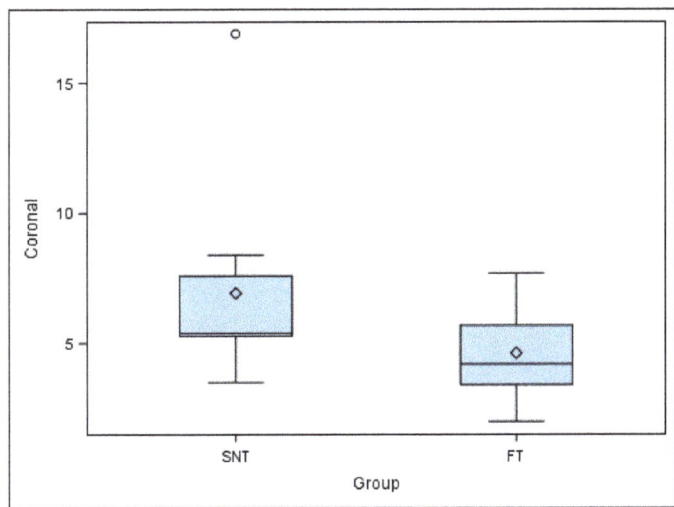

Figure 6. Box plot of the coronal deviation of the autotransplanted teeth. The horizontal line in each box represents the respective median value of the study groups. ◊: Mean value of the box plots. ○: Means and extreme value.

Mean comparison of the apical deviation of the autotransplanted teeth randomly assigned to the SNT study group did not show a normal distribution; therefore, the comparative analysis was performed again with a Mann–Whitney non-parametric test. Median comparison of the autotransplanted teeth revealed statistically significant differences at the apical deviation ($p = 0.038$) between SNT (5.65 ± 2.81 mm) and FT (3.90 ± 1.99 mm) study groups (Figure 7).

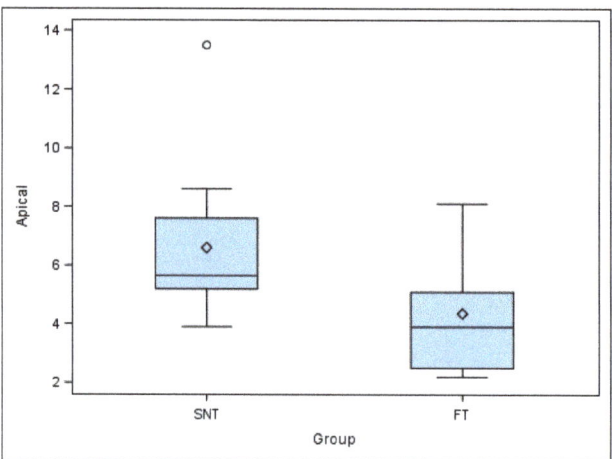

Figure 7. Box plot of the apical deviation of the autotransplanted teeth. The horizontal line in each box represents the respective median value of the study groups. ◊: Mean value of the box plots. ○: Means and extreme value.

A mean comparison of the angular deviation of the autotransplanted teeth randomly assigned to the SNT study group showed a normal distribution; therefore, the comparative analysis was performed using Student's *t*-test. Mean comparison of the autotransplanted teeth revealed no statistically significant differences at the angular deviation ($p = 0.208$) between SNT (5.65 ± 2.81 mm) and FT (3.90 ± 1.99 mm) study groups (Figure 8).

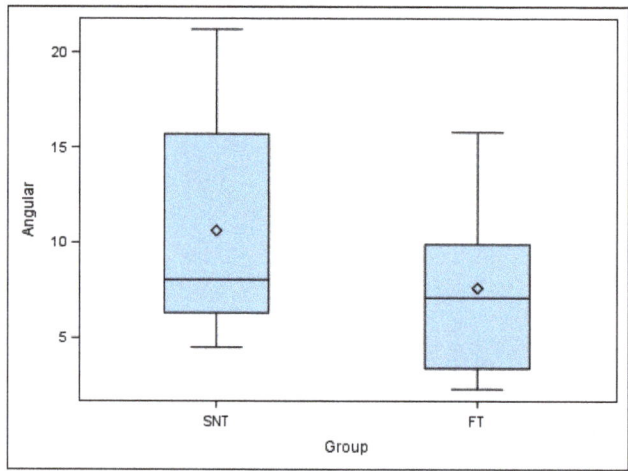

Figure 8. Box plot of the angular deviation of the autotransplanted teeth. The horizontal line in each box represents the respective median value of the study groups. ◊: Mean value of the box plots.

4. Discussion

The present study reported that the coronal and angular deviations between the SNT and FT study groups did not show statistically significant differences; however, statistically significant differences were observed between the apical deviation of the SNT and FT study groups. One of the main problems in dentistry is the premature loss of teeth resulting from trauma, caries or malformations, especially in growing patients [33]. With this in mind, the clinician can choose from various treatment options depending on the patient's age [23]. The most common restorative approaches for adults include fixed or removable partial dentures, implants or orthodontics. However, in paediatric and adolescent patients, implant placement is totally contraindicated [34]. Accordingly, in determined patients, autologous transplantation offers an effective treatment option with the potential to restore masticatory function and aesthetics [10]. Unlike implants, transplanted teeth behave in the same way as any natural tooth, both of which maintain the alveolar bone and occlusion during growth. The benefit of this procedure is that it allows the replacement of a hopeless or missing tooth with another tooth from the same patient [34].

Depending on the time of autotransplantation, the technique can be performed in either fresh extraction sockets or surgically created sockets [33]. In an immediate autotransplantation, fibroblasts and PDL remaining in the socket wall proliferate and migrate to the blood clot, promoting bone and connective tissue reconstruction and significantly aiding the revascularization of the root surface of the donor tooth [35]. One potential drawback to immediate autotransplantation is that the donor tooth may not fit perfectly into the recipient socket, which results in a discrepancy between the tooth surface and the alveolar wall. For bone formation to take place, it is essential for the root surface of the donor tooth to be near the cervical level of the adjacent bone, since the underlying tissue acts like a closed wound, reducing the possibility of infection and complications [2]. There are some indications for late autotransplantation placement according to patient- or site-specific reasons. These include patients with congenitally missing teeth or premature tooth loss, or when there is insufficient mesio-distal space in the recipient area, for which subsequent orthodontic treatment is needed [33]. Although this technique is more challenging, no significant difference in outcomes compared to autotransplantation in fresh extraction sockets have been observed [36,37]. After tooth extraction, the buccal and lingual walls of the alveolus resorb significantly [38]. In this situation, the root of the donor tooth can be rotated or even resected to fit within the new socket. The clinician may choose from surgical drrills, implant drills or even trephines to surgically create the new socket [21]. The main factors determining a successful autotransplantation involve preserving the PDL and correctly adapting tissue [39]. Hence, it is crucial to avoid excessive manipulation of the tooth and minimize both the extra-alveolar time (should not exceed 12 min) and the distance between the alveolus and the root of the tooth [24,25,34]. This is particularly relevant in surgically created sockets, in which revascularization is delayed, leading to insufficient nutrition of the apical tissues, negatively affecting the vitality of Hertwig's epithelial root sheath (HERS) [40,41]. This is a highly technical and sensitive surgical procedure that demands all the clinician's experience and skill [25]. In the conventional autotransplantation technique, whose first clinical application dates to 1950 [41], the donor tooth served as a template to prepare the socket, which involved excessive manipulation of the donor tooth, greater chemical and physical trauma to the PDL and more extra-alveolar time. However, with the advent of CBCT and digital planning, the complexity and failure rate of this technique has been substantially reduced [4,18,22]. In 2001, Lee et al. described the use of computer-assisted replicas of the donor tooth, making it possible to prepare the recipient socket without having to use the donor tooth itself [22]. In addition, available surgical planning software allows the clinician to design and manufacture 3D-printed surgical guides. These guides approximate autotransplantation surgery to guided surgery, but the literature analysed has shown that certain inaccuracies between the original digitally planned position and the final position of the donor tooth remain frequent. For a guided surgery to be closer to its original digital planning, it is essential to achieve a precise osteotomy that produces minimal trauma to the recipient area [4]. Trauma is directly related to overheating of the bone during osteotomy, which can lead to cell death, preventing new bone formation. In addition, an overlarge alveoloplasty increases the discrepancy between the donor tooth and the recipient area, causing instability of the blood clot and impeding periodontal regeneration [1,7]. Given the limited studies in which personalized, and 3D-designed surgical appliances are used in guided autotransplantation, the authors of the present study evaluated the accuracy and success of this surgical approach. Anssari Moin et al. in their study using guided autotransplantation with surgical splints and customized surgical instruments on human mandibular cadaver jaws reported a mean coronal deviation of 3.15 +/− 1.16 mm, a mean apical deviation of 2.61 +/− 0.78 mm and a mean angular deviation of 5.6–5.4° between the digitally planned position and the definitive position of the transplanted teeth [24]. These values are within the generally accepted ranges for surgical guides in implant treatment; however, they may be clinically relevant for autotransplantation, and thus these results should be improved. Moreover, Wu et al. also reported a high accuracy of the static surgical guides for dental implant placement [42]. Impacted teeth are often considered candidates for tooth autotransplantation and Cavuoti et al. highlighted the risk of root resorption in impacted teeth and recommended repositioning the impacted tooth to prevent root resorption [43]. However, our results are difficult to compare with those of Anssari Moin et al., who expressed the results as means and standard deviation [24]. Due to the fact that the mean comparison of both the coronal and apical deviations of the autotransplanted teeth in our study showed no normal distribution, a statistical analysis was performed by median comparison using a Mann–Whitney non-parametric test. The inherent deficiencies in the digital workflow were related to the lack of precision regarding the result. Ender et al. reported less statistical accuracy ($p < 0.05$) of the digital impressions of the partial-arch than of the digital impressions of the total-arch [44]. In the present study, the imprecision of the manual segmentation may have influenced the choice of bur size, which may have resulted in inadequate drilling. In addition, the sockets were surgically created using a single bur, but the oval section of the autotransplanted teeth required additional manual drilling to adapt the root anatomy of the donor tooth to the socket, which may have influenced the definitive position. In addition, it is essential to analyse the root morphology to avoid fractures during dental extraction manoeuvres and complications during the autotransplantation procedure (especially in dislacerated roots or divergent roots of multirooted teeth). Likewise, it is necessary to evaluate the mesio-distal size of the edentulous space to be rehabilitated by the tooth to be autotransplanted and the occlusal contacts. The authors recommend evaluating these parameters in the surgical planning phase. Moreover, the trueness of the intraoral scanner has been highlighted as a relevant factor, since it can induce the appearance of a clinically relevant cumulative error; however, the present study used powder-dependent intraoral scanners, which are significantly better ($p < 0.05$) than non-powder-dependent scanners as the translucency they produce shows fewer errors in the images [45].

Finally, the authors of the present study suggest there is a need to conduct a study on cryopreserved cadavers to evaluate the precision and reproducibility of the technique using different splints and customized surgical instruments, given the dearth of studies on guided surgery to create neo-alveolus in autotransplantations. Furthermore, the deviation between the planned and final position of the surgically guided autotransplantation in this study should also be assessed. Additionally, the experimental nature of the study allows for better 3D visibility and perception compared to a clinical situation.

5. Conclusions

Within the limitations of this in vitro study, the results show that the computer aided SNT was less reliable than FT and the use of SNT in the clinic should be suspended until further research is conducted. Specifically, coronal and angular deviations between the computer aided SNT and FT study groups did not show statistically significant differences;

however, statistically significant differences were observed between the apical deviation of the SNT and FT study groups.

Author Contributions: Conceptualization, E.R.D., N.Z.L.T. and Á.Z.-M., design, D.G.M.; data acquisition, M.B.P.; formal analysis, A.G.C.; performed all statistical analyses, Á.Z.-M. and F.A.S.; review and editing, S.H.M. All authors have read and agreed to the published version of the manuscript.

Funding: This research received no external funding.

Institutional Review Board Statement: Not applicable.

Informed Consent Statement: Not applicable.

Data Availability Statement: Data available on request due to restrictions, e.g., privacy or ethical.

Acknowledgments: The authors would like to express their thanks to Carmen Caballero for his advice, guidance and help during this study.

Conflicts of Interest: The authors declare no conflict of interest.

References

1. Natiella, J.R.; Armitage, J.E.; Greene, G.W. The replantation and transplantation of teeth. A review. *Oral Surg. Oral Med. Oral Pathol.* **1970**, *29*, 397–419. [CrossRef]
2. Andreasen, J.O.; Paulsen, H.U.; Yu, Z.; Bayer, T.; Schwartz, O. A long-term study of 370 autotransplanted premolars. Part II. Tooth survival and pulp healing subsequent to transplantation. *Eur. J. Orthod.* **1990**, *12*, 14–24. [CrossRef] [PubMed]
3. Tsukiboshi, M. Autotransplantation of teeth: Requirements for predictable success. *Dent. Traumatol.* **2002**, *18*, 157–180. [CrossRef] [PubMed]
4. Park, J.H.; Tai, K.; Hayashi, D. Tooth autotransplantation as a treatment option: A review. *J. Clin. Pediatr. Dent.* **2010**, *35*, 129–135. [CrossRef] [PubMed]
5. Kim, S.; Lee, S.J.; Shin, Y.; Kim, E. Vertical bone growth after autotransplantation of mature third molars: 2 case reports with long-term follow-up. *J. Endod.* **2015**, *41*, 1371–1374. [CrossRef]
6. Chung, W.C.; Tu, Y.K.; Lin, Y.H.; Lu, H.K. Outcomes of autotransplanted teeth with complete root formation: A systematic review and meta-analysis. *J. Clin. Periodontol.* **2014**, *41*, 412–423. [CrossRef]
7. Almpani, K.; Papageorgiou, S.N.; Papadopoulos, M.A. Autotransplantation of teeth in humans: A systematic review and meta-analysis. *Clin. Oral Investig.* **2015**, *19*, 1157–1179. [CrossRef]
8. Apfel, H. Autoplasty of enucleated prefunctional third molars. *J. Oral Surg.* **1950**, *8*, 289–296.
9. Miller, H.M. Transplantation; a case report. *J. Am. Dent. Assoc.* **1950**, *40*, 237.
10. Lundberg, T.; Isaksson, S. A clinical follow-up study of 278 autotransplanted teeth. *Br. J. Oral Maxillofac. Surg.* **1996**, *34*, 181–185. [CrossRef]
11. Mejàre, B.; Wannfors, K.; Jansson, L. A prospective study on transplantation of third molars with complete root formation. *Oral Surg. Oral Med. Oral Pathol. Oral Radiol. Endod.* **2004**, *97*, 231–238. [CrossRef]
12. Kumar, R.; Khambete, N.; Priya, E. Successful immediate autotransplantation of tooth with incomplete root formation: Case report. *Oral Surg. Oral. Med. Oral Pathol. Oral Radiol. Endod.* **2013**, *115*, e16–e21. [CrossRef] [PubMed]
13. Slagsvold, O.; Bjercke, B. Applicability of autotransplantation in cases of missing upper anterior teeth. *Am. J. Orthod.* **1978**, *74*, 410–421. [CrossRef]
14. Slagsvold, O.; Bjercke, B. Indications for autotransplantation in cases of missing premolars. *Am. J. Orthod.* **1978**, *74*, 241–257. [CrossRef]
15. Kristerson, L.; Lagerstrom, L. Autotransplantation of teeth in cases with agenesis or traumatic loss of maxillary incisors. *Eur. J. Orthod.* **1991**, *13*, 486–492. [CrossRef] [PubMed]
16. Nethander, G. Autogenous free tooth transplantation with a two-stage operation technique. *Swed. Dent. J.* **2003**, *161*, 1–51.
17. Kitahara, T.; Nakasima, A.; Shiatuschi, Y. Orthognathic treatment with autotransplantation of impacted maxillary third molar. *Angle Orthod.* **2009**, *79*, 401–406. [CrossRef]
18. Czochrowska, E.M.; Stenvik, A.; Bjercke, B.; Zachrisson, B.U. Outcome of tooth transplantation: Survival and success rates 17-41 years posttreatment. *Am. J. Orthod. Dent. Orthop.* **2002**, *121*, 110–119. [CrossRef]
19. Bae, J.H.; Choi, Y.H.; Cho, B.H.; Kim, Y.K.; Kim, S.G. Autotransplantation of teeth with complete root formation: A case series. *J. Endod.* **2010**, *36*, 1422–1426. [CrossRef]
20. Sugai, T.; Yoshizawa, M.; Kobayashi, T.; Ono, K.; Takagi, R.; Kitamura, N.; Okiji, K.; Saito, C. Clinical study on prognostic factors for autotransplantation of teeth with complete root formation. *Int. J. Oral Maxillofac. Surg.* **2010**, *39*, 1193–1203. [CrossRef]
21. Yu, H.J.; Jia, P.; Lv, Z.; Qiu, L.X. Autotransplantation of third molars with completely formed roots into surgically created sockets and fresh extraction sockets: A 10-year comparative study. *Int. J. Oral Maxillofac. Surg.* **2017**, *46*, 531–538. [CrossRef] [PubMed]
22. Lee, S.J.; Jung, I.Y.; Lee, C.Y.; Choi, S.Y.; Kum, K.Y. Clinical application of computer-aided rapid prototyping for tooth transplantation. *Dent. Traumatol.* **2001**, *17*, 114–119. [CrossRef]

23. Strbac, G.D.; Schnappauf, A.; Giannis, K.; Bertl, M.H.; Moritz, A.; Ulm, C. Guided autotransplantation of teeth: A novel method using virtually planned 3-dimensional templates. *J. Endod.* **2016**, *42*, 1844–1850. [CrossRef] [PubMed]
24. Anssari Moin, D.; Verweij, J.P.; Waars, H.; van Merkesteyn, R.; Wismeijer, D. Accuracy of computer-assisted template-guided autotransplantation of teeth with custom three-dimensional designed/printed surgical tooling: A cadaveric study. *J. Oral Maxillofac. Surg.* **2017**, *75*, 925.e1–925.e7. [CrossRef] [PubMed]
25. Verweij, J.P.; Jongkees, F.A.; Anssari Moin, D.; Wismeijer, D.; van Merkesteyn, J.P.R. Autotransplantation of teeth using computer-aided rapid prototyping of a three-dimensional replica of the donor tooth: A systematic literature review. *Int. J. Oral Maxillofac. Surg.* **2017**, *46*, 1466–1474. [CrossRef] [PubMed]
26. Pogrel, M.A. Evaluation of over 400 autogenous tooth transplants. *J. Oral Maxillofac. Surg.* **1987**, *45*, 205–211. [CrossRef]
27. Tahmaseb, A.; Wismeijer, D.; Coucke, W.; Derksen, W. Computer technology applications in surgical implant dentistry: A systematic review. *Int. J. Oral Maxillofac. Implant.* **2014**, *29*, 25–42. [CrossRef]
28. Zubizarreta-Macho, Á.; Muñoz, A.P.; Deglow, E.R.; Agustín-Panadero, R.; Álvarez, J.M. Accuracy of Computer-Aided Dynamic Navigation Compared to Computer-Aided Static Procedure for Endodontic Access Cavities: An in Vitro Study. *J. Clin. Med.* **2020**, *9*, 129. [CrossRef]
29. Nagendrababu, V.; Murray, P.E.; Ordinola-Zapata, R.; Peters, O.A.; Rôças, I.N.; Siqueira, J.F., Jr.; Priya, E.; Jayaraman, J.; Pulikkotil, S.J.; Dummer, P.M.H.; et al. PRILE 2021 guidelines for reporting laboratory studies in Endodontology: A consensus-based development. *Int. Endod. J.* **2021**, *54*, 1482–1490. [CrossRef]
30. Nagendrababu, V.; Murray, P.E.; Ordinola-Zapata, R.; Peters, O.A.; Rôças, I.N.; Siqueira, J.F., Jr.; Priya, E.; Jayaraman, J.; Pulikkotil, S.J.; Dummer, P.M.H.; et al. PRILE 2021 guidelines for reporting laboratory studies in Endodontology: Explanation and elaboration. *Int. Endod. J.* **2021**, *54*, 1491–1515. [CrossRef]
31. Renne, W.; Ludlow, M.; Fryml, J.; Schurch, Z.; Mennito, A.; Kessler, R.; Lauer, A. Evaluation of the accuracy of 7 digital scanners: An in vitro analysis based on 3-dimensional comparisons. *J. Prosthet. Dent.* **2017**, *118*, 36–42. [CrossRef] [PubMed]
32. Medina-Sotomayor, P.; Pascual-Moscardo, A.; Camps, A.I. Accuracy of 4 digital scanning systems on prepared teeth digitally isolated from a complete dental arch. *J. Prosthet. Dent.* **2019**, *121*, 811–820. [CrossRef] [PubMed]
33. Abella Sans, F.; Ribas, F.; Doria, G.; Roig, M.; Durán-Sindreu, F. Guided tooth autotransplantation in edentulous areas post-orthodontic treatment. *J. Esthet. Restor. Dent.* **2021**, *33*, 685–691. [CrossRef] [PubMed]
34. Plotino, G.; Abella Sans, F.; Duggal, M.S.; Grande, N.M.; Krastl, G.; Nagendrababu, V.; Gambarini, G. Clinical procedures and outcome of surgical extrusion, intentional replantation and tooth autotransplantation—A narrative review. *Int. Endod. J.* **2020**, *53*, 1636–1652. [CrossRef] [PubMed]
35. Jang, Y.; Choi, Y.J.; Lee, S.J.; Roh, B.D.; Park, S.H.; Kim, E. Prognosis factors for clinical outcomes in autotransplantation in teeth with complete root formation: Survival analysis for up to 12 years. *J. Endod.* **2016**, *42*, 198–205. [CrossRef]
36. Bauss, O.; Engelke, W.; Fenske, C.; Schilke, R.; Schwestka-Polly, R. Autotransplantation of immature third molars into edentulous and atrophied jaw sections. *Int. J. Oral Maxillofac. Surg.* **2004**, *33*, 558–563. [CrossRef]
37. Bauss, O.; Zonios, I.; Rahman, A. Root development of immature third molars transplanted to surgically created sockets. *J. Oral Maxillofac. Surg.* **2008**, *66*, 1200–1211. [CrossRef]
38. Kim, E.; Jung, J.Y.; Cha, I.H.; Kum, K.Y.; Lee, S.J. Evaluation of the prognosis and causes of failure in 182 cases of autogenous tooth transplantation. *Oral Surg. Oral Med. Oral Pathol. Oral Radiol. Endod.* **2005**, *100*, 112–119. [CrossRef]
39. Kafourou, V.; Tong, H.J.; Day, P.; Houghton, N.; Spencer, R.J.; Duggal, M. Outcomes and prognostic factors that influence the success of tooth autotransplantation in children and adolescents. *Dent. Traumatol.* **2017**, *33*, 393–399. [CrossRef]
40. Kristerson, L.; Andreasen, J.O. Autotransplantation and replantation of tooth germs in monkeys. Effect of damage to the dental follicle and position of transplant in the alveolus. *Int. J. Oral Surg.* **1984**, *13*, 324–333. [CrossRef]
41. Andreasen, J.O.; Kristerson, L.; Andreasen, F.M. Damage of the Hertwig's epithelial root sheath: Effect upon root growth after autotransplantation of teeth in monkeys. *Endod. Dent. Traumatol.* **1988**, *4*, 145–151. [CrossRef]
42. Wu, D.; Zhou, L.; Yang, J.; Zhang, B.; Lin, Y.; Chen, J.; Huang, W.; Chen, Y. Accuracy of dynamic navigation compared to static surgical guide for dental implant placement. *Int. J. Implant. Dent.* **2020**, *6*, 78. [CrossRef] [PubMed]
43. Cavuoti, S.; Matarese, G.; Isola, G.; Abdolreza, J.; Femiano, F.; Perillo, L. Combined orthodontic-surgical management of a transmigrated mandibular canine. *Angle Orthod.* **2016**, *86*, 681–691. [CrossRef] [PubMed]
44. Ender, A.; Zimmermann, M.; Mehl, A. Accuracy of complete- and partial-arch impressions of actual intraoral scanning systems in vitro. *Int. J. Comput. Dent.* **2019**, *22*, 11–19. [PubMed]
45. Zimmermann, M.; Koller, C.; Rumetsch, M.; Ender, A.; Mehl, A. Precision of guided scanning procedures for full-arch digital impressions in vivo. *J. Orofac. Orthop.* **2017**, *78*, 466–471. [CrossRef] [PubMed]

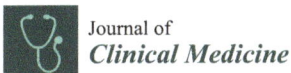

Article

Short-Term Pain Evolution and Treatment Success of Pulpotomy as Irreversible Pulpitis Permanent Treatment: A Non-Randomized Clinical Study

Julien Beauquis [1,2,*], Hugo M. Setbon [2,3], Charles Dassargues [1,2,4], Pierre Carsin [1,2,5], Sam Aryanpour [1,2,6], Jean-Pierre Van Nieuwenhuysen [1,2] and Julian G. Leprince [1,2,*]

1. Adult and Child Dentistry, Cliniques Universitaires Saint-Luc, 1200 Brussels, Belgium; charlesdassargues@hotmail.com (C.D.); pierre.carsin@saintluc.uclouvain.be (P.C.); samaryanpour@gmail.com (S.A.); vannieuwenhuysen@me.com (J.-P.V.N.)
2. DRIM Research Group & Advanced Drug Delivery and Biomaterials, Louvain Drug Research Institute, UCLouvain, 1200 Brussels, Belgium; hugosetbon@gmail.com
3. Private Practice, Av. Louise 391, 1050 Brussels, Belgium
4. Private Practice, Rue Edmond Laffineur 9, 1300 Wavre, Belgium
5. Private Practice, All. de la Minerva 2, 1150 Brussels, Belgium
6. Private Practice, Rte du Lion 10, 1420 Braine-l'Alleud, Belgium
* Correspondence: julien.beauquis@saintluc.uclouvain.be (J.B.); julian.leprince@saintluc.uclouvain.be (J.G.L.)

Abstract: The objective of this work was to evaluate (1) the short-term evolution of pain and (2) the treatment success of full pulpotomy as permanent treatment of irreversible pulpitis in mature molars. The study consisted of a non-randomized comparison between a test group ($n = 44$)—full pulpotomy performed by non-specialist junior practitioners, and a control group ($n = 40$)—root canal treatments performed by specialized endodontists. Short-term pain score (Heft–Parker scale) was recorded pre-operatively, then at 24 h and 7 days post-operatively. Three outcomes were considered for treatment success: *radiographic*, *clinical* and *global* success. For short-term evolution of pain, a non-parametric Wilcoxon test was performed (significance level = 0.05). For treatment success, a Pearson Chi square or Fisher test were performed (significance level = 0.017–Bonferroni correction). There was no significant difference between *test* and control groups neither regarding short term evolution of pain at each time point, nor regarding *clinical* (80% and 90%, respectively) or *global* success (77% and 67%, respectively). However, a significant difference in *radiographic* success was observed (94% and 69%, respectively). The present work adds to the existing literature to support that pulpotomy as permanent treatment could be considered as an acceptable and conservative treatment option, potentially applied by a larger population of dentists.

Keywords: pulpotomy; pulpitis; endodontics; toothache; treatment outcome; tricalcium silicate

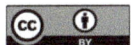

1. Introduction

Dental pulp pathologies are often associated with high levels of pain, requiring appropriate local treatment to effectively relieve the patient [1]. While reversible pulpitis is currently managed by vital pulp therapies [2], the treatment of cases diagnosed clinically as irreversible pulpitis is more invasive. It indeed consists in a pulpotomy as emergency procedure [3], followed by complete root canal treatment.

However, a trend towards more conservative strategies has been observed in recent years notably the consideration of pulpotomy as a permanent treatment [4–7]. This evolution is related to improved knowledge in pulp biology and biomaterials. First, histological studies of teeth with pulpitis have highlighted the existence of a gradient of inflammation within the pulp tissue. Healthy pulp tissue was shown to persist underneath areas with high levels of inflammation and sometimes necrosis [8]. Second, tricalcium-silicate cements were reported in histological studies to have the potential of inducing more favorable pulp responses compared to previous calcium-hydroxide pulp capping materials [9]. A trend in favor of these materials was also identified in clinical studies [9,10].

Preserving pulp tissue by pulpotomies followed by pulp capping has several potential benefits. These include preservation of immunocompetent tissue, reduction in the cost of treatment for both the patient and healthcare systems, and reduction in the treatment complexity and duration. It has nevertheless been stated that additional prospective works are necessary to confirm the positive trend in favor of this treatment strategy [2,11]. Moreover, apart from a few studies [12–14], most available works have a rather limited follow-up time ($\leq$12 months).

While some works consider pulpotomy as a treatment of teeth with carious exposures [15,16], regardless of clinical symptoms, others, like the present one, focused on the treatment of clinically-diagnosed irreversible pulpitis. In the latter case, it is important to consider not only long-term outcomes, but also the effectiveness of short-term pain relief. For this purpose, numerical rating scales and/or category judgments that are subsequently converted into numerical values have been widely used as they are easily understood by patients and considered suitable for the measurement of dental pain [17–19]. With regard to appropriate times for assessing post-endodontic treatment pain, one day and one week have been described as key time points [20].

Finally, the level of experience of practitioners has, to our knowledge, never been considered in the design of the studies evaluating these procedures. However, as mentioned above, the pulpotomy as permanent treatment is referred to as an easier procedure, therefore potentially accessible to less experienced practitioners, including non-specialists. To take this aspect into account, we designed a non-randomized clinical study to compare the alternative strategy to what is considered as "best available therapy". Two groups were considered: (1) pulpotomy as permanent treatment performed by non-specialist junior practitioners (test group), and (2) root canal treatment performed by specialized endodontists in private practice (control group).

The objective of the present work was to evaluate (1) the short-term evolution of pain and (2) the treatment success of full pulpotomy as permanent treatment of irreversible pulpitis in mature molars.

2. Materials and Methods
2.1. Patient Selection

The present prospective study conformed to STROBE guidelines and received approval from the ethics committee of Cliniques universitaires Saint-Luc (Brussels, Belgium) (Reference# 2016/19JAN/016) and was registered at clinicaltrials.gov with registration number NCT02920606.

The study included adult patients with a diagnosis of irreversible pulpitis in mature molar teeth, respecting eligibility criteria for inclusion and exclusion (Table 1). Irreversible pulpitis was defined as spontaneous, radiating pain that lingers after removal of cold stimulus [2]. The inclusion period was from June 2016 to June 2020. An information letter was given to all patients, and informed consent was signed.

In the design of the present study, a difficulty in including patients was expected, due to aspects such as patient motivation (emergency cases) or predictable heterogeneity between groups (population consulting specialists compared to those visiting a dental emergency department). In this context, the present study was initially designed as a pilot study with 50 patients per group as a realistic target.

Systematic forms were used to collect the data for each patient on the day of inclusion.

The study consisted of a non-randomized comparison between two groups (test and control) (Figure 1).

Table 1. Eligibility criteria for inclusion in the clinical study.

Pre-Operative Criteria:	Intra-Operative Criteria:
INCLUSION	EXCLUSION
- Adult patient ($\geq$18 years) - Molar teeth - Irreversible pulpitis diagnosis (spontaneous pain, radiating pain that lingers after removal of cold stimulus) EXCLUSION - Internal/External resorption - Root and crown fracture - Presence of a sinus tract - Anormal mobility - Immature apex - Swelling - Systemic condition - Non-independent patient - Non-restorable tooth - Periodontal pocket $\geq$ 6 mm - Participation in other medical studies	- Pulp necrosis in at least one root canal (both groups) - Need of intra-pulpal injection (test group only) - Impossibility to achieve pulp hemostasis at the root canal entrance (test group only)

The test group included patients treated in the dental department of Cliniques universitaires St-Luc (Brussels, Belgium). The treatment consisted in a full pulpotomy as permanent treatment, and was performed by non-specialist junior practitioners ($\leq$3 years residents).

The control group included patients treated in private specialist dental practice. The treatment, considered as gold standard, consisted in a root canal treatment performed by specialized endodontists in two different practices.

2.2. Clinical Procedure

Following patient inclusion and prior to anesthesia, pain and pre-operative data were collected. Bitewing and a periapical radiographs were taken systematically.

Test group—The tooth was then anesthetized using either Scandonest (3%) or Septanest (4%, 1:200,000 adrenalin) (Septodont, Saint-Maur-des-Fossés, France), respectively, for inferior alveolar nerve block (lower molars) and infiltration anesthesia (upper molars); complementary intra-ligament injections were performed with Scandonest when required. Rubber dam was placed, and the carious lesion was thoroughly excavated when present. The pulp chamber was then accessed with a new sterile bur, and the coronal pulp was completely eliminated. The pulp chamber was rinsed with NaCl, and hemostasis was obtained with a sterile cotton pellet soaked in NaCl. The cavity was gently dried with air spray, and the pulp tissue was capped with a tricalcium-silicate cement (Biodentine, Septodont, Saint-Maur-des-Fossés, France), which was left to set for 15 min. Whenever possible, a permanent composite restoration was placed on the same appointment using a combination of Clearfil SE Bond 2 (Kuraray-Noritake, Japan) and a highly filled composite, either GrandioSO (VOCO, Germany) or Clearfil Majesty Posterior (Kuraray-Noritake, Japan). When permanent restoration could not be placed directly, it was performed within the four weeks after the procedure. All permanent restorations were placed by the investigating team within the dental department. The use of magnification was systematic, mostly loupes, and sometimes microscopes, to properly evaluate pulpal status and compliance with inclusion/exclusion criteria (Table 1).

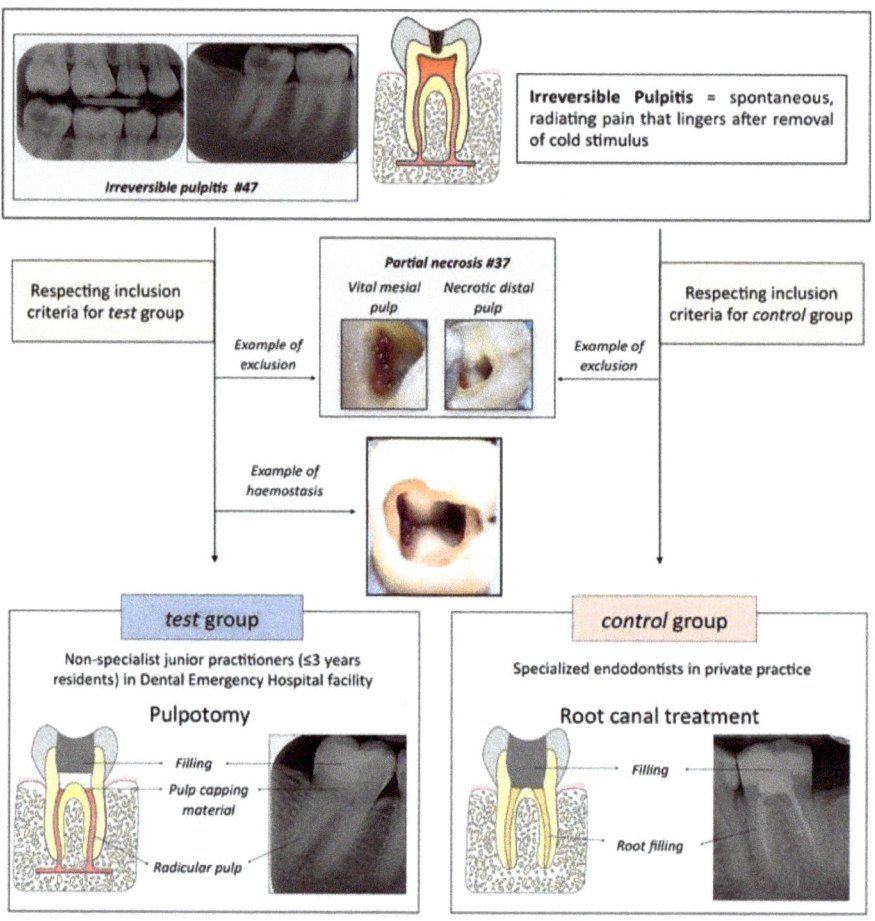

Figure 1. Experimental design.

Control group—No specific recommendations were given on how to perform root canal procedures, considering that the treatments were performed based on the ESE quality guidelines [21]. The aim was to let the specialist practitioners carry out their treatments according to their usual procedure, to be as close as possible to their routine work. The use of operative microscope was systematic, and allowed to evaluate compliance with inclusion/exclusion criteria corresponding to control group (Table 1). They were encouraged to perform their treatments in one appointment whenever possible, but were allowed to delay root canal obturation when time was lacking. A temporary glass ionomer restoration was placed between the appointments. A permanent coronal restoration was placed within the four weeks after the procedure by the referring dentist (either composite, crown or onlay/overlay).

2.3. Short-Term Evolution of Pain

Pain score was measured using the Heft–Parker scale [22]. The latter is based on verbal descriptors of clinical pain (used with patients), which are then converted into numerical values (by the investigators) (see Supplementary Materials Figure S1). The Heft–Parker scale has the specificity of presenting the clinical pain levels with an unequal numerical spacing between pain descriptors, in order to better reflect the differences in word meaning [17].

Besides pre-operative measurement of pain intensity, the investigators conducted a telephone follow-up at 24 h (24 h) and 7 days (7 d) for patients in both groups. The pain scale (verbal descriptors only) was given to patients at the initial appointment to facilitate their evaluation at each timepoint.

In the control group, if the treatment was performed in more than one appointment, pain score was recorded after each appointment and the highest pain level was taken into account for the analysis.

2.4. Treatment Success

The evaluation of treatment success was performed in both groups based on similar criteria. One or more controls were performed depending on patient availability and compliance. Bitewing and periapical radiographs were taken systematically at each follow-up appointment. Three outcomes were considered.

Global success was defined as the combination of *clinical* and *radiographic* success.

Clinical success was defined as the absence of clinical signs (swelling, sinus tract, tooth mobility or deep periodontal probing) and symptoms (pain or discomfort). Therefore, any documented endodontic re-intervention or extraction for endodontic reasons at any time was considered as *clinical* failure.

Radiographic success was considered for cases with ≥12 months follow-up. It was determined as follows: first, no root resorption or furcal bone loss shall be observed; second, the periapical index (PAI) evolution shall either be a maintenance or return to healthy status (PAI 1 or 2), a maintenance of PAI 3 or a decrease in PAI if a true periapical lesion was pre-existing (PAI > 3).

The radiographs were submitted to two independent evaluators for analysis (JPVNH and SA). They were previously calibrated on 30 cases selected outside the present study based on the PAI scoring system defined by Ørstavik et al. [23]. The analysis of all radiographs were performed in a random order, under the same light conditions and on the same screen. Since multi-rooted teeth were studied, the highest PAI score at the root level was attributed to the tooth. In case of hesitation between two PAI scores, evaluators were asked to favor the higher one. The evaluation was repeated in a similar manner 3 weeks later. At the end of each session, disagreements were identified by the principal investigators (JB and JGL) and discussed between both evaluators to reach a consensus. Cohen's kappa coefficient was calculated to assess evaluator agreement.

2.5. Histological Analysis

For any successful case extracted for non-endodontic reasons in the *test* group (e.g., non-restorable factures or prosthetic reasons), teeth were placed in paraformaldehyde 4% for fixation and processed for histological evaluation according to the procedure described in [24].

2.6. Statistical Analysis

The data were submitted to analysis of normality using the Shapiro–Wilk test.

For short-term evolution of pain, a non-parametric Wilcoxon test was performed to test the effect of group (at each timepoint). For the effect of time, since normality could not be demonstrated, a Wilcoxon signed rank test was used.

For treatment success, a Pearson chi square or Fisher test were performed to compare *clinical*, *radiographic* and *global* success between test and control groups.

A logistic regression or test of independence was performed to test the impact of several variables, on the one hand on attribution of patients to both groups, and on the other hand on treatment success. A significance level of 0.05 was chosen for short-term analyses and sample distribution. Since three outcomes were considered for treatment success, a Bonferroni correction was applied and a significance level of 0.017 was chosen.

3. Results

A total of 57 and 41 patients were eligible to participate in the study in the test and control groups respectively (Figure 2), which were subsequently reduced to 44 and 41 patients due to intra-operative exclusion criteria (Table 1).

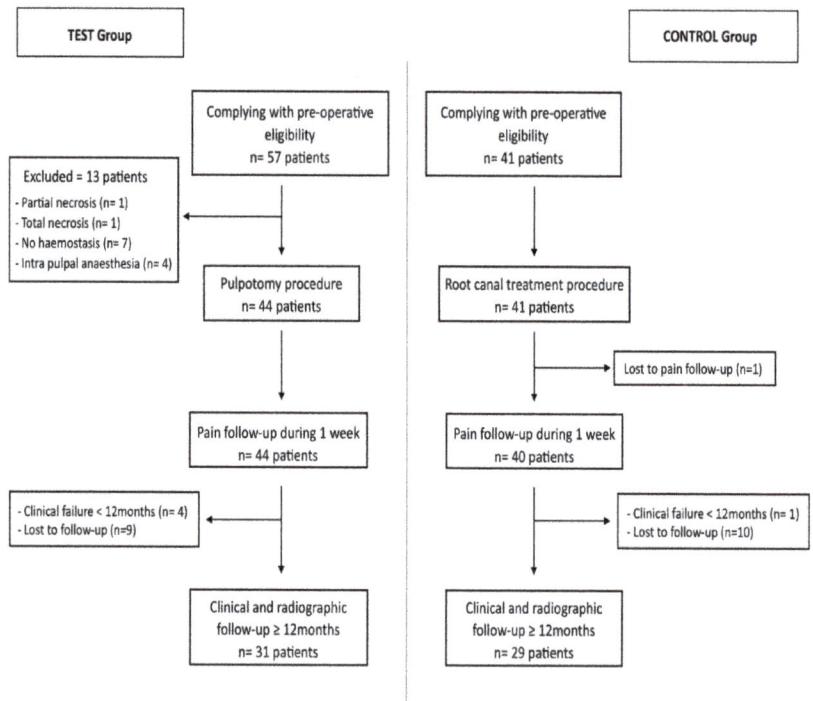

Figure 2. Flowchart for test and control groups based on STROBE recommendations.

3.1. Short-Term Evolution of Pain

This analysis could be performed for 44 and 40 patients in the test and control groups respectively. There was no significant difference ($p > 0.05$) between both groups at each time point (T0, 24 h, 7 d) (Figure 3). However, a significant reduction in pain was observed between each time point ($p < 0.0001$).

3.2. Treatment Success

Follow-up for global success evaluation was possible for 79.5% and 75% of the patients, with a median follow-up of 24 and 20.5 months, and a mean follow-up of 25.9 and 25.6 months, respectively, in test and control groups. The characteristics of the population in both groups are presented in Table 2. The logistic regression (univariate) regarding patient distribution between both groups based on these variables revealed the following significant differences: pre-operative pain to percussion ($p = 0.049$), patient age ($p = 0.0004$) and presence of a carious cavity ($p < 0.0001$).

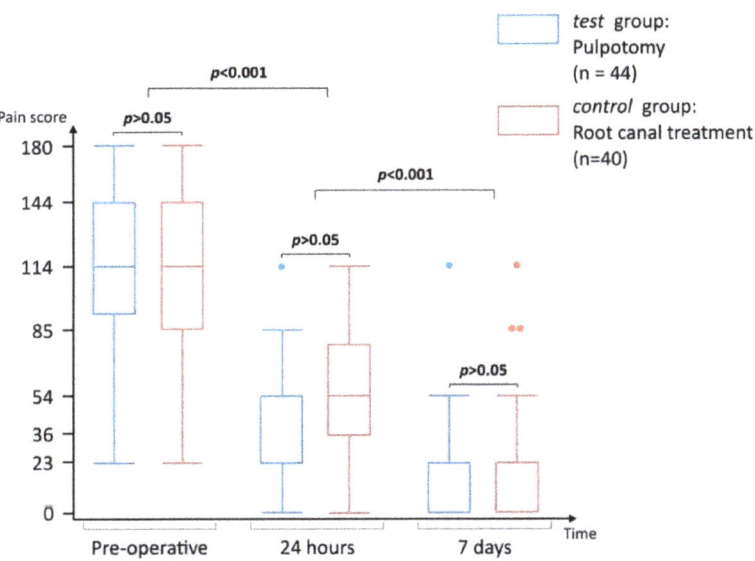

Figure 3. Boxplots of short-term pain evolution for test and control groups; the dots correspond to outliers.

Table 2. Characteristics of cases included in treatment success evaluation ($N = 65$).

Variables	Total n (%)	Test Group (Pulpotomy) n (%)	Control Group (Root Canal Treatment) n (%)
Patients (n)	65 (100)	35 (100)	30 (100)
Age (years)			
Mean	39.4	34.8	46.7
Median	38.5	29	49
Male	22 (33.8)	9 (25.7)	13 (43.3)
Dental arch			
Maxillary teeth			
First molar	8 (12.3)	5 (14.3)	3 (10)
Second molar	10 (15.4)	4 (11.4)	6 (20)
Mandibular teeth			
First molar	17 (26.2)	11 (31.4)	6 (20)
Second molar	29 (44.6)	14 (40)	15 (50)
Third molar	1 (1.5)	1 (2.9)	0 (0)
Pre-operative masticatory pain	38 (58.5)	18 (51.4)	20 (66.7)
Pre-operative pulsatile pain	40 (61.5)	18 (51.4)	22 (73.3)
Pre-operative percussion pain	37 (57)	16 (45.7)	21 (70)
Duration of pre-operative pain			
≤2 days	19 (29.2)	13 (37.2)	6 (20)
>2 days–≤ 7 days	15 (23.1)	6 (17.1)	9 (30)
>7 days–≤14 days	5 (7.7)	0 (0)	5 (16.7)
>14 days	26 (40)	16 (45.7)	10 (33.3)
Pre-operative PAI			
1	30 (46.2)	18 (51.5)	12 (40)
2	22 (33.8)	13 (37.1)	9 (30)
3	10 (14.4)	4 (11.4)	6 (20)
4	3 (4.6)	/	3 (10)
Presence of carious cavity	25 (38.5)	21 (63.4)	4 (13.3)

Five patients experienced *clinical* failure <12 months, four in test group (managed by root canal treatment) and one in control group, which led to tooth extraction due to vertical root fracture.

For patients with follow-up ≥12 months, the evaluation of the radiographs by two independent observers resulted in a consensus PAI scoring, characterized by a Cohen's kappa coefficient of 0.72 between the two evaluation sessions. The PAI evolution for each patient according to their follow-up duration is available in the Supplementary Material (Tables S1 and S2). Representative examples of the radiographic evolution can be observed in Figure 4a–h for test group and Figure 4i–p for control group.

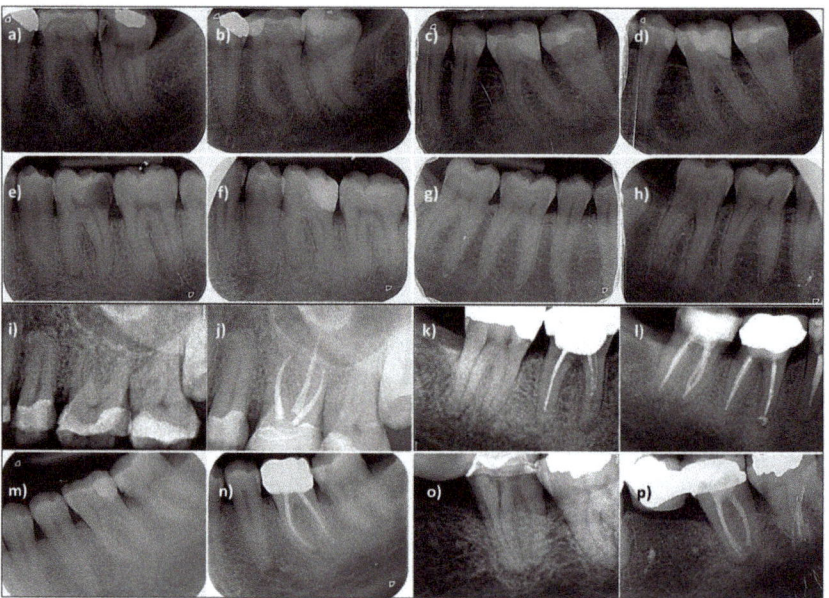

Figure 4. (**a–h**) test group—4 clinical cases of pulpotomy. (**a,b**) #37 Healthy status quo, follow-up at 46 months; (**c,d**) #36 peri-apical healing, follow-up at 20 months; (**e,f**) #36 peri-apical healing, follow-up at 16 months; (**g–h**) #47 peri-apical aggravation, follow-up at 20 months. (**i–p**) control group—4 clinical cases of root canal treatment. (**i,j**) #26 Healthy status quo, follow-up at 47 months; (**k,l**) #47 peri-apical status quo, follow-up at 50 months; (**m,n**) #36 peri-apical aggravation, follow-up at 24 months; (**o,p**) #37 peri-apical healing, follow-up at 12 months.

No significant difference was observed between test and control groups regarding *clinical* ($p = 0.32$) or *global* success ($p = 0.347$). However, a significant difference in *radiographic* success was observed ($p = 0.014$) (Table 3).

Table 3. Characteristics of cases included in treatment success evaluation ($N = 65$).

Variables	Test Group (Pulpotomy) % (n)	Control Group (Root Canal Treatment) % (n)
Clinical success	80 (28/35)	90 (27/30)
Radiographic success *	94 ** (29/31)	69 ** (20/29)
Global success	77 (27/35)	67 (20/30)

* excluding clinical failures <12 months. ** Significant difference ($p < 0.017$).

None of the variables listed in Table 2 were found to have a significant effect on either *global*, *radiographic* or *clinical* success (univariate analysis; $p > 0.017$).

Among the *clinical* failures in the test group (<12 months, $n = 4$; ≥12 months, $n = 3$), six cases presented evidence of pulp vitality in all canals. A pronounced inflammation was observed, indicated by intense bleeding. One case was re-treated in another practice.

3.3. Histological Analysis

One case classified as global success in the test group at 45 months had to be extracted for restorative reasons, i.e., non-restorable fracture (Figure 5a–c). The tooth was processed for histological evaluation (Figure 5d–g), which revealed a vital pulp tissue present in the root canals without any sign of inflammation and with an odontoblastic layer lining the canal walls. It must be noted that difficulties in sectioning were encountered. While demineralized, the collagen remained hard in some areas, preventing serial sectioning throughout the whole sample.

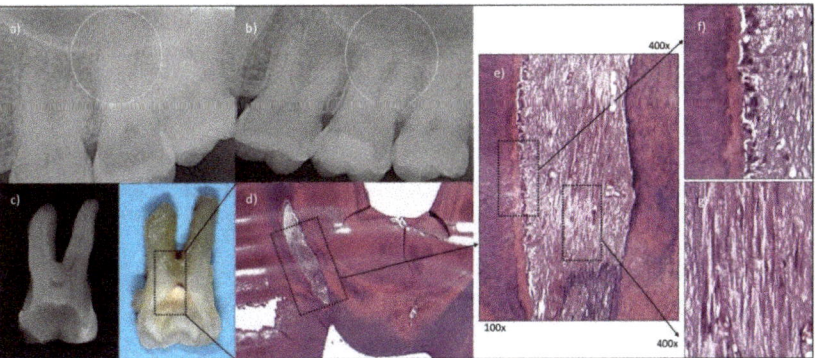

Figure 5. Histological analysis of a case considered as global success, extracted for restorative reason, performed by Domenico Ricucci. (**a**) #27 pre-operative situation, PAI score:1; (**b**) #27 healthy status quo, follow-up at 45 months; (**c**) radiographic and clinical images of extracted tooth; (**d–g**) histological sections (H&E staining) at various magnifications, revealing the presence of a vital pulp tissue in the root canals without any sign of inflammation or tissue disruption. An odontoblastic layer lining the canal walls can be observed.

4. Discussion

The first major finding was the efficiency of the pulpotomy procedure as permanent treatment in terms of short-term pain relief. A comparable pain reduction at 24 h and 7 d between both treatment procedures was indeed observed. This is in accordance with a randomized clinical study comparing full pulpotomy, selective pulpectomy (restricted to one canal) and full pulpectomy [25]. Another randomized trial reported an even higher and significant pain reduction in the pulpotomy group as compared to the root-canal treatment [26]. The evolution of pain at 24 h and 7 d follows a previously described trend following root-canal treatment, with a moderate drop within one day, and a substantial reduction to minimal levels in 7 days [20]. Hence, pulpotomy as permanent treatment of irreversible pulpitis using tricalcium-silicate cements is at least as efficient as the gold standard procedure in terms of short-term pain relief. Pain relief is an essential component of an endodontic procedure, with pathologies that can lead to very high levels of pain [1,17–19], in the same range as those observed in other painful diseases such as renal colic [27,28]. Such levels of dental pain can severely affect patient quality of life during the acute phase, and were, also, shown to be a major cause of acute medical admission following unintentional paracetamol overdose [29,30].

The second major finding was the equivalent efficiency of the pulpotomy procedure as permanent treatment regarding *global* success, as compared to the gold standard procedure.

A higher trend was even observed in the test group (77%) but not significantly ($p > 0.017$) compared to the control group (67%). This is in line with a similar observation made in a randomized clinical trial [12]. The latter is currently the most robust study available on the topic, with confirmed irreversible pulp status, >12 months mean follow-up and including a control group.

The incidence (11.4%) of *clinical* failure observed within the first 12 months following the test procedure is in line with the data available in the literature [4–7]. The overall *clinical* success rate was 80% in our work, all *clinical* failures were related to pain and not to other clinical signs, and lead to re-intervention via standard root-canal treatment. It is important to mention that the location of root canals required the use of magnification, which was possible in all cases. Moreover, the evidence of pulp vitality associated with pronounced inflammation observed in most failed cases connects to the possible interest of quantifying biomarkers such as MMP-9, TNF-α or IL-8 as predictors of the procedure prognosis [4,31–33].

The significant difference in *radiographic* success observed in favor of the test group (94% vs. 69%; $p < 0.017$) could be considered unexpected. It cannot be excluded that the higher percentage pre-operative PAI $\geq$ 3 in the control group affects such finding, but this variable was not identified as statistically significant ($p > 0.05$). Nevertheless, the trend is consistent with the one reported in the literature at two years [13], even considering cases with pre-existing periapical involvement. This trend, illustrated in Figure 4c,d may indicate the positive effect of preserving a living, immunocompetent pulp tissue within the root canal on periapical healing. It is worth noticing that while the presence of a periapical radiolucency (PAI > 3) is not expected in case of an inflamed pulp, some cases were classified as PAI = 4 in the present work and in another [6]. This is due to the fact that the PAI score was not considered in the inclusion/exclusion criterion, which are mainly clinical. Since the radiographic interpretation is performed by independent observers, some cases with PAI > 3 can therefore be reported.

The survival of healthy radicular pulp tissue in successful cases following a pulpotomy as permanent treatment remains unknown. Histology is indeed required to determine the exact status of the pulp tissue, and only few short-term studies provided such information for pulpotomies as permanent treatment in case of irreversible pulpitis. A two-month report on 12 molars reported the presence of healthy radicular pulp devoid of inflammatory signs [34] and a 10-month case report made similar observations in a premolar [35]. In the present work, the histology performed on the successful case provided similar evidence but at 45 months follow-up. In the absence of histology, the observation of a hard tissue barrier underneath the capping material has been considered by some authors as indicator of pulp vitality, as mentioned in a recent review [36]. However, the latter, also, underlines the low reliability of such observation. It is indeed not trivial to determine accurately on a radiograph if an actual barrier has formed, since there is no standardized definition nor are the X-ray images taken in a reproducible manner. Despite the level of evidence regarding the ability of materials to induce mineral bridge formation, it was reported that either pure calcium hydroxide powder or tricalcium-silicate cements are likely the most appropriate materials to cover the pulp [37,38], which was performed here (Biodentine, Septodont, Saint-Maur-des-Fossés, France). The remaining pulp tissue must be free of inflammation, which can be assessed clinically by obtaining a hemostasis. This was a prerequisite in the present work, since it was demonstrated in the context of a direct pulp capping following carious exposure that the degree of pulp bleeding was associated with treatment success [39]. Furthermore, compared to carious exposures, the success rate of pulp capping in traumatic exposures, associated with little or no pulp inflammation, is known to be higher [40]. Nevertheless, it must be noted again that clinical criteria are unfortunately associated with little level of evidence to correlate to histological pulp status [41]. More recently, other intra-operative parameters were subject to discussion, such as the time required to achieve hemostasis [42] or the type and concentration of irrigants [43], without identifying clear trends with regards to treatment outcome. In addition, it was recently shown that in presence of low levels of pulp inflammation (evaluated by MMP-9 quantification), the irrigant (saline vs. 2.5% NaOCl) had little impact on the direct pulp capping outcome [44].

One of the limitations of the study is the modest sample size in each group, but it is relatively in the same range as most available studies on the topic of vital pulp therapy of irreversible pulpitis [4–6], except one works with a much larger sample size [12]. In terms of follow-up, apart from the latter providing results at five years, the present study provides the longest duration with an average of 25 months. The recall rate is reasonable given the difficulties associated with this specific topic, although it should ideally be higher given the limited sample size. Emergency patients are indeed quite difficult to follow over time, as they often consult irregularly and/or tend to return to their regular dentist once the emergency is over, both in test and control groups. The number of patients was balanced between test and control groups. Both groups were also shown to be equivalent in terms of initial pain intensity ($p > 0.05$), but not for three other variables. Among these, none had a significant impact on treatment success ($p > 0.017$). However, based on the differences of distribution between both groups, we cannot exclude the existence of a selection bias. The latter, combined with the limited sample size, could account for the lower success rate in the control group. It can also explain the lower *global* success rate in that group compared to those reported in the literature [45,46]. However, these reported success rates shall be compared with those of irreversible pulpitis with caution, as they correspond to cases with "vital pulp", without further distinction regarding pulpal diagnosis. To our knowledge, the endodontic treatment success rates available regarding irreversible pulpitis are 65.8% at five years [12], which is lower than the rates usually reported for vital pulp cases as a whole.

Another limitation of the work is the restriction to molar cases only. This was determined based on two main criteria: The ease to identify the anatomical transition between coronal and radicular pulp, and the level of treatment complexity. The first criteria was in fact a methodological decision in order to make the procedure more easily reproducible. The second criteria was related to clinical relevance, since both European and American endodontic associations have identified molar teeth as a criteria for treatment complexity [47,48]. Hence, it was the point of the present work to consider the more conservative pulpotomy strategy (test group) as one potentially applied by a larger population of dentists, whereas the gold standard root canal treatment may be restricted to specialized endodontists. It was interesting to assess whether a strict protocol for performing the vital pulp therapy procedure (facilitated by use of magnification) could compensate for the lesser experience of non-specialist practitioners.

Regarding study design, it has been described in the past that while randomized clinical trials are ideal for evaluating the effect of drugs, it is not easily the case for surgical interventions such as endodontic procedures [49]. A double-blind system or the use of a placebo is generally not possible. Moreover, the preference of using "best available therapy" control group rather than a placebo has been described [50] with reference to the World Medical Association Declaration of Helsinki. In the context of irreversible pulpitis, the "best available therapy" would be defined as root canal treatment, but no study to date has considered practitioner experience as an important part of the definition. Both AAE and ESE clearly identify "best available therapy" as one performed by specialized endodontists [47,48]. Hence, it was the purpose of this study to take this aspect into account in the group design, with specialists performing the procedures in the control group, and non-specialists in the test group. In order to be as relevant as possible, specialists working in private practice were selected for control cases, which therefore resulted in a non-randomized study design. While the latter certainly introduces biases on the one hand, it potentially increases the usefulness of the study on the other hand, which is to be taken into account in a study quality aspect [51].

5. Conclusions

To conclude, within the limitations of the present work, this prospective non-randomized study tends to support that pulpotomy is an acceptable and more conservative permanent treatment option for irreversible pulpitis in mature molars. Additionally, re-intervention with the gold standard procedure remains possible in case of failure. Hence, despite its non-randomized design and relatively low sample size, the present work adds to the existing literature to support the fact that pulpotomy as permanent treatment could be considered as first line treatment. The latter could be applied by a larger population of dentists, provided that strict inclusion/exclusion criteria and a rigorous clinical protocol are respected. Ideally, the present findings should be confirmed by a multi-centric practice-based study with larger sample size.

Supplementary Materials: The following supporting information can be downloaded at: https://www.mdpi.com/article/10.3390/jcm11030787/s1, Figure S1: Practitioner and patient pain scales; Table S1: Detailed follow-up evaluation for each patient in test group; Table S2. Detailed follow-up evaluation for each patient in control group.

Author Contributions: Conceptualization, J.B., H.M.S. and J.G.L.; Methodology, J.B., H.M.S. and J.G.L.; Software, J.B., H.M.S. and J.G.L.; Validation, J.B. and J.G.L.; Formal Analysis, J.B., J.-P.V.N. and J.G.L.; Investigation, J.B., C.D., P.C., S.A., J.-P.V.N. and J.G.L.; Resources, J.B. and J.G.L.; Data Curation, J.B. and J.G.L.; Writing—Original Draft Preparation, J.B. and J.G.L.; Writing—Review & Editing, J.B., H.M.S., C.D., P.C., S.A., J.-P.V.N. and J.G.L.; Visualization, J.B., S.A., J.-P.V.N. and J.G.L.; Supervision, J.B. and J.G.L.; Project Administration, J.B. and J.G.L.; Funding Acquisition, J.G.L. All authors have read and agreed to the published version of the manuscript.

Funding: This research received no external funding.

Institutional Review Board Statement: The study was conducted according to the guidelines of the Declaration of Helsinki and approved by the Institutional Review Board (or Ethics Committee) of Cliniques universitaires Saint-Luc (Brussels, Belgium) which received full accreditation from the Association for Accreditation of Human Research Protection Program. Reference #2016/19JAN/016 approved on 4 February 2016.

Informed Consent Statement: Informed consent was obtained from all subjects involved in the study.

Data Availability Statement: The data presented in this study are available on request from the corresponding authors.

Acknowledgments: The authors thank the staff of the School of Dental Medicine (Cliniques universitaires Saint-Luc, UCLouvain, Brussels, Belgium) from the department of Adult and Child Dentistry who performed the treatments in the test group: Gaëtan Larondelle, Julien Beauquis, Jean-Philippe Marien, Laure Spinhayer, Marco Macri, Martin Stalla, Nicolas Martin, Romane Dewaele, Thomas Chiarini, Valentin Michaux. We thank the specialized endodontists who performed the treatments in the control group: Arman Gazi, Charles Dassargues, Pierre Carsin. We thank Lieven Desmet for his assistance in statistical analyses (SMCS, UCLouvain). The authors are extremely grateful to Domenico Ricucci for performing the histological sections and analyses. J.G. Leprince thanks Cliniques universitaires Saint-Luc (Brussels, Belgium) for his FRC fellowship.

Conflicts of Interest: Julien Beauquis and Julian G. Leprince on behalf of the co-authors declare no potential conflicts of interest with respect to the research, authorship, and/or publication of this article.

References

1. Beauquis, J.; Petit, A.E.; Michaux, V.; Sagué, V.; Henrard, S.; Leprince, J.G. Dental Emergencies Management in COVID-19 Pandemic Peak: A Cohort Study. *J. Dent. Res.* **2021**, *100*, 352–360. [CrossRef] [PubMed]
2. Duncan, H.F.; Galler, K.M.; Tomson, P.L.; Simon, S.; El Karim, I.; Kundzina, R.; Krastl, G.; Dammaschke, T.; Fransson, H.; Markvart, M.; et al. European Society of Endodontology position statement: Management of deep caries and the exposed pulp. *Int. Endod. J.* **2019**, *52*, 923–934. [CrossRef] [PubMed]
3. Hasselgren, G.; Reit, C. Emergency pulpotomy: Pain relieving effect with and without the use of sedative dressings. *J. Endod.* **1989**, *15*, 254–256. [CrossRef]

4. Sharma, R.; Kumar, V.; Logani, A.; Chawla, A.; Mir, R.A.; Sharma, S.; Kalaivani, M. Association between concentration of active MMP-9 in pulpal blood and pulpotomy outcome in permanent mature teeth with irreversible pulpitis—A preliminary study. *Int. Endod. J.* **2020**, *54*, 479–489. [CrossRef]
5. R, R.; Aravind, R.; Kumar, V.; Sharma, S.; Chawla, A.; Logani, A. Influence of occlusal and proximal caries on the outcome of full pulpotomy in permanent mandibular molar teeth with partial irreversible pulpitis: A prospective study. *Int. Endod. J.* **2021**, *54*, 1699–1707. [CrossRef] [PubMed]
6. Taha, N.A.; Abdelkhader, S.Z. Outcome of full pulpotomy using Biodentine in adult patients with symptoms indicative of irreversible pulpitis. *Int. Endod. J.* **2018**, *51*, 819–828. [CrossRef] [PubMed]
7. Asgary, S.; Eghbal, M.J.; Ghoddusi, J.; Yazdani, S. One-year results of vital pulp therapy in permanent molars with irreversible pulpitis: An ongoing multicenter, randomized, non-inferiority clinical trial. *Clin. Oral Investig.* **2013**, *17*, 431–439. [CrossRef]
8. Ricucci, D.; Loghin, S.; Siqueira, J.F., Jr. Correlation between Clinical and Histologic Pulp Diagnoses. *J. Endod.* **2014**, *40*, 1932–1939. [CrossRef]
9. Parirokh, M.; Torabinejad, M. Mineral trioxide aggregate: A comprehensive literature review–Part I: Chemical, physical, and antibacterial properties. *J. Endod.* **2010**, *36*, 16–27. [CrossRef]
10. Hilton, T.J.; Ferracane, J.; Mancl, L.; Baltuck, C.; Barnes, C.; Beaudry, D.; Shao, J.; Lubisich, E.; Gilbert, A.; Lowder, L.; et al. Comparison of CaOH with MTA for Direct Pulp Capping: A PBRN randomized clinical trial. *J. Dent. Res.* **2013**, *92*, S16–S22. [CrossRef]
11. Cushley, S.; Duncan, H.F.; Lappin, M.J.; Tomson, P.L.; Lundy, F.T.; Cooper, P.; Clarke, M.; El Karim, I.A. Pulpotomy for mature carious teeth with symptoms of irreversible pulpitis: A systematic review. *J. Dent.* **2019**, *88*, 103158. [CrossRef] [PubMed]
12. Asgary, S.; Eghbal, M.J.; Fazlyab, M.; Baghban, A.A.; Ghoddusi, J. Five-year results of vital pulp therapy in permanent molars with irreversible pulpitis: A non-inferiority multicenter randomized clinical trial. *Clin. Oral Investig.* **2015**, *19*, 335–341. [CrossRef]
13. Asgary, S.; Eghbal, M.J.; Ghoddusi, J. Two-year results of vital pulp therapy in permanent molars with irreversible pulpitis: An ongoing multicenter randomized clinical trial. *Clin. Oral Investig.* **2014**, *18*, 635–641. [CrossRef] [PubMed]
14. Taha, N.A.; Al-Khatib, H. 4-Year Follow-up of Full Pulpotomy in Symptomatic Mature Permanent Teeth with Carious Pulp Exposure Using a Stainproof Calcium Silicate–based Material. *J. Endod.* **2022**, *48*, 87–95. [CrossRef]
15. Linsuwanont, P.; Wimonsutthikul, K.; Pothimoke, U.; Santiwong, B. Treatment Outcomes of Mineral Trioxide Aggregate Pulpotomy in Vital Permanent Teeth with Carious Pulp Exposure: The Retrospective Study. *J. Endod.* **2017**, *43*, 225–230. [CrossRef] [PubMed]
16. Taha, N.A.; Abdulkhader, S.Z. Full Pulpotomy with Biodentine in Symptomatic Young Permanent Teeth with Carious Exposure. *J. Endod.* **2018**, *44*, 932–937. [CrossRef]
17. Chapman, C.R.; Casey, K.L.; Dubner, R.; Foley, K.M.; Gracely, R.H.; Reading, A.E. Pain measurement: An overview. *Pain* **1985**, *22*, 1–31. [CrossRef]
18. Sharav, Y.; Leviner, E.; Tzukert, A.; McGrath, P.A. The spatial distribution, intensity and unpleasantness of acute dental pain. *Pain* **1984**, *20*, 363–370. [CrossRef]
19. Seymour, R.A.; Simpson, J.M.; Charlton, E.J.; Phillips, M.E. An evaluation of length and end-phrase of visual analogue scales in dental pain. *Pain* **1985**, *21*, 177–185. [CrossRef]
20. Pak, J.G.; White, S.N. Pain Prevalence and Severity before, during, and after Root Canal Treatment: A Systematic Review. *J. Endod.* **2011**, *37*, 429–438. [CrossRef]
21. European Society of Endodontology. Quality guidelines for endodontic treatment: Consensus report of the European Society of Endodontology. *Int. Endod. J.* **2006**, *39*, 921–930. [CrossRef] [PubMed]
22. Heft, M.W.; Parker, S.R. An experimental basis for revising the graphic rating scale for pain. *Pain* **1984**, *19*, 153–161. [CrossRef]
23. Orstavik, D.; Kerekes, K.; Eriksen, H.M. The periapical index: A scoring system for radiographic assessment of apical periodontitis. *Dent. Traumatol.* **1986**, *2*, 20–34. [CrossRef] [PubMed]
24. Ricucci, D.; Siqueira, J.F., Jr.; Rôças, I.N. Pulp Response to Periodontal Disease: Novel Observations Help Clarify the Processes of Tissue Breakdown and Infection. *J. Endod.* **2021**, *47*, 740–754. [CrossRef]
25. Eren, B.; Onay, E.O.; Ungor, M. Assessment of alternative emergency treatments for symptomatic irreversible pulpitis: A randomized clinical trial. *Int. Endod. J.* **2018**, *51*, e227–e237. [CrossRef]
26. Asgary, S.; Eghbal, M.J. The effect of pulpotomy using a Calcium-Enriched Mixture cement versus one-visit root canal therapy on postoperative pain relief in irreversible pulpitis: A randomized clinical trial. *Odontology* **2010**, *98*, 126–133. [CrossRef]
27. Collaborative Group of the Spanish Society of Clinical Pharmacology; Garcća-Alonso, F. Comparative study of the efficacy of dipyrone, diclofenac sodium and pethidine in acute renal colic. *Eur. J. Clin. Pharmacol.* **1991**, *40*, 543–546. [CrossRef]
28. Sasmaz, M.I.; Kirpat, V. The relationship between the severity of pain and stone size, hydronephrosis and laboratory parameters in renal colic attack. *Am. J. Emerg. Med.* **2019**, *37*, 2107–2110. [CrossRef]
29. Siddique, I.; Mahmood, H.; Mohammed-Ali, R. Paracetamol overdose secondary to dental pain: A case series. *Br. Dent. J.* **2015**, *219*, E6. [CrossRef]
30. O'Sullivan, L.M.; Ahmed, N.; Sidebottom, A.J. Dental pain management-a cause of significant morbidity due to paracetamol overdose. *Br. Dent. J.* **2018**, *224*, 626. [CrossRef]
31. Rechenberg, D.-K.; Galicia, J.C.; Peters, O.A. Biological Markers for Pulpal Inflammation: A Systematic Review. *PLoS ONE* **2016**, *11*, e0167289. [CrossRef]

32. Zanini, M.; Meyer, E.; Simon, S. Pulp Inflammation Diagnosis from Clinical to Inflammatory Mediators: A Systematic Review. *J. Endod.* **2017**, *43*, 1033–1051. [CrossRef] [PubMed]
33. Rechenberg, D.-K.; Bostanci, N.; Zehnder, M.; Belibasakis, G.N. Periapical fluid RANKL and IL-8 are differentially regulated in pulpitis and apical periodontitis. *Cytokine* **2014**, *69*, 116–119. [CrossRef] [PubMed]
34. Eghbal, M.J.; Asgary, S.; Baglue, R.A.; Parirokh, M.; Ghoddusi, J. MTA pulpotomy of human permanent molars with irreversible pulpitis. *Aust. Endod. J.* **2009**, *35*, 4–8. [CrossRef] [PubMed]
35. Chueh, L.-H.; Chiang, C.-P. Histology of Irreversible Pulpitis Premolars Treated with Mineral Trioxide Aggregate Pulpotomy. *Oper. Dent.* **2010**, *35*, 370–374. [CrossRef] [PubMed]
36. Zanini, M.; Hennequin, M.; Cousson, P.-Y. A Review of Criteria for the Evaluation of Pulpotomy Outcomes in Mature Permanent Teeth. *J. Endod.* **2016**, *42*, 1167–1174. [CrossRef] [PubMed]
37. Fransson, H.; Wolf, E.; Petersson, K. Formation of a hard tissue barrier after experimental pulp capping or partial pulpotomy in humans: An updated systematic review. *Int. Endod. J.* **2016**, *49*, 533–542. [CrossRef]
38. Pedano, M.S.; Li, X.; Yoshihara, K.; Van Landuyt, K.; Van Meerbeek, B. Cytotoxicity and Bioactivity of Dental Pulp-Capping Agents towards Human Tooth-Pulp Cells: A Systematic Review of In-Vitro Studies and Meta-Analysis of Randomized and Controlled Clinical Trials. *Materials* **2020**, *13*, 2670. [CrossRef]
39. Matsuo, T.; Nakanishi, T.; Shimizu, H.; Ebisu, S. A clinical study of direct pulp capping applied to carious-exposed pulps. *J. Endod.* **1996**, *22*, 551–556. [CrossRef]
40. Krastl, G.; Weiger, R.; Filippi, A.; Van Waes, H.; Ebeleseder, K.; Ree, M.; Connert, T.; Widbiller, M.; Tjäderhane, L.; Dummer, P.H.M.; et al. Endodontic management of traumatized permanent teeth–a comprehensive review. *Int. Endod. J.* **2021**, *54*, 1221–1245. [CrossRef]
41. Mejàre, I.A.; Axelsson, S.; Davidson, T.; Frisk, F.; Hakeberg, M.; Kvist, T.; Norlund, A.; Petersson, A.; Portenier, I.; Sandberg, H.; et al. Diagnosis of the condition of the dental pulp: A systematic review. *Int. Endod. J.* **2012**, *45*, 597–613. [CrossRef] [PubMed]
42. Qudeimat, M.A.; Alyahya, A.; Hasan, A.A.; Barrieshi-Nusair, K.M. Mineral trioxide aggregate pulpotomy for permanent molars with clinical signs indicative of irreversible pulpitis: A preliminary study. *Int. Endod. J.* **2016**, *50*, 126–134. [CrossRef] [PubMed]
43. Munir, A.; Zehnder, M.; Rechenberg, D.-K. Wound Lavage in Studies on Vital Pulp Therapy of Permanent Teeth with Carious Exposures: A Qualitative Systematic Review. *J. Clin. Med.* **2020**, *9*, 984. [CrossRef]
44. Ballal, N.V.; Duncan, H.F.; Wiedemeier, D.B.; Rai, N.; Jalan, P.; Bhat, V.; Belle, V.S.; Zehnder, M. MMP-9 Levels and NaOCl Lavage in Randomized Trial on Direct Pulp Capping. *J. Dent. Res.* **2021**, 220345211046874. [CrossRef] [PubMed]
45. Ng, Y.-L.; Mann, V.; Rahbaran, S.; Lewsey, J.; Gulabivala, K. Outcome of primary root canal treatment: Systematic review of the literature–Part 2. Influence of clinical factors. *Int. Endod. J.* **2008**, *41*, 6–31. [CrossRef] [PubMed]
46. Ricucci, D.; Russo, J.; Rutberg, M.; Burleson, J.A.; Spångberg, L.S. A prospective cohort study of endodontic treatments of 1369 root canals: Results after 5 years. *Oral Surg. Oral Med. Oral Pathol. Oral Radiol. Endodontol.* **2011**, *112*, 825–842. [CrossRef] [PubMed]
47. Ree, M.H.; Timmerman, M.F.; Wesselink, P.R. Factors influencing referral for specialist endodontic treatment amongst a group of Dutch general practitioners. *Int. Endod. J.* **2003**, *36*, 129–134. [CrossRef]
48. AAE. AAE Endodontic Case Difficulty Assessment Form and Guidelines. Available online: https://www.aae.org/specialty/wp-content/uploads/sites/2/2019/02/19AAE_CaseDifficultyAssessmentForm.pdf (accessed on 9 November 2021).
49. Bergenholtz, G.; Kvist, T. Evidence-based endodontics. *Endod. Top.* **2014**, *31*, 3–18. [CrossRef]
50. Castro, M. Placebo versus Best-Available-Therapy Control Group in Clinical Trials for Pharmacologic Therapies: Which Is Better? *Proc. Am. Thorac. Soc.* **2007**, *4*, 570–573. [CrossRef]
51. Bergenholtz, G.; Kvist, T. Call for improved research efforts on clinical procedures in endodontics. *Int. Endod. J.* **2013**, *46*, 697–699. [CrossRef]

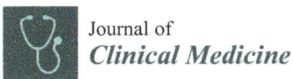

Article

Comparative Analysis of Root Canal Dentin Removal Capacity of Two NiTi Endodontic Reciprocating Systems for the Root Canal Treatment of Primary Molar Teeth. An In Vitro Study

Vicente Faus-Llácer [1], Dalia Pulido Ouardi [1], Ignacio Faus-Matoses [1], Celia Ruiz-Sánchez [1], Álvaro Zubizarreta-Macho [2,3,4,*], Anabella María Reyes Ortiz [5] and Vicente Faus-Matoses [1]

[1] Department of Stomatology, Faculty of Medicine and Dentistry, University of Valencia, 46010 Valencia, Spain; fausvj@uv.es (V.F.-L.); dapuou@alumni.uv.es (D.P.O.); ignacio.faus@uv.es (I.F.-M.); ceruizsan@gmail.com (C.R.-S.); vicente.faus@uv.es (V.F.-M.)
[2] Department of Endodontics, Faculty of Health Sciences, Alfonso X El Sabio University, 28691 Madrid, Spain
[3] Department of Surgery, Faculty of Medicine and Dentistry, University of Salamanca, 37008 Salamanca, Spain
[4] Department of Implant Surgery, Faculty of Health Sciences, Alfonso X El Sabio University, Avenida Universidad, 1, Villanueva de la Cañada, 28691 Madrid, Spain
[5] Department of Pediatric Dentistry, Faculty of Health Sciences, Alfonso X El Sabio University, 28691 Madrid, Spain; areyeort@uax.es
* Correspondence: amacho@uax.es

Abstract: The objective of the present study was to evaluate and compare the dentin removal capacity of Endogal Kids and Reciproc Blue NiTi alloy endodontic reciprocating systems for root canal treatments in primary second molar teeth via a micro-computed tomography (micro-CT) scan. Materials and Methods: Sixty root canal systems in fifteen primary second molar teeth were chosen and classified into one of the following study groups: A: EK3 Endogal Kids (n = 30) (EDG) and B. R25 Reciproc Blue (n = 30) (RB). Preoperative and postoperative micro-CT scans were uploaded into image processing software to analyze the changes in the volume of root canal dentin using a mathematical algorithm that enabled progressive differentiation between neighboring pixels after defining and segmenting the root canal systems in both micro-CT scans. Volumetric variations in the root canal system and the root canal third were calculated using a t-test for independent samples or a nonparametric Mann–Whitney–Wilcoxon test. Results: Statistically significant differences (p = 0.0066) in dentin removal capacity were found between the EDG (2.89 ± 1.26 mm^3) and RB (1.22 ± 0.58 mm^3) study groups for the coronal root canal third; however, no statistically significant differences were found for the middle (p = 0.4864) and apical (p = 0.6276) root canal thirds. Conclusions: Endogal and Reciproc Blue NiTi endodontic reciprocating systems showed similar capacity for the removal of root canal dentin, except for the coronal root canal third, in which the Reciproc Blue NiTi endodontic reciprocating system preserved more root canal dentin tissue.

Keywords: endodontics; endodontic reciprocating file; micro-computed tomography scan; root canal dentin removal; primary molar teeth

1. Introduction

The presence of bacteria within the root canal system poses a risk factor for the appearance of pulp and periapical diseases in both primary and permanent dentition [1,2]. The biomechanical preparation of the root canal system is therefore considered to be a fundamental step in the root canal treatment process in order to adequately eliminate bacteria, necrotic tissue, and infected dentin [3]. In addition, the root canal system must be funnel shaped, becoming narrower in the apical direction in order to maintain the original anatomy and enable sufficient obturation [4,5]. A pulpectomy is widely recommended for primary teeth so as to preserve arch length, maintain primary teeth, including their functional and aesthetic properties, and guide the proper eruption of permanent dentition [6]. Hand files are widely used to work with the root canal system in primary dentition; however, the root anatomy makes successful endodontic treatment difficult [7,8]. In primary teeth, the root canal system is characterized by high anatomical variability, including accessory and curved canals, as well as physiological root resorption that can alter the formation of the root canal system [9]. Nickel–titanium (NiTi) endodontic rotary instruments enable clinicians to maintain the original anatomy of curved canals, reducing the likelihood of potential mishaps during root canal system preparation [10]. Recently, novel NiTi endodontic rotary files have been specifically developed for the root canal treatment of primary teeth. Endogal Kids Rotary can be used either with a rotary or reciprocating motion; however, this latter movement is recommended for use in children, since it reduces the working time. This endodontic reciprocating system is manufactured in a NiTi alloy with heat treatment, and has a 17 mm length, 4% taper, 300μm apical diameter, and triangular cross-section design. Moreover, Reciproc Blue NiTi endodontic pediatric files also performs a reciprocating motion and is manufactured in a CM-Blue Wire NiTi alloy with heat treatment, and has a 17 mm length, 300μm apical diameter, and double-S cross-section design. The heat treatment improves the physical properties of NiTi endodontic rotary files, increasing their cyclic fatigue resistance and helping them adapt to different curvatures and angulations. Some studies have described the use of single files in a reciprocating motion for the root canal treatment of primary molars and reported significant advantages in pediatric dentistry, such as a decrease in working time, low risk of iatrogenic errors, or the prevention of cross-contamination [11–13]. That being said, root canal treatments can be affected by various factors, including anatomical design, diameter, kinematics, taper, and the number of files used during the procedure [14,15]. In addition, several techniques have been used to measure the amount of dentin removal, including plastic models, histologic sections, serial sectioning, scanning electron microscopic studies, radiographic comparison, and the silicone impression of un-instrumented root canal systems [15]. However, few studies have used the micro-CT with primary molars, which is a conservative, accurate, and nondestructive measurement procedure [11]. Micro-computed tomography (micro-CT) analysis has become a conservative measurement technique for obtaining an accurate 3D analysis, enabling both the quantitative and qualitative assessment of the root canal system anatomy after the shaping procedures [6,16].

The objective of the present study was to evaluate and compare the dentin removal capacity of Endogal Kids and Reciproc Blue NiTi endodontic reciprocating systems for the root canal treatment of primary second molar teeth via a micro-CT scan, with a null hypothesis (H_0) that there are no differences in root dentin removal capacity between the Endogal Kids and Reciproc Blue NiTi endodontic reciprocating systems for root canal treatments in primary molar teeth.

2. Materials and Methods

2.1. Study Design

Sixty root canal systems were chosen from a total of fifteen primary second molar teeth (8 upper and 7 lower) that had been extracted for orthodontic or restorative reasons. Between January and March 2021, around three root canal systems were selected for study from cases at the Department of Stomatology at the University of Valencia in Valencia, Spain. All of the selected root canal systems presented no prior root canal filling materials or root resorption. A power of 80.00% was calculated using the bilateral Student's t-test for two independent samples. When used to calculate the variation from the null hypothesis $H_0: \mu_1 = \mu_2$, the significance level of 5.00% and power of 80.00% meant that 60 root canal systems were necessary for the purposes of this study. The study was carried out as a randomized controlled experimental trial, in keeping with the norms outlined by the statement of the German Ethics Committee on the use of organic tissues as part of medical research (Zentrale Ethikkommission, 2003). Additionally, the study was reviewed and approved by

2.2. Experimental Procedure

The sixty root canal systems in the fifteen selected primary second molar teeth were assigned randomly (Epidat 4.1, Galicia, Spain) to one of the following NiTi endodontic reciprocating systems: A. EK3 Endogal Kids (Endogal, Galician Endodontics Company, Lugo, Spain) (n = 30) (EDG) or B. R25 Reciproc Blue (VDW, Baillagues, Switzerland) (n = 30) (RB). Impressions of the teeth were taken using polyvinyl siloxane material (Ref.: 7000054992, Express™ 2 Putty Soft, 3M ESPE™, Saint Paul, MN, USA) to enable the access cavity to be prepared using the technique described by Rover et al. [17]. The root canal working length was determined with a stainless steel #10 K-file (Dentsply Maillefer, Ballaigues, Switzerland) and observed under magnification (OPMI pico, Zeiss Dental Microscopes, Oberkochen, Germany) until the far end of the file became visible through the epical foramen. Each root canal system was manually prepared with up to a #25 K-file (Dentsply Maillefer, Ballaigues, Switzerland) before being performed upon according to the NiTi endodontic reciprocating system to which it had been assigned. Root canal systems randomly assigned to the EDG study group were prepared with a reciprocating movement, and the root canal systems randomly assigned to the RB study group were also prepared with a reciprocating motion. In addition, the root canal systems were irrigated using a 5 mL sterile saline solution (Braun, Jaén, Spain) with 5 mL of 17% EDTA (SmearClear; SybronEndo, CA, USA) and 5 mL of 5.25% NaOCl (Clorox; Oakland, CA, USA), administered using a 0.3 mm endodontic needle (Miraject Endo Luer; Hager & Werken, Duisburg, Germany) inserted into the working length up to 1 mm. The teeth were kept in an incubator (mco-18aic, Sanyo, Moriguchi, Osaka, Japan) and stored at 37 °C with 100% relative humidity. A single clinician performed all the root canal procedures.

2.3. Micro-CT Scanning

Preoperative and postoperative micro-CT scans (Micro-CAT II, Siemens Preclinical Solutions, Knoxville, TN, USA) were performed to analyze and compare the amount of root canal dentin removed by the Endogal Kids and Reciproc Blue NiTi endodontic reciprocating systems subsequent to the root canal treatment of the primary second molar teeth. The scans were taken using the following exposure parameters: 88 µA, 90 kV, 360° rotation, and 50 µm isotropic resolution. Tomographic 3D images of the entire tooth showed a total of 512 slices, with an isotropic voxel size of 50 microns and a 512 × 512-pixel resolution for each slice (Figure 1A–F).

2.4. Measurement Procedure

The analysis of the change in the volume of dentin removed after the root canal procedures was carried out using image processing software (ImageJ, National Institutes of Health, Bethesda, MD, USA) after the root canal systems had been defined and segmented (ROI: 10 × 10 × 10 mm) using the preoperative and postoperative micro-CT scans (Micro-CAT II, Siemens Preclinical Solutions, Knoxville, TN, USA). In addition, transverse section images were also analyzed in the apical, middle, and coronal root thirds (Figure 2).

2.5. Statistical Tests

Statistical analysis was carried out using SAS 9.4 (SAS Institute Inc., Cary, NC, USA). The mean and standard deviation (SD) were used for the descriptive analysis of quantitative data. For each of the variables, the difference between the pre- and postoperative values was analyzed using a t-test for independent samples or a nonparametric Mann–Whitney–Wilcoxon test based on compliance with the application criteria. $p < 0.05$ was determined to be the level for statistical significance.

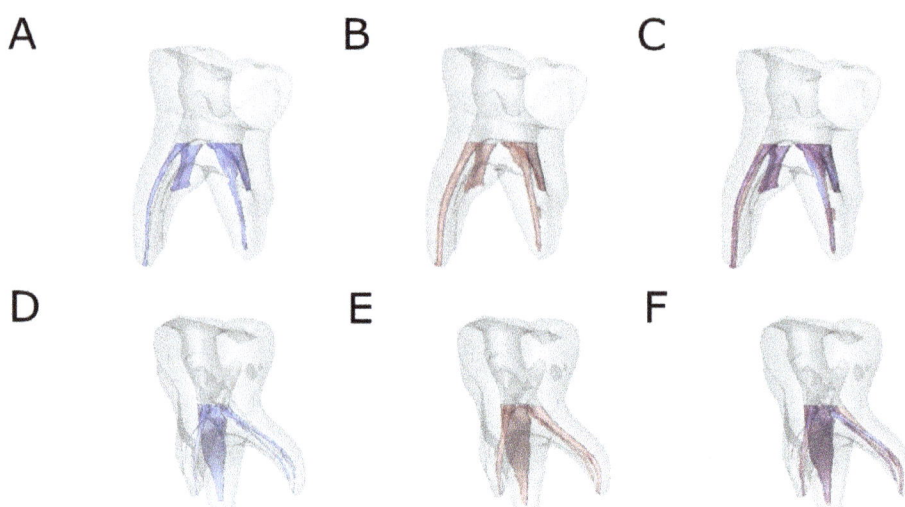

Figure 1. Reconstructed 3D micro-CT images of (**A**) preoperative (blue), (**B**) postoperative (red), and (**C**) superimposed pre- and postoperative images of the EDG study group (blue and red) and (**D**) preoperative (blue), (**E**) postoperative (red), and (**F**) superimposed pre- and postoperative images of the RB study group (blue and red).

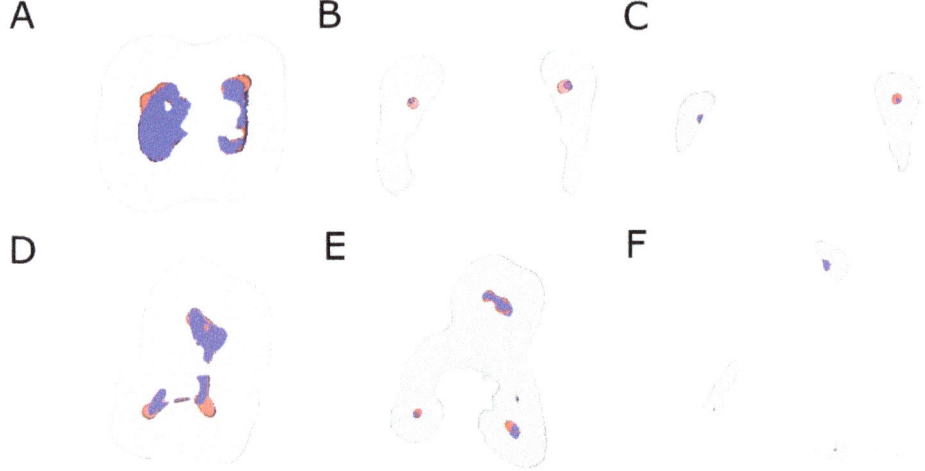

Figure 2. Transverse section images after aligning preoperative (blue) and postoperative (red) micro-CT scans of the EDG study group at the (**A**) coronal, (**B**) middle, and (**C**) apical root third and (**D**) coronal, (**E**) middle, and (**F**) apical root third of the RB study group.

3. Results

Table 1 and Figure 2 show the mean and standard deviation values for the volume of root canal system (mm^3) between EDG and RB NiTi endodontic files at coronal, middle and apical root canal third.

Table 1. Descriptive analysis of the volume of root canal system (mm^3) between EDG and RB NiTi endodontic files at coronal, middle and apical root canal third.

Study Group	Root Third	Time	n	Mean	SD	Minimum	Maximum
EDG	Coronal	Preoperative	30	7.61 [a]	4.81	3.58	18.20
		Postoperative	30	10.50 [a]	5.78	4.13	22.95
	Middle	Preoperative	30	1.74 [a]	1.23	0.22	4.20
		Postoperative	30	2.94 [a]	1.58	0.83	5.81
	Apical	Preoperative	30	0.33 [a]	0.36	0.00	1.17
		Postoperative	30	0.53 [a]	0.39	0.00	1.19
RB	Coronal	Preoperative	30	6.53 [b]	1.08	5.22	8.58
		Postoperative	30	7.75 [b]	1.48	6.07	10.63
	Middle	Preoperative	30	1.71 [a]	1.10	0.05	3.04
		Postoperative	30	2.56 [a]	1.38	0.95	3.91
	Apical	Preoperative	30	0.40 [a]	0.23	0.03	0.68
		Postoperative	30	0.66 [a]	0.25	0.41	1.15

EDG: Endogal; RB: Reciproc Blue; [a,b]: statistical significance.

The paired *t*-test found no statistically significant differences ($p = 0.0767$) in the volume of root canal dentin removed between the EDG (4.30 ± 2.58 mm^3) and RB (2.32 ± 1.07 mm^3) study groups. However, the paired *t*-test found statistically significant differences ($p = 0.0066$) between the EDG (2.89 ± 1.26 mm^3) and RB (1.22 ± 0.58 mm^3) study groups in the volume of root canal dentin removed at the coronal root canal third (Figure 3).

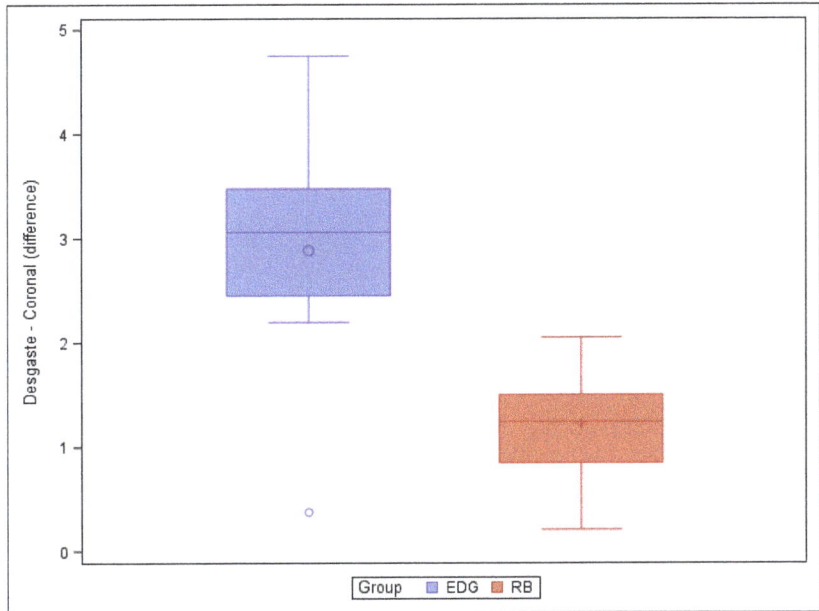

Figure 3. Box plot of the difference in dentin volume pre- and post-root canal procedure between the EDG and RB study groups at the coronal level.

However, the paired *t*-test did not find any statistically significant differences ($p = 0.4864$) in the volume of root canal dentin removed between the EDG (1.20 ± 1.27 mm^3) and RB (0.85 ± 0.47 mm^3) study groups at the middle root canal third (Figure 4).

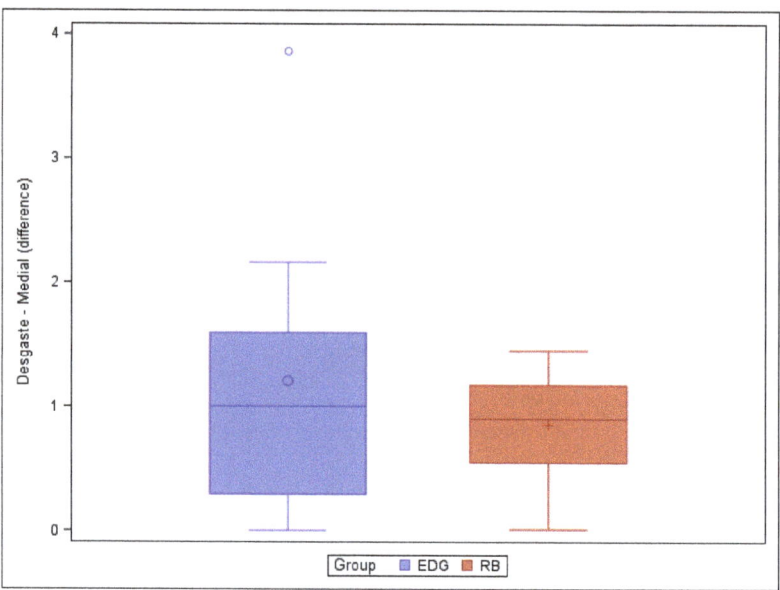

Figure 4. Box plot of the difference in dentin volume pre- and post-root canal procedure between the EDG and RB study groups at the middle level.

Moreover, the paired *t*-test did not reveal any statistically significant differences ($p = 0.6276$) in the volume of root canal dentin removed between the EDG (0.20 ± 0.25 mm^3) and RB (0.26 ± 0.17 mm^3) study groups at the apical root canal third (Figure 5).

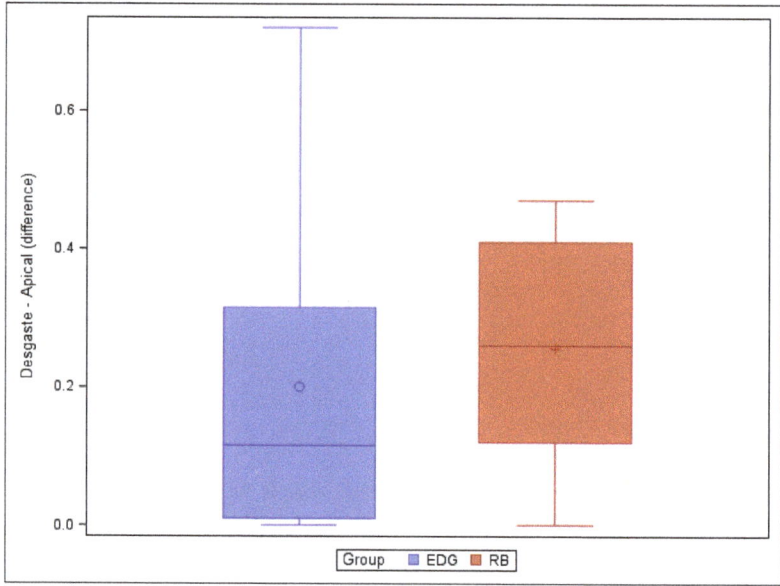

Figure 5. Box plot of the difference in dentin volume pre- and post-root canal procedure between the EDG and RB study groups at the apical level.

4. Discussion

The results of the present study refute the null hypothesis (H_0) that there is no difference in root dentin removal capacity between the Endogal Kids and Reciproc Blue NiTi endodontic reciprocating systems for the root canal treatment of primary molar teeth.

Various methods have previously been used to evaluate root canal instrumentation, including plastic models, serial sectioning, scanning electron microscopic studies, and radiographic comparisons [18]. More recently, noninvasive 3D techniques, such as CBCT or micro-CT scans, have been used to assess the efficiency of cleaning and dentin removal after root canal treatment procedures [19]. In addition, high-resolution 3D micro-CT images are the gold standard for evaluating the root canal system anatomy and root canal instrumentation [20,21]. In the present study, micro-CT scans were used to examine the internal anatomy of the root canal system and evaluate the effectiveness of root canal instrumentation on the root canal system of primary second molar teeth. The authors selected the primary second molars because the anatomy of this tooth is very similar to that of the permanent first molar, which allows a comparison to be made between them. In addition, the eruption chronology of the second premolars is usually later than that of the first premolars, which leads to less root resorption of the primary second molars compared to the primary first molars [22].

Micro-CT scan measurement techniques have previously been used to analyze the amount of root canal dentin removed from permanent teeth after root canal treatment. Yilmaz et al. reported no statistically significant differences between the amount of dentin removed by ProTaper Next (Dentsply Maillefer, Ballaigues, Switzerland), OneShape (MicroMega, Besançon, France), and EdgeFile (Edge Endo, Albuquerque, NM) NiTi alloy endodontic rotary files for the whole canal length ($p > 0.05$) [23]. Moreover, de Albuquerque et al. reported that the Protaper Next, Wave One Gold, Predesign Logic, and Vortex Blue NiTi alloy endodontic systems caused a greater dentin removal at the coronal third (9 mm), decreasing at the apical one (3 mm) [24]. These findings are aligned with the results shown in the present study.

The root canals in primary teeth are not always easy to shape and obturate during treatments. In fact, many characteristics of the root canal anatomy make endodontic treatment difficult, potentially resulting in apical transportation, zipping, perforations, or gaps [18,21]. Esentürk et al. observed that 60% of the root canal system was left uninstrumented upon after root canal preparation due to the anatomical complexity of the primary molars, highlighting a need for NiTi alloy endodontic rotary instruments to be developed for use in primary teeth [25]. Prabhakar et al. found that the Wave One NiTi alloy endodontic reciprocal system enabled quicker and safer instrumentation compared with the One Shape NiTi alloy endodontic rotary system, because the former reduces levels of both torsional and flexural stress, as well as the number of instruments required for the sequence [11]. According to their findings, Katge et al. reported that the Wave One NiTi alloy endodontic reciprocal system had a statistically greater cleaning capability than the Protaper NiTi alloy endodontic rotary system at the coronal and middle third due to the benefits of reciprocating motion [12]. However, the risk of root perforation and root canal transportation is more correlated with a high taper value than a reciprocating or continuous motion, which means that the NiTi alloy endodontic system should be selected primarily based on the taper [21]. Ramazani et al. assessed the efficiency of Mtwo NiTi alloy endodontic rotary files and Reciproc NiTi alloy endodontic reciprocating files when cleaning, finding no statistically significant differences between the two study groups, although the Reciproc NiTi alloy endodontic reciprocating files required less preparation time [13]. Azar et al. found no statistically significant differences in cleaning capabilities between Mtwo NiTi alloy endodontic rotary files, Protaper NiTi alloy endodontic rotary files, and manual K files in the three root thirds of the root canal system, measuring the differences using ink and stereo microscopes [26]. These results were corroborated by the findings of Ramazani et al. for Mtwo NiTi alloy endodontic rotary files and K files [13]; Moghaddam et al. for Master NiTi alloy endodontic rotary files, Rotary Flex NiTi alloy endodontic rotary files, and K files [8]; and Mehalawat et al. for Profile NiTi alloy endodontic rotary files and K files [27]. However, Madan et al. did observe statistically significant differences between Profile NiTi alloy endodontic rotary files and K files when using the same ink removal method, during which the Profile NiTi alloy endodontic rotary files were more efficient at cleaning the coronal root third, while the manual files were better at cleaning the apical root third [28].

Some studies have compared the cleaning capacity of both manual and NiTi alloy endodontic rotary files in permanent teeth [23], but not as many included primary teeth, and only a few of the studies used micro-CT scan assessments. The volume of dentin removed reveals the remaining dentin thickness, which is needed to provide enough resistance for root canal treatments. The force with which root canal instruments are used is in direct proportion to the amount of dentin removed [29]. Although manual instrumentation is commonly used in primary teeth, many studies have found that more dentin is removed using manual files than rotary instrumentation [19,20,29,30]. Selvakumar et al. used K3 NiTi alloy endodontic rotary files (with a 0.02 taper) and found significantly lower dentin removal when compared with manual K files and K3 NiTi alloy endodontic rotary files (with a 0.04 taper), which were shown to remove more dentin tissue in the coronal and apical root thirds in comparison with K files and K3 NiTi alloy endodontic rotary files (with a 0.02 taper) [19]. On the other hand, Zameer et al. observed no statically significant differences when using either the 2% or 4% taper rotary files to remove dentin, without damaging the dentinal walls and achieving an improved canal shape for root canal filling material [31]. In addition, Moghaddam found that a continuous rotation movement with up to a #30 apical diameter enabled better instrumentation and safer results when used with primary teeth without excessive dentin removal [8]. However, Zameer et al. observed a greater number of root perforations when dentin removal was performed using 4% taper NiTi alloy endodontic rotary files compared with 2% NiTi alloy endodontic rotary files and manual K files [31]. This result corroborates the findings of Kummer et al., who used rotary 6% taper NiTi alloy endodontic rotary files with a #30 apical diameter and found three root perforations, concluding that the mesial and distal roots of lower molars and mesiobuccal roots of upper molars had a higher risk of root perforation [30]. In addition, Barasuol et al. observed two perforations in the apical and middle root third, as well as root canal transportation, when using 8% taper Reciproc NiTi alloy endodontic reciprocating files [21]. Files with a larger taper can result in the reduced thickness of the dentinal wall, leading to greater fragility of the teeth and a higher risk of root perforation [20]. Madan et al. found that instrumentation failure was reduced when using 0.04 taper Profile NiTi alloy endodontic rotary files, which were also less damaging for primary teeth [28].

The strengths and innovation of the current study are that not many studies analyze the effect of specific pediatric instrumentation systems on primary teeth, even though pulpectomy is a widely performed dental treatment. Furthermore, the instrumentation systems compared are very novel; especially the Reciproc Blue system, which has not been released on the market. Finally, the micro-CT scan measurement technique for dentin removal analysis is very accurate and innovative.

The present findings are limited by the constraints of an in vitro study. The use of instrumentation with primary teeth is not subject to any universal guidelines, and clinical trials are needed to obtain clinical results. Additional studies should be carried out on a larger sample size, as well as using pediatric files.

5. Conclusions

To summarize, within the constraints of this in vitro study, the results indicate that the Endogal and Reciproc Blue NiTi endodontic reciprocating systems are similarly capable of removing root canal dentin, except for in the coronal root canal third, in which the Reciproc Blue NiTi endodontic reciprocating system preserved more root canal dentin tissue.

Author Contributions: All authors aided in the research, supervision, writing, review, and editing of the study. Conceptualization, V.F.-L. and Á.Z.-M.; data curation, I.F.-M. and D.P.O.; formal analysis, V.F.-M.; visualization, C.R.-S. and A.M.R.O. All authors have read and agreed to the published version of the manuscript.

Funding: No external funding was applied to this research.

Institutional Review Board Statement: Not applicable.

Informed Consent Statement: Not applicable.

Data Availability Statement: Information is available on request in accordance with any relevant restrictions (e.g., privacy or ethical).

Conflicts of Interest: The authors declare no conflict of interest.

References

1. Jensen, A.L.; Abbott, P.V.; Castro Salgado, J. Interim and temporary restoration of teeth during endodontic treatment. *Aust. Dent. J.* **2007**, *52*, S83–S99. [CrossRef]
2. Amato, M.; Pantaleo, G.; Abtellatif, D.; Blasi, A.; Gagliani, M.; Iandolo, A. An in vitro evaluation of the degree of pulp tissue dissolution through different root canal irrigation protocols. *J. Conserv. Dent.* **2018**, *21*, 175–179. [PubMed]
3. Manchanda, S.; Sardana, D.; Yiu, C.K.Y. A systematic review and meta-analysis of randomized clinical trials compar-ing rotary canal instrumentation techniques with manual instrumentation techniques in primary teeth. *Int. Endod. J.* **2020**, *53*, 333–353. [CrossRef] [PubMed]
4. Siqueira Junior, J.F.; Rôças, I.D.N.; Marceliano-Alves, M.F.; Pérez, A.R.; Ricucci, D. Unprepared root canal surface areas: Causes, clinical implications, and therapeutic strategies. *Braz. Oral Res.* **2018**, *32*, e65. [CrossRef] [PubMed]
5. van der Vyver, P.J.; Paleker, F.; Vorster, M.; de Wet, F.A. Root Canal Shaping Using Nickel Titanium, M-Wire, and Gold Wire: A Micro-computed Tomographic Comparative Study of One Shape, ProTaper Next, and WaveOne Gold In-struments in Maxillary First Molars. *J. Endod.* **2019**, *45*, 62–67. [CrossRef] [PubMed]
6. Johnson, M.S.; Britto, L.R.; Guelmann, M. Impact of a biological barrier in pulpectomies of primary molars. *Pediatr. Dent.* **2006**, *28*, 506–510.
7. Jeevanandan, G.; Govindaraju, L. Clinical comparison of Kedo-S paediatric rotary files vs manual instrumentation for root canal preparation in primary molars: A double blinded randomised clinical trial. *Eur. Arch. Paediatr. Dent.* **2018**, *19*, 273–277. [CrossRef]
8. Nazari Moghaddam, K.; Mehran, M.; Farajian Zadeh, H. Root canal cleaning efficacy of rotary and hand files in-strumentation in primary molars. *Iran. Endod. J.* **2009**, *4*, 53–57.
9. Ahmed, H.M.A.; Musale, P.K.; El Shahawy, O.I.; Dummer, P.M.H. Application of a new system for classifying tooth, root and canal morphology in the primary dentition. *Int. Endod. J.* **2020**, *53*, 27–35. [CrossRef]
10. Pathak, S. In vitro comparison of K-file, Mtwo, and WaveOne in cleaning efficacy and instrumentation time in primary molars. *CHRISMED J. Health Res.* **2016**, *3*, 60–64. [CrossRef]
11. Prabhakar, A.R.; Yavagal, C.; Dixit, K.; Naik, S.V. Reciprocating vs Rotary Instrumentation in Pediatric Endodontics: Cone Beam Computed Tomographic Analysis of Deciduous Root Canals using Two Single-file Systems. *Int. J. Clin. Pediatr. Dent.* **2016**, *9*, 45–49. [CrossRef]
12. Katge, F.; Patil, D.; Poojari, M.; Pimpale, J.; Shitoot, A.; Rusawat, B. Comparison of instrumentation time and cleaning efficacy of manual instrumentation, rotary systems and reciprocating systems in primary teeth: An in vitro study. *J. Indian Soc. Pedod. Prev. Dent.* **2014**, *32*, 311–316. [CrossRef]
13. Ramazani, N.; Mohammadi, A.; Amirabadi, F.; Ramazani, M.; Ehsani, F. In vitro investigation of the cleaning efficacy, shaping ability, preparation time and file deformation of continuous rotary, reciprocating rotary and manual in-strumentations in primary molars. *J. Dent. Res. Dent. Clin. Dent. Prospect.* **2016**, *10*, 49–56. [CrossRef]
14. Silva, L.A.; Leonardo, M.R.; Nelson-Filho, P.; Tanomaru, J.M. Comparison of rotary and manual instrumentation tech-niques on cleaning capacity and instrumentation time in deciduous molars. *J. Dent. Child (Chic)* **2004**, *71*, 45–47.
15. Espir, C.G.; Nascimento-Mendes, C.A.; Guerreiro-Tanomaru, J.M.; Cavenago, B.C.; Hungaro Duarte, M.A.; Tanomaru-Filho, M. Shaping ability of rotary or reciprocating systems for oval root canal preparation: A micro-computed to-mography study. *Clin. Oral. Investig.* **2018**, *22*, 3189–3194. [CrossRef]
16. Sousa-Neto, M.D.; Silva-Sousa, Y.C.; Mazzi-Chaves, J.F.; Carvalho, K.K.T.; Barbosa, A.F.S.; Versiani, M.A.; Jacobs, R.; Leoni, G.B. Root canal preparation using micro-computed tomography analysis: A literature review. *Braz. Oral Res.* **2018**, *18*, e66. [CrossRef] [PubMed]
17. Rover, G.; Belladonna, F.G.; Bortoluzzi, E.A.; De-Deus, G.; Silva, E.J.N.L.; Teixeira, C.S. Influence of Access Cavity Design on Root Canal Detection, Instrumentation Efficacy, and Fracture Resistance Assessed in Maxillary Molars. *J. Endod.* **2017**, *43*, 1657–1662. [CrossRef] [PubMed]
18. Selvakumar, H.; Kavitha, S.; Thomas, E.; Anadhan, V.; Vijayakumar, R. Computed Tomographic Evaluation of K3 Rotary and Stainless Steel K File Instrumentation in Primary Teeth. *J. Clin. Diagn. Res.* **2016**, *10*, ZC05–ZC8. [CrossRef] [PubMed]

19. Musale, P.K.; Jain, K.R.; Kothare, S.S. Comparative assessment of dentin removal following hand and rotary instru-mentation in primary molars using cone-beam computed tomography. *J. Indian Soc. Pedod. Prev. Dent.* **2019**, *37*, 80–86. [CrossRef]
20. Kaya, E.; Elbay, M.; Yiğit, D. Evaluation of the Self-Adjusting File system (SAF) for the instrumentation of primary molar root canals: A micro-computed tomographic study. *Eur. J Paediatr. Dent.* **2017**, *18*, 105–110.
21. Barasuol, J.C.; Alcalde, M.P.; Bortoluzzi, E.A.; Duarte, M.A.H.; Cardoso, M.; Bolan, M. Shaping ability of hand, rotary and reciprocating files in primary teeth: A micro-CT study in vitro. *Eur. Arch. Paediatr. Dent.* **2020**, *22*, 195–201. [CrossRef]
22. Azar, M.R.; Mokhtare, M. Rotary Mtwo system versus manual K-file instruments: Efficacy in preparing primary and per-manent molar root canals. *Indian J. Dent. Res.* **2011**, *22*, 363. [CrossRef]
23. Yılmaz, F.; Eren, İ.; Eren, H.; Badi, M.A.; Ocak, M.; Çelik, H.H. Evaluation of the Amount of Root Canal Dentin Removed and Apical Transportation Occurrence after Instrumentation with ProTaper Next, OneShape, and EdgeFile Rotary Systems. *J. Endod.* **2020**, *46*, 662–667. [CrossRef]
24. de Albuquerque, M.S.; Nascimento, A.S.; Gialain, I.O.; de Lima, E.A.; Nery, J.A.; de Souza Araujo, P.R.; de Menezes, R.F.; Kato, A.S.; Braz, R. Canal Transportation, Centering Ability, and Dentin Removal after Instrumentation: A Micro-CT Eval-uation. *J. Contemp. Dent. Pract.* **2019**, *20*, 806–811. [CrossRef] [PubMed]
25. Esentürk, G.; Akkas, E.; Cubukcu, E.; Nagas, E.; Uyanik, O.; Cehreli, Z.C. A micro-computed tomographic assessment of root canal preparation with conventional and different rotary files in primary teeth and young permanent teeth. *Int. J. Paediatr. Dent.* **2020**, *30*, 202–208. [CrossRef] [PubMed]
26. Azar, M.R.; Safi, L.; Nikaein, A. Comparison of the cleaning capacity of Mtwo and Pro Taper rotary systems and manual instruments in primary teeth. *Dent. Res. J. (Isfahan)* **2012**, *9*, 146–151. [CrossRef]
27. Mehlawat, R.; Kapoor, R.; Gandhi, K.; Kumar, D.; Malhotra, R.; Ahuja, S. Comparative evaluation of instrumentation timing and cleaning efficacy in extracted primary molars using manual and NiTi rotary technique—Invitro study. *J. Oral Biol. Craniofac. Res.* **2019**, *9*, 151–155. [CrossRef]
28. Madan, N.; Rathnam, A.; Shigli, A.L.; Indushekar, K.R. K-file vs ProFiles in cleaning capacity and instrumentation time in primary molar root canals: An in vitro study. *J. Indian Soc. Pedod. Prev. Dent.* **2011**, *29*, 2–6. [CrossRef]
29. Seema, T.; Ahammed, H.; Parul, S.; Cheranjeevi, J. Comparative Evaluation of Dentin Removal and Taper of Root Canal Preparation of Hand K File, ProTaper Rotary File, and Kedo S Rotary File in Primary Molars Using Cone-beam Computed Tomography. *Int. J. Clin. Pediatr. Dent.* **2020**, *13*, 332–336.
30. Kummer, T.R.; Calvo, M.C.; Cordeiro, M.M.; de Sousa Vieira, R.; de Carvalho Rocha, M.J. Ex vivo study of manual and rotary instrumentation techniques in human primary teeth. *Oral Surg. Oral Med. Oral Pathol. Oral Radiol. Endod.* **2008**, *105*, e84–e92. [CrossRef]
31. Zameer, M. Evaluation of radicular dentin remaining and risk of perforation after manual and rotary instrumen-tations in root canals of primary teeth: An in vitro study. *J. Pediatr. Dent.* **2016**, *4*, 57–65. [CrossRef]

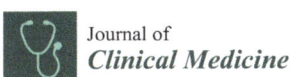

Article

Fatigue Analysis of NiTi Rotary Endodontic Files through Finite Element Simulation: Effect of Root Canal Geometry on Fatigue Life

Victor Roda-Casanova [1], Antonio Pérez-González [1], Álvaro Zubizarreta-Macho [2,3,*] and Vicente Faus-Matoses [4]

1. Department of Mechanical Engineering and Construction, Universitat Jaume I, 12071 Castelló de la Plana, Spain; vroda@uji.es (V.R.-C.); aperez@uji.es (A.P.-G.)
2. Department of Dentistry, Alfonso X el Sabio University, 28691 Madrid, Spain
3. Department of Orthodontics, University of Salamanca, 37008 Salamanca, Spain
4. Department of Stomatology, Faculty of Medicine and Dentistry, University of Valencia, 46010 Valencia, Spain; vicente.faus@uv.es
* Correspondence: amacho@uax.es

Abstract: This article describes a numerical procedure for estimating the fatigue life of NiTi endodontic rotary files. An enhanced finite element model reproducing the interaction of the endodontic file rotating inside the root canal was developed, which includes important phenomena that allowed increasing the degree of realism of the simulation. A method based on the critical plane approach was proposed for extracting significant strain results from finite element analysis, which were used in combination with the Coffin–Manson relation to predict the fatigue life of the NiTi rotary files. The proposed procedure is illustrated with several numerical examples in which different combinations of endodontic rotary files and root canal geometries were investigated. By using these analyses, the effect of the radius of curvature and the angle of curvature of the root canal on the fatigue life of the rotary files was analysed. The results confirm the significant influence of the root canal geometry on the fatigue life of the NiTi rotary files and reveal the higher importance of the radius of curvature with respect to the angle of curvature of the root canal.

Keywords: endodontic rotary files; finite element analysis; fatigue analysis

Citation: Roda-Casanova, V.; Pérez-González, A.; Zubizarreta-Macho, A.; Faus-Matoses, V. Fatigue Analysis of NiTi Rotary Endodontic Files through Finite Element Simulation: Effect of Root Canal Geometry on Fatigue Life. *J. Clin. Med.* **2021**, *10*, 5692. https://doi.org/10.3390/jcm10235692

Academic Editors: Massimo Amato, Giuseppe Pantaleo and Alfredo Iandolo

Received: 5 November 2021
Accepted: 29 November 2021
Published: 3 December 2021

Publisher's Note: MDPI stays neutral with regard to jurisdictional claims in published maps and institutional affiliations.

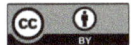

Copyright: © 2021 by the authors. Licensee MDPI, Basel, Switzerland. This article is an open access article distributed under the terms and conditions of the Creative Commons Attribution (CC BY) license (https://creativecommons.org/licenses/by/4.0/).

1. Introduction

The use of nickel-titanium (NiTi) rotary files for shaping root canals has spread in endodontics during the last decades, in detriment of manual preparation with traditional stainless-steel instruments. The superelasticity of NiTi and its lower Young's modulus reduce the risk of canal transportation and ledging in the treatment of curved root canals [1]. The superelasticity of the NiTi refers to the capacity of the material for undergoing large elastic deformations that can be restored after the forces producing the deformation are released. During these large deformations of the superelastic material, a phase transformation is induced within the material from austenite to martensite at a nearly constant stress. Due to this superelastic behaviour, files made of NiTi can adapt easily to strongly curved root canals. Successive modifications introduced during the last two decades in these instruments have allowed improving the quality of the cleaning and shaping, as well as saving time for both clinicians and patients [2–4]. However, the main problem that persists is the fracture of the files inside the root canal [5].

Fracture of rotary instruments occurs mainly by two different mechanisms, usually referred to as torsion overload and flexural fatigue [6,7]. A torsion overload mechanism corresponds to a static failure and occurs when a section of the file is locked within the canal, and the shank continues to rotate. In this static failure, the file fails because the stress value reaches the elastic limit of the material, and the file undergoes permanent deformations and finally it fractures. Flexural fatigue is a failure mechanism produced mainly by the alternating compressive and tensile stresses and strains that appear in any point of a file rotating inside a curved root canal. This fatigue failure results in a sudden fracture of the file after a certain number of rotations, even if the stress levels are far below the elastic limit of the material due to the nucleation and progression of small cracks in some stressed sections of the file. The typical number of cycles to failure (NCF) is between some hundreds to several thousands [8]. This is equivalent to an expected life below some few minutes if a typical speed of rotation of 300 rpm is considered.

There is no definitive conclusion about which is the predominant mechanism of failure in the clinical practice [6]. Satappan et al. [9] indicated a higher prevalence of torsional fracture (55.7%) than flexural fatigue (44.3%). However, Peng et al. [10] and Wei et al. [11] observed the opposite, with a clear preponderance of flexural fatigue. Notwithstanding, flexural fatigue seems to be the main concern for clinicians, because there is no easy method to avoid or anticipate this failure [7], resulting in a common practice of discarding the files after a certain number of uses to prevent it. However, there is no clear rule about the recommended number of uses, mainly due to the variety of factors potentially affecting NCF, such as root canal anatomy, file geometry or the operator's experience, among others [12]. Therefore, a better understanding of the independent and combined effect of the different parameters on the flexural fatigue failure mechanism is desirable and additional research should be addressed to this end.

Experimental and simulated approaches have been used in the literature to analyse the effect of clinical and design parameters on the expected life of NiTi rotary files. Experimental approach has been mainly tackled by using in vitro studies in order to improve reproducibility. In general, those studies make the file rotate inside a curved path, reproducing the root canal geometry and registering NCF [6]. However, the differences among previous studies in the methodology and the setup used to bend the file hamper the comparability of results and limit their clinical relevance [6,12]. Due to this, a call for an international standard on the cyclic fatigue testing of rotary endodontic instruments is recurrent in the literature [6,13]. Despite these difficulties, the results from previous experimental studies on experimental fatigue tests on NiTi wires, or directly on endodontic files, have allowed drawing some conclusions about the fatigue behaviour of NiTi:

- The strain–life relationship is similar to that observed in low-cycle fatigue for metals, with a decrease in NCF for higher strain amplitudes, corresponding to highly curved canals [14].
- The fatigue life increases for files with a higher fraction of martensite, both by initial composition of the material or induced by phase transformation under deformation [15,16].
- The oral temperature and other parameters affecting the file temperature, such as rotational speed, can change the expected life, because they influence the phase fractions present in different points of the file in clinical use [17–19].
- Apart from the 'structural fatigue' resulting in the final fracture, NiTi exhibits 'functional fatigue', a significant and asymptotic change in the stress–strain curve and the phase transformation stresses during the first 100–140 cycles, resulting in a reduction in hysteresis cycle area and an increase in residual permanent strains after cycling [20].

These previous experimental studies have shown that, under constant value for other parameters, strain amplitude and NCF for NiTi wires are correlated, and this correlation can be adequately represented by the Coffin–Manson relation [14,16,20].

The simulated approach for analysing flexural fatigue has been mainly undertaken through the use of finite element (FE) models. FE analysis is a mathematical technique that can be used for predicting the state of stress and strain in a body or group of bodies under applied external loads and constraints. It is based on a fine discretisation of the geometry of bodies in a high number of small finite elements. This method allows gaining some insight into the stress and strain distributions inside the file, helping gain a better understanding of the failure mechanism. A recent study made a critical review of the use of this method applied to NiTi endodontic instruments [21] and highlighted some of the main limitations of the analyses performed to date. According to this study, very few studies modelled cyclic fatigue using FE simulation. The authors cited those of Lee et al. [8], Scattina et al. [7] and Ha et al. [22].

In [8] the authors performed a simulation of four different file models on three root canal geometries with different curvature and compared the results with those obtained from in vitro tests on equivalent systems. In the FE model, the file was rotated inside the simulated FE model of the root canal, and the maximum von Mises stress on the file nodes was analysed. They found that the location of the maximum von Mises stress in the FE model is a good predictor of the fractured section observed experimentally. Additionally, they confirmed a negative correlation between the maximum von Mises stress in the file and the NCF. The authors cited computational problems that forced them to reduce the rotational speed to 240 rpm and to consider a friction coefficient of 0.01 in order to avoid nodal binding. The non-linear behaviour of the material was considered by using data from [23], which did not include the lower plateau in the stress–strain curve characteristic of the phase transformation for the unloading path, which corresponds to a lower stress level than that observed for the loading phase.

Scattina et al. [7] tried to predict NCF using FE simulations. They compared in vitro tests and FE simulations for three file models on a single root canal geometry. The model considered the contact between the file and the root canal, represented with rigid shell elements, and the simulation included the rotation of the file and the analysis of the stress state every 0.2 s during 2 s at a rotation speed of 300 rpm. The authors used a multiaxial random fatigue criterion [24] to predict the NCF based on the stress history. They tuned the material properties with an optimisation procedure to match NCF predictions with experimental results on two of the file models and used these properties to predict NCF for the third model, finding a good agreement with experiments in both NCF and fracture location. However, the paper neither cited the final material parameters obtained from this optimisation nor the specific parameters considered.

In [22], the authors used FE simulation to develop a new file model intermediate between G-1 and G-2 models (Dentsply Maillefer, Ballaigues, Switzerland), but in this case the FE model did not include a fatigue simulation.

Cheung et al. [25] also performed an FE based fatigue analysis for comparing two different cross section geometries for the file, NiTi and steel based on a fully reversed bending analysis without including the root canal in the model. They applied the Coffin–Manson equation for predicting NCF.

The objective of the present study is to contribute to a better understanding of the effect of root canal geometry on the expected life of NiTi rotary files using FE simulation. To our knowledge, only Lee et al. [8] attempted a similar study, but they only considered three canal geometries with a different curvature, without changing the length of the straight part at the entrance of the root canal. Moreover, they based their analysis on the von Mises stress instead of analysing strain, which is the relevant parameter for predicting the fatigue life for low-cycle fatigue, according to the Coffin–Manson relation [25]. They also used a constitutive material model that did not include the hysteresis cycle formed in the stress–strain cycle due to the different stress levels corresponding to the phase transformation during loading and unloading.

In the present study, we used transient FE simulation for analysing the fatigue behaviour of a NiTi endodontic file with two different pitch values on a greater variety of root canal geometries, with changes in both the angle between the initial part and the apical part of the root and the radius of curvature in the connection between both sections. The model also includes a more comprehensive constitutive model for NiTi material and a very detailed discretisation of the file into quadratic finite elements. It simulates the introduction of the file into the canal and its rotation, including contact and friction. With this model, we calculated the strain range during a cycle for each point of the file. We used the Coffin–Manson relation to predict the expected NCF of the file in each root canal geometry.

2. Materials and Methods

The present investigation was conducted by using finite element analysis of a set of cases of study in which several combinations of endodontic rotary files and root canal geometries were studied.

Two different geometries of endodontic rotary file were considered, which are denoted as P2 (Figure 1a) and P3 (Figure 1b). Both of them have a convex ProTaper cross section shown in Figure 1c, their total length being $L_{total} = 25$ mm, the length of their active part is $L_{ap} = 16$ mm and the diameter of their shaft and their tip is $d_{sh} = 1.20$ mm and $d_{ap} = 0.25$ mm, respectively. The only difference between P2 and P3 resides in their axial pitch: $p_z = 2$ mm for P2 and $p_z = 3$ mm for P3.

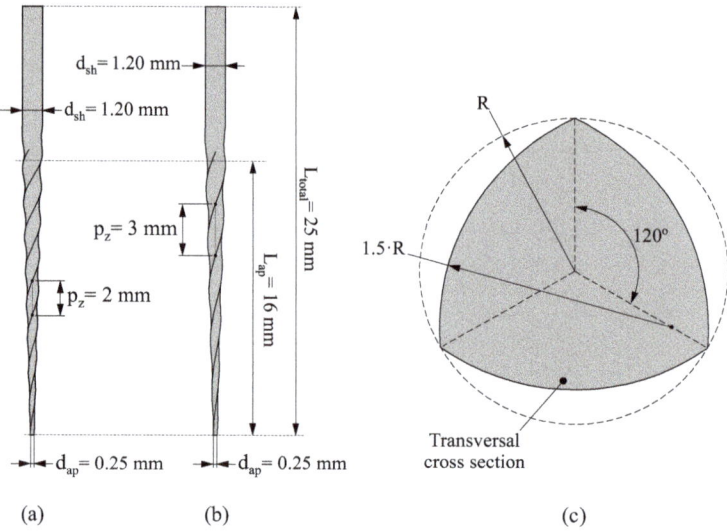

Figure 1. Geometry of the endodontic files P2 (**a**) and P3 (**b**) and normalised transversal cross section for both of them (**c**).

On the other hand, the geometry of the root canal was constructed as follows (Figure 2):

1. Segment AB has a length of $AB_{RC} = 10$ mm, and it is perpendicular to the external surface, as indicated in Figure 2a. Line L_1 passes through point B, and it is inclined at angle θ_{RC} with respect to segment AB.
2. A fillet, for which its radius is given by r_{RC}, is defined between segment AB and line L_1, as illustrated in Figure 2b. The tangency points of the fillet with the existing segments are denoted by D and E.
3. Point F is located over line L_1 in such a manner that the total length from point A to point F is $L_{RC} = 16$ mm. By performing this, the entire active part of the endodontic rotary files can be inserted within the canal. The resulting curve ADEF is the neutral axis of the root canal.
4. Finally, a conic surface is created by sweeping a circumference along the neutral axis of the root canal, as illustrated in Figure 2c. At the entrance of the canal, the diameter of this circumference is $D_{RC} = 1.26$ mm, and at the end of the canal it is $d_{RC} = 0.26$ mm.

The resulting geometry of the root canal depends on two parameters: the angle of curvature θ_{RC} and the radius of curvature r_{RC}, according to the method proposed by Pruett [26]. The variation of these parameters allows us to consider different geometries for the root canal. In this study, three different values for the angle of curvature $\theta_{RC} = [30°, 45°, 60°]$ and three different radii of curvature $r_{RC} = [5 \text{ mm}, 10 \text{ mm}, 15 \text{ mm}]$

were considered. Combining these variables, 9 different geometries of the root canal were obtained, which are shown in Figure 3 (denoted as RC1, RC2, ..., RC9).

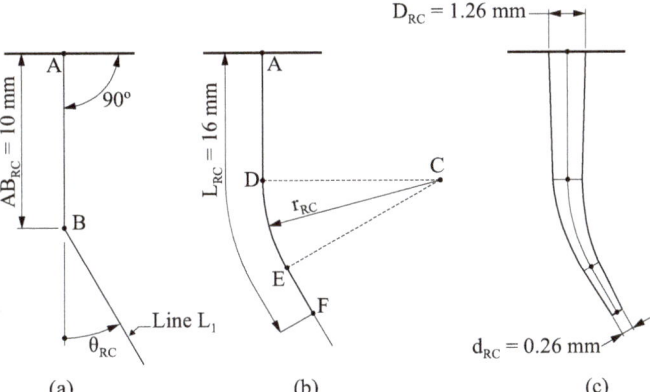

Figure 2. Parametrisation of the geometry of the root canal: (a) definition of the segment AB_{RC} and line L_1, (b) definition of the fillet and (c) definition of the root canal surface.

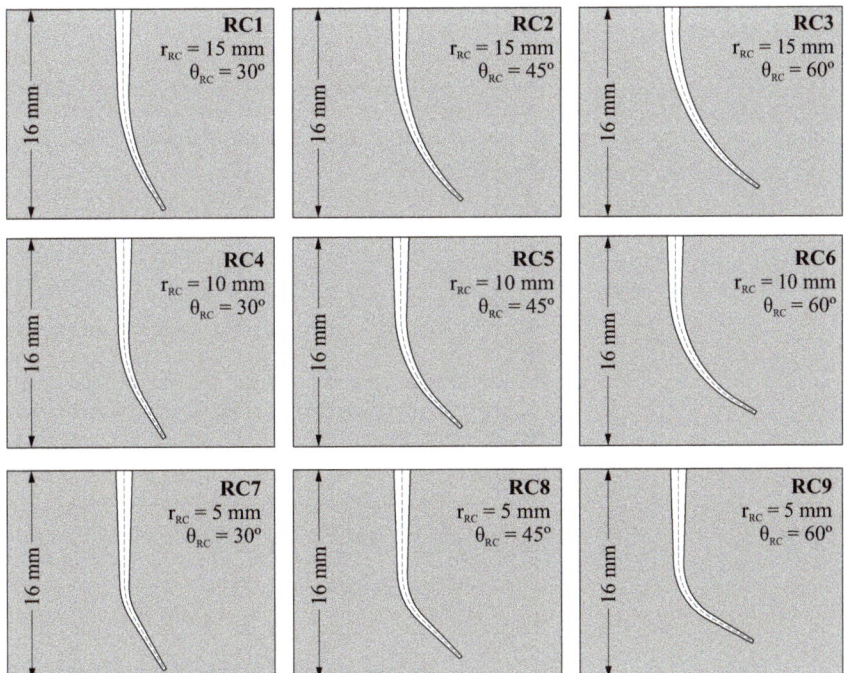

Figure 3. Geometries of root canal considered for the study.

2.1. Definition of the Finite Element Model

Figure 4 shows the finite element model used in this study, which consists of an endodontic rotary file and a root canal. The root canal is modelled as a rigid surface under the assumption that its deformations are so small compared to the deformations of the endodontic rotary file that they can be neglected. The root canal remains immovable during the analysis.

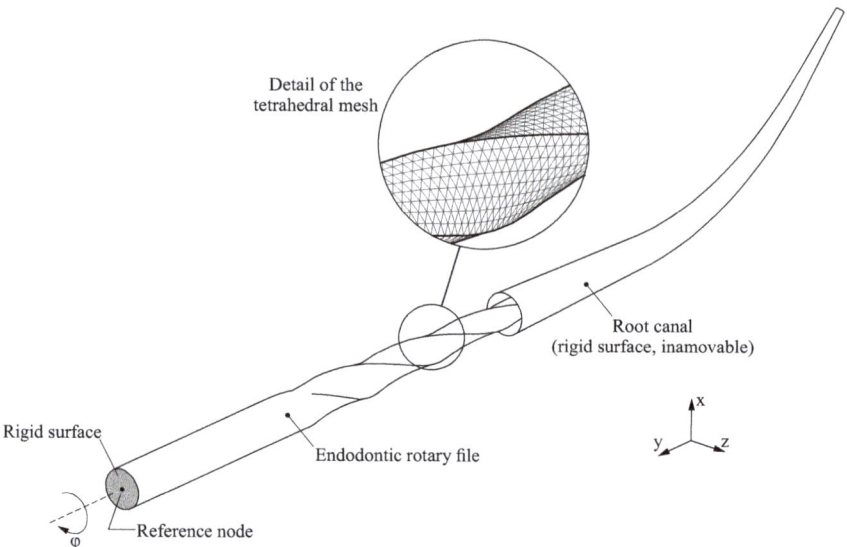

Figure 4. Definition of the finite element model.

The geometry of the endodontic file is generated and then discretised into quadratic finite element tetrahedrons following the ideas provided in [27]. The average element size has been set to 0.1 mm, which has proven to provide a good compromise between accuracy and computational cost. The resulting finite element model has 103,609 nodes and 68,367 elements.

The top surface of the endodontic rotary file is defined as a rigid surface (shaded in grey in Figure 4), and its movements are coupled to the movements of a reference node that is used to define the boundary conditions of the endodontic rotary file.

The superelastic behaviour of the NiTi alloy was modelled by using the material model developed by Auricchio [28], which is summarized in Figure 5. Here, E_A and E_M represent the Young's modulus of austenite and martensite, respectively. The beginning and the end of the loading transformation phase are given by σ_L^S and σ_L^E, respectively, whereas the beginning and the end of the unloading transformation phase are given by σ_U^S and σ_U^E. Finally, ε_L represents the uniaxial transformation strain, and σ_{ME}^E indicates the end of the martensitic elastic regime. In this work, the material properties that characterise this material model were extracted from [29].

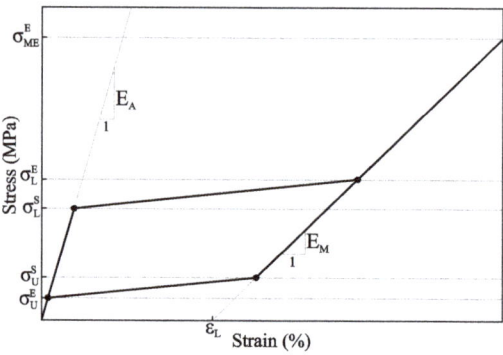

Figure 5. Definition of the stress–strain curve for the constitutive model of the superelastic NiTi alloy.

The mechanical interaction between the root canal and the endodontic rotary file was considered by using a node-to-surface contact. A penalty-based constraint enforcement method was selected in order to enhance the convergency of the numerical solution. The tangential behaviour of the contact was also taken into account in the finite element model, with a constant coefficient of friction $\mu = 0.1$ [30].

The finite element model was solved by using transient analysis, which was conducted by using a large displacement formulation, and performed in two sequential steps:

1. Insertion step: In the first step, the endodontic rotary file is inserted into the root canal. This is performed by prescribing a displacement at its reference node, which takes place along the y axis and has a magnitude equal to the length of the active part of the endodontic rotary file (L_{ap}). The rest of the movements of the reference node (displacements in x and y directions and all the rotations) are restricted in this step.
2. Rotation step: In the second step, after the active part of the endodontic rotary file is inserted in the root canal, the endodontic rotary file performs a complete revolution along its axis of rotation. This is performed by prescribing a 360° rotation along the y axis, while the rest of the movements of the reference node are restricted (rotations along x and z axes and all the displacements). The rotated angle is denoted by φ.

2.2. Fatigue Life Estimation from the Results of the Finite Element Analysis

The objective of this study was to predict the fatigue life of NiTi rotary files as they are rotating inside the root canal. For such a purpose, the strain results obtained from the rotation step of the finite element analysis were used in combination with the Coffin–Manson relation. This relation is conveniently expressed by the following equation:

$$\frac{\Delta\varepsilon}{2} = \varepsilon'_F \cdot N_f^c + \frac{\sigma'_F}{E} \cdot N_f^b \quad (1)$$

where N_f is equivalent to NCF, ε'_F is the fatigue ductility coefficient, σ'_F is the fatigue strength coefficient, c is the fatigue ductility exponent, b is the fatigue strength exponent, $\Delta\varepsilon$ is the total strain range and $\Delta\varepsilon/2$ is the strain amplitude. The prime in the equation indicates that the properties correspond to the cyclic properties, i.e., those after the initial 100–140 cycles.

In this equation, the first addend of the right side corresponds to the plastic strain amplitude $\Delta\varepsilon_p/2$ and the second one to the elastic strain amplitude $\Delta\varepsilon_e/2$. Figure 6 shows a logarithmic plot of the Equation (1), showing the contribution of these two terms, with the parameters for NiTi used in the present study, taken from [25]. The exponents b and c in the equation are negative, because the number of cycles correlates negatively with the strain amplitude. For high strain amplitudes, the plastic strain is much higher than the elastic strain, and the number of cycles to failure is low (low-cycle fatigue, LCF); for very low strain amplitudes, the second term of the equation is dominant because there is no significant plastic strain, and the number of cycles to failure is high (high-cycle fatigue, HCF). The transition between LCF and HCF can be observed as a change in the slope of the curve, which is typically located close to 10^3–10^4 cycles.

Since the Coffin–Manson relation is based on a uniaxial strain, a criterion to reduce the obtained multiaxial strain state to an equivalent uniaxial strain condition is required. The critical plane concept has been extensively used for such a purpose, with successful results both for high and low cycle fatigue [31]. In the critical plane approach, the assessment of the fatigue failure is carried out in the material plane where the amplitude of some stress/strain components (or a combination of them) exhibits a maximum [24]. In the discretised finite element model of the endodontic rotary file, each node i on the surface will have an associated critical plane Π_i characterised by its normal direction $\vec{n}_i$.

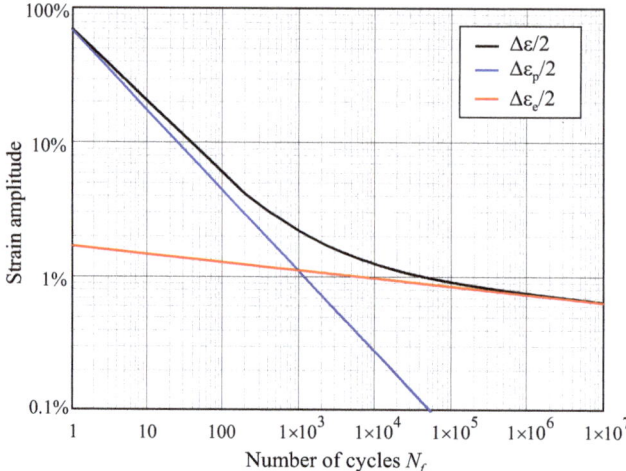

Figure 6. Coffin–Manson relation between strain amplitude and number of cycles to failure (NCF). Parameters for NiTi from [25]: $\varepsilon'_F = 0.68$, $\sigma'_F = 705$ MPa, $E = 42.5$ GPa, $c = -0.6$, $b = -0.06$.

In this study, the critical plane Π_i was defined in such a manner that its normal direction $\vec{n}_i$ is parallel to the direction of the maximum principal strain produced in node i, when the amplitude of this maximum principal strain reaches its maximum value. The direction $\vec{n}_i$ could be determined by observing the maximum principal strain at each frame of the analysis. However, in order to speed up the calculations, in this study it will be assumed that this maximum principal strain is normal to the plane that contains the trajectory of the observed node, as illustrated in Figure 7. Hence, $\vec{n}_i$ will be normal to the plane of rotation of node i.

After the critical plane Π_i is determined for node i, a bending strain value $\varepsilon_{i,j}$ can be then obtained for that node at each analysis frame j by transforming the strain tensor and selecting the strain component in the direction of $\vec{n}_i$. Finally, the total strain range $\Delta\varepsilon_i$ for node i is defined as follows.

$$\Delta\varepsilon_i = \max_{j=1\ldots n}\left(\varepsilon_{i,j}\right) - \min_{j=1\ldots n}\left(\varepsilon_{i,j}\right) \quad (2)$$

This total strain range $\Delta\varepsilon_i$ can be used in the Coffin–Manson relation to assess the fatigue life associated to node i. The material parameters considered for the application of the Coffin–Manson relation were extracted from [25].

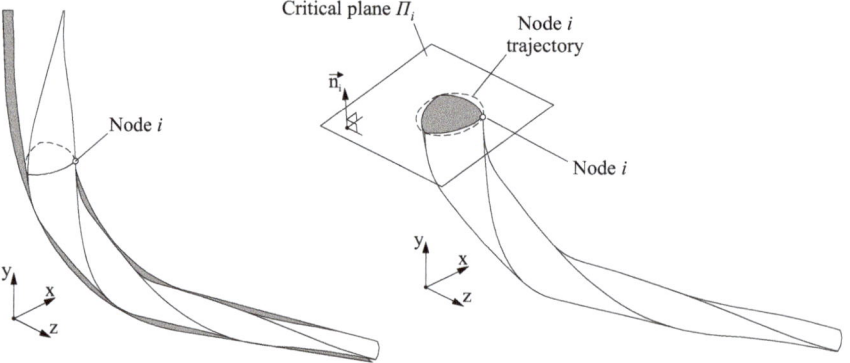

Figure 7. Determination of the critical plane and bending strain for node i.

The fatigue life of the endodontic rotary file was defined by the minimum value of fatigue life considering all the nodes in the surface of the endodontic rotary file. The node where $\Delta\varepsilon_i$ reaches a maximum value is the critical node, and it is denoted as $i = crit$.

3. Results

Figure 8 shows the strain results for endodontic rotary files P2 and P3 when they are rotating inside the most curved root canal RC9. Figure 8a shows the maximum principal strain plot for the case of study P2/RC9 in the instant of the rotation step of the analysis where the bending strain at the critical node reaches its maximum value. Figure 8b shows the minimum principal strain plot, for the same case of study, in the instant of the rotation step of the analysis where the bending strain at the critical node reaches its minimum value. The figure also shows the location of the critical node in both instants of time, as well as the critical plane for such a node. Figure 8c,d show the equivalent results for case P3/RC9 in which the file has a different pitch. The highest strains, both in tension and compression, are located at the edge in the surface of the file.

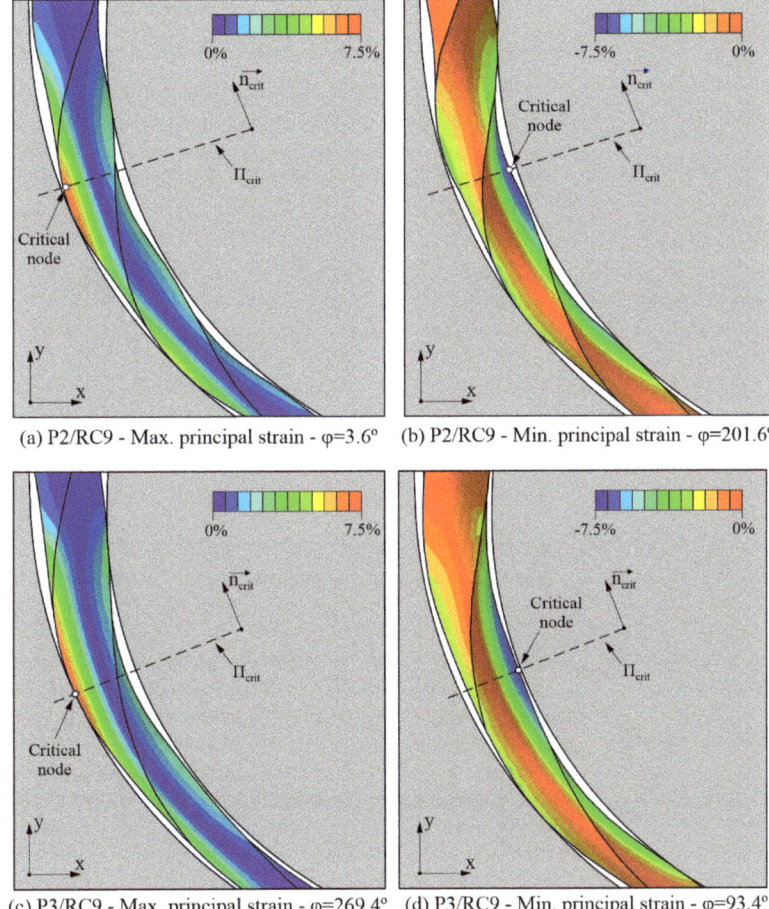

(a) P2/RC9 - Max. principal strain - φ=3.6° (b) P2/RC9 - Min. principal strain - φ=201.6°

(c) P3/RC9 - Max. principal strain - φ=269.4° (d) P3/RC9 - Min. principal strain - φ=93.4°

Figure 8. Principal strains in two different analysis frames for cases of study P2/RC9 and P3/RC9.

The evolution of the bending strain and the maximum and minimum principal strains during an entire rotation of the file are shown in Figure 9 for P2/RC9 and P3/RC9, reflecting a similar pattern for both files, but with a slightly higher strain range for the file with pitch 3 mm. The phase shift is due to a different orientation of the edges of the file in the critical plane. The points marked with a star correspond to the frames of maximum and minimum bending strain values, shown in Figure 8.

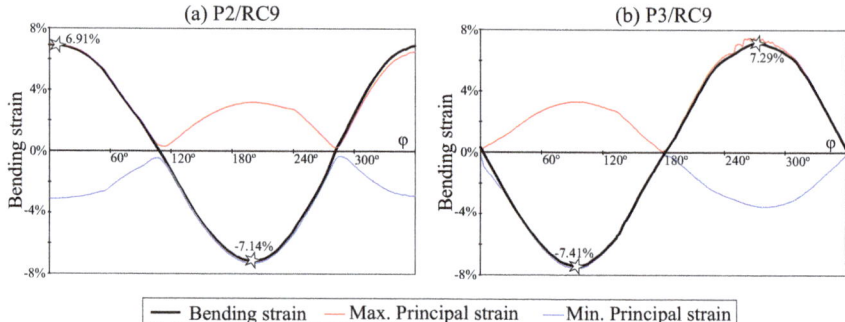

Figure 9. Strain history at critical nodes of cases of study P2/RC9 (**a**) and P3/RC9 (**b**).

The strain ranges obtained for all the studied cases are summarised in Figure 10. In these plots, the horizontal axis indicates the angle of curvature of the root canal and the vertical axis indicates the radius of curvature. The black dots indicate the combinations of radius and angle of curvature that have been studied, and the isolines are interpolated from these results.

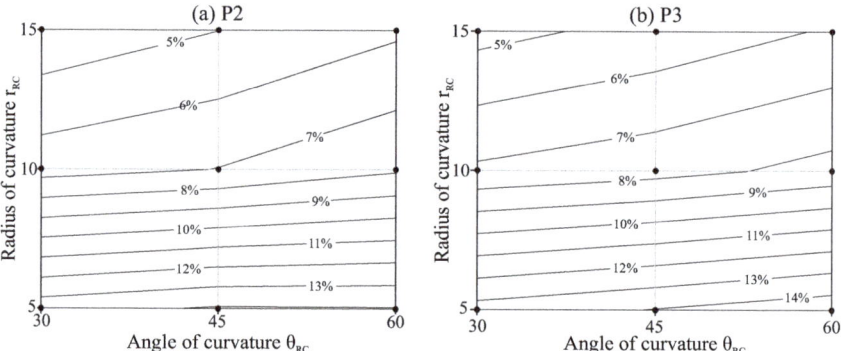

Figure 10. Maximum bending strain range as a function of the geometry of the root canal. (**a**) P2 and (**b**) P3.

Figure 11 shows the expected life for each file as a function of the radius and the angle of curvature of the root canal, calculated as indicated in Section 2.2, also with interpolated isolines.

The results in Figures 10 and 11 indicate that root canals with higher curvatures (higher angles of curvature or/and smaller radii of curvature) force the files to a higher strain range and reduce their fatigue life. The effect of the angle of curvature is less significant for smaller radii of curvature, as indicated by the lower inclination of the isolines in the bottom of the figures. The file with pitch 3 mm (P3) showed higher strain and shorter fatigue life as compared with that of pitch 2 mm (P2), but this effect is slight, especially for less curved canals.

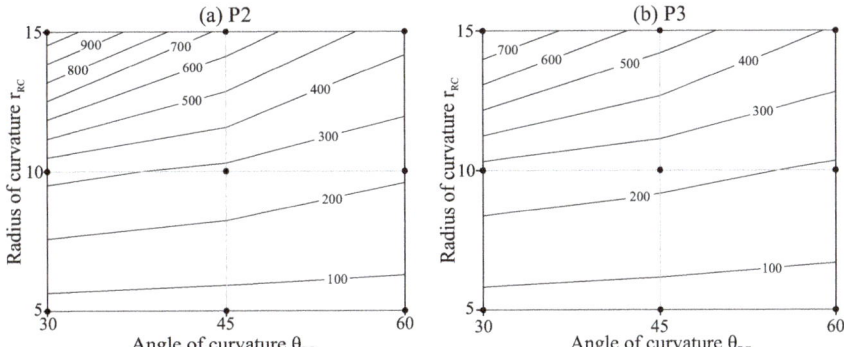

Figure 11. Expected life in number of fatigue cycles N_f as a function of the geometry of the root canal. (**a**) P2 and (**b**) P3.

Finally, Figure 12 summarizes the effect of the degree of insertion of the endodontic rotary file inside the root canal for the case of study P2/RC9. Here, the degree of insertion of the rotary file inside the root canal is expressed as the percentage of the active part that is inserted. Figure 12a shows the evolution of the bending strain at the critical node during a entire revolution of the file for different degrees of insertion of the file inside the root canal (70%, 85% and 100%).

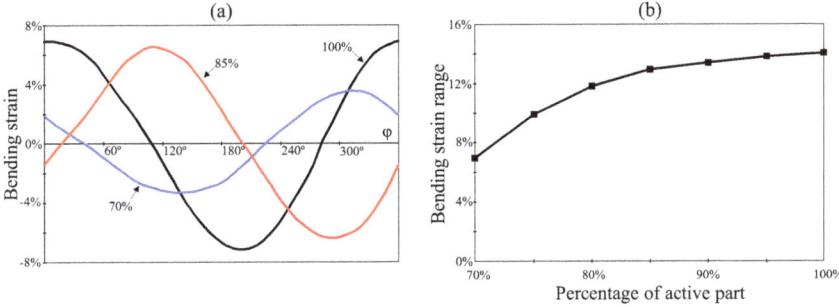

Figure 12. Effect of the degree of insertion of the endodontic file within the root canal. (**a**) Bending strain history at critical nodes and (**b**) bending strain range as a function of the degree of insertion.

Figure 12b shows the evolution of the bending strain range with the degree of insertion of the endodontic rotary file inside the root canal. Here, additional data points are considered for a better observation of the evolution of this magnitude. This figure shows that the bending strain range is reduced as the degree of insertion of the endodontic rotary file inside the root canal is decreased.

4. Discussion

This study analysed numerically the effect of the root canal geometry on the bending fatigue life of NiTi rotary instruments. Some previous studies have shown the predictive capacity of this simulated approach based on the use of FE models to predict the location of the file fracture [7,8]. However, a recent review highlighted some limitations introduced in previous FE studies in this field, especially in the representation of the boundary conditions, the accuracy of the mesh to represent the real file geometry or the lack of consideration of friction in the FE analysis [21]. Our investigation solved these main limitations, with a very accurate mesh of quadratic elements for the file, and undertook a transient non-linear simulation of the introduction of the file inside the root canal and its rotation inside the canal, including contact and friction simulation. We also used the Coffin–Manson relation to estimate the expected life for the file working on a representative set of root canal geometries, proposing an adequate methodology for translating FE results to clinically relevant variables, which can be useful for manufacturers of NiTi rotary instruments.

Our results confirm that more curved canals are prone to reduce fatigue life, which was also previously observed in several in vitro studies [5,8,14]. We also found that the radius of curvature of the canal has a higher effect than the angle between the shaft and the apical portion of the file, especially for the lower radii of curvature. Changing the radius of curvature from 15 mm to 5 mm multiplies the strain amplitude by a factor of close to three for curvature angles of 30° and by a factor close to 2.5 for curvature angles of 60°. Due to the logarithmic relationship between strain and NCF, this effect is higher in the expected life, which is reduced by a factor close to ten for 30° of curvature angle and by a factor six for 60°. This result is in agreement with the experimental study by Chi et al. [5], although their setup was different because the curved part of the file reached the apical end for all conditions.

In most of the experimental studies, NCF is represented against a theoretical bending strain value obtained from geometrical approximations of the radius of curvature of the file and its diameter at the failure section using Equation (3) [14,16,17]:

$$\varepsilon_a = \frac{d}{2R} \quad (3)$$

where d is the file diameter, and R is the approximate radius of curvature of the file. Thus, the higher effect of the radius of curvature is expected from a theoretical point of view, because the ideal strain amplitude in bending is defined by Equation (3), depending only on the diameter of the file and the radius of curvature. However, the angle between the entrance and the apical portion of the root canal and also the clearance between the file and the canal walls affect the actual deformation of the file, which can be different to that defined by the geometrical approximation indicated by Equation (3), as observed in Figure 8. This would explain the effect observed for the angle of curvature.

The difference in strain amplitude and fatigue life for the files with pitch 2 mm and 3 mm is limited, with a slightly higher fatigue life for P2 and more pronounced for less curved root canals. Ha et al. [30] also observed lower stresses for closer pitch when analysing the screw-in tendency of NiTi rotary files with a transient FE model.

In Figure 12, we also studied the effect that the degree of insertion of the rotary file has on bending strain range. We observed that the bending strain range at the critical node decreases with a reduction in the degree of insertion. According to the Coffin–Manson relation, this increases the fatigue life of the rotary file. This reduction in the bending strain range could be explained because the diameter d of the rotary file at the curved part of the root canal is smaller with partial insertion and, according to Equation (3), this results in a reduction in the bending strain. Additionally, the greater clearance between the rotary file and root canal implies that the effective curvature radius of the file is higher than that of the root canal. Again, according to Equation (3), this implies an additional contribution to the reduction in bending strain range.

In this study, we based the analysis of file behaviour on the strain values observed, as recommended for LCF with significant strain values and fatigue life below some thousands of cycles [25]. We also proposed a method for calculating the strain amplitude during the cyclic rotation of the file, based on the use of a critical plane defining the direction of the maximum and minimum principal strains in the critical points. The results shown in Figure 9 reveal that the method proposed here for defining the critical plane is correct, because when the bending strain reaches its maximum and minimum points, its values coincide with the maximum and minimum principal strains, respectively.

This study has some limitations. We only considered a geometry of the file section, with a constant taper and pitch through its length. We also limited the analysis to root canals for which its geometrical axis can be represented by a planar curve. Moreover, despite our work trying to be as representative as possible of the clinical situation of the file rotating inside the root canal, some possible improvements remain and are commented in the following paragraphs. They can be observed as challenges for future studies trying to improve the accuracy of the model.

The material model used in this study is non-linear and included the phase transformation plateaus in the stress–strain curve and the different Young's modulus of martensite and austenite. However, heat dissipated due to the hysteresis loop in the loading–unloading curve, and heat generated by sliding friction between the file and the canal can also induce phase transformations from martensite to austenite due to the shape memory effect of the material, adding a complex thermal–mechanical coupling that is not considered here. On the other hand, we have made estimations of the fatigue life based on the Coffin–Manson equation, but the fatigue ductility coefficient and fatigue ductility exponent were taken from the literature. We have not considered the effect of the phase transformations between austenite and martensite on fatigue response and, hence, on these parameters. Previous studies have shown that higher strains did not necessarily imply less cycles to failure, because a higher fraction of martensite results in a better response under cyclic loads [16]. To our knowledge, there is no clear approach for the moment to include this effect in the FE simulations.

In this study, we considered a transient simulation, but this simulation does not include the dynamical effects, which are dependent on the rotational speed of the file. Moreover, our model included normal and shear contact between the file and root canal walls, but these walls are simplified as rigid elements. Considering the dentine properties for the walls would be necessary for estimating the risk of canal transportation or ledging.

We have proposed a method for dealing with the multiaxial strain state in order to predict fatigue life, but the fatigue phenomenon in shape memory alloys is still under investigation [32], and there is no clearly established fatigue criterion for analysing multiaxial fatigue in those materials [7,32].

In addition, since the first introduction of NiTi rotary instruments in the last decade of the twentieth century, several changes have been introduced to new families of files in terms of composition, manufacturing methods and thermomechanical treatments, which is not always publicly known, affecting greatly the percentage of martensite or austenite present in the file in clinical use and also the fatigue life of instruments [15,33].

5. Conclusions

This numerical study confirms that the geometry of the root canal affects the fatigue life of rotary NiTi instruments. More curved root geometries, either by a higher inclination of the apical part of the canal with respect to the initial part at the entrance or by a lower radius of curvature, result in higher strain amplitudes in the file surface and to lower fatigue life. The radius of curvature in the curves of the root canal has a greater effect than the angle of curvature. Changes in the radius of curvature from 15 mm to 5 mm in the root canal can reduce fatigue life by factors close to ten. A change in the file pitch between 2 mm and 3 mm does not have an important effect on the fatigue life for the root canal geometries analysed, although the higher pitch exhibited a slightly lower life for root canals with low curvature. The degree of insertion of the file inside the root canal significantly affects the strain range obtained in the critical point of the file, and the strain range is reduced when the file is partially inserted within the file.

Author Contributions: Conceptualization, A.P.-G. and V.R.-C.; methodology, A.P.-G. and V.R.-C.; software, V.R.-C.; investigation, A.P.-G. and V.R.-C.; resources, Á.Z.-M. and V.F.-M.; writing—original draft preparation, A.P.-G.; writing—review and editing, V.R.-C.; supervision, Á.Z.-M. and V.F.-M.; project administration, Á.Z.-M. and V.F.-M. All authors have read and agreed to the published version of the manuscript.

Funding: This research received no external funding.

Institutional Review Board Statement: Not applicable.

Informed Consent Statement: Not applicable.

Conflicts of Interest: The authors declare no conflicts of interest.

References

1. Bürklein, S.; Schäfer, E. Critical evaluation of root canal transportation by instrumentation. *Endod. Top.* **2013**, *29*, 110–124. [CrossRef]
2. Iandolo, A.; Amato, A.; Martina, S.; Latif, D.A.; Pantaleo, G. Management of severe curvatures in root canal treatment with the new generation of rotating files using a safe and predictable protocol. *Open Dent. J.* **2020**, *14*, 421–425. [CrossRef]
3. Iandolo, A.; Abdellatif, D.; Pantaleo, G.; Sammartino, P.; Amato, A. Conservative shaping combined with three-dimensional cleaning can be a powerful tool: Case series. *J. Conserv. Dent.* **2020**, *23*, 648–652. [CrossRef]
4. Kuzekanani, M. Nickel-titanium rotary instruments: Development of the single-file systems. *J. Int. Soc. Prev. Community Dent.* **2018**, *8*, 386–390. [CrossRef]
5. Chi, C.W.; Li, C.C.; Lin, C.P.; Shin, C.S. Cyclic fatigue behavior of nickel–titanium dental rotary files in clinical simulated root canals. *J. Formos. Med. Assoc.* **2017**, *116*, 306–312. [CrossRef] [PubMed]
6. Plotino, G.; Grande, N.M.; Cordaro, M.; Testarelli, L.; Gambarini, G. A Review of Cyclic Fatigue Testing of Nickel-Titanium Rotary Instruments. *J. Endod.* **2009**, *35*, 1469–1476. [CrossRef]
7. Scattina, A.; Alovisi, M.; Paolino, D.S.; Pasqualini, D.; Scotti, N.; Chiandussi, G.; Berutti, E. Prediction of cyclic fatigue life of nickel-titanium rotary files by virtual modeling and finite elements analysis. *J. Endod.* **2015**, *41*, 1867–1870. [CrossRef]
8. Lee, M.H.; Versluis, A.; Kim, B.M.; Lee, C.J.; Hur, B.; Kim, H.C. Correlation between experimental cyclic fatigue resistance and numerical stress analysis for nickel-titanium rotary files. *J. Endod.* **2011**, *37*, 1152–1157. [CrossRef] [PubMed]
9. Sattapan, B.; Nervo, G.J.; Palamara, J.E.; Messer, H.H. Defects in rotary nickel-titanium files after clinical use. *J. Endod.* **2000**, *26*, 161–165. [CrossRef] [PubMed]
10. Peng, B.; Shen, Y.; Cheung, G.S.; Xia, T.J. Defects in ProTaper S1 instruments after clinical use: Longitudinal examination. *Int. Endod. J.* **2005**, *38*, 550–557. [CrossRef] [PubMed]
11. Wei, X.; Ling, J.; Jiang, J.; Huang, X.; Liu, L. Modes of Failure of ProTaper Nickel-Titanium Rotary Instruments after Clinical Use. *J. Endod.* **2007**, *33*, 276–279. [CrossRef]
12. McGuigan, M.B.; Louca, C.; Duncan, H.F. Endodontic instrument fracture: Causes and prevention. *Br. Dent. J.* **2013**, *214*, 341–348. [CrossRef] [PubMed]
13. Lo Savio, F.; Rosa, G.L.; Bonfanti, M.; Alizzio, D.; Rapisarda, E.; Pedullà, E. Novel Cyclic Fatigue Testing Machine for Endodontic Files. *Exp. Tech.* **2020**, *44*, 649–665. [CrossRef]
14. Cheung, G.S.; Darvell, B.W. Fatigue testing of a NiTi rotary instrument. Part 1: Strain-life relationship. *Int. Endod. J.* **2007**, *40*, 612–618. [CrossRef]
15. Tabassum, S.; Zafar, K.; Umer, F. Nickel-titanium rotary file systems: What's new? *Eur. Endod. J.* **2019**, *4*, 111–117. [CrossRef]
16. Figueiredo, A.M.; Modenesi, P.; Buono, V. Low-cycle fatigue life of superelastic NiTi wires. *Int. J. Fatigue* **2009**, *31*, 751–758. [CrossRef]
17. Eggeler, G.; Hornbogen, E.; Yawny, A.; Heckmann, A.; Wagner, M. Structural and functional fatigue of NiTi shape memory alloys. *Mater. Sci. Eng. A* **2004**, *378*, 24–33. [CrossRef]
18. Vilaverde Correia, S.; Nogueira, M.T.; Silva, R.J.C.; Pires Lopes, L.; Braz Fernandes, F.M. Phase Transformations in NiTi Endodontic Files and Fatigue Resistance. In *European Symposium on Martensitic Transformations*; EDP Sciences: Les Ulis, France, 2009; p. 07004. [CrossRef]
19. Dornelas Silva, J.; Lopes Buono, V.T. Effect of the initial phase constitution in the low-cycle fatigue of NiTi wires. *SN Appl. Sci.* **2019**, *1*, 1591. [CrossRef]
20. Maletta, C.; Sgambitterra, E.; Furgiuele, F.; Casati, R.; Tuissi, A. Fatigue properties of a pseudoelastic NiTi alloy: Strain ratcheting and hysteresis under cyclic tensile loading. *Int. J. Fatigue* **2014**, *66*, 78–85. [CrossRef]
21. Chien, P.Y.; Walsh, L.J.; Peters, O.A. Finite element analysis of rotary nickel-titanium endodontic instruments: A critical review of the methodology. *Eur. J. Oral Sci.* **2021**, *129*, e12802. [CrossRef]
22. Ha, J.H.; Lee, C.J.; Kwak, S.W.; El Abed, R.; Ha, D.; Kim, H.C. Geometric optimization for development of glide path preparation nickel-titanium rotary instrument. *J. Endod.* **2015**, *41*, 916–919. [CrossRef] [PubMed]
23. Xu, X.; Eng, M.; Zheng, Y.; Eng, D. Comparative study of torsional and bending properties for six models of nickel-titanium root canal instruments with different cross-sections. *J. Endod.* **2006**, *32*, 372–375. [CrossRef] [PubMed]
24. Carpinteri, A.; Spagnoli, A.; Vantadori, S.; Bagni, C. Structural integrity assessment of metallic components under multiaxial fatigue: The C-S criterion and its evolution. *Fatigue Fract. Eng. Mater. Struct.* **2013**, *36*, 870–883. [CrossRef]
25. Cheung, G.S.; Zhang, E.W.; Zheng, Y.F. A numerical method for predicting the bending fatigue life of NiTi and stainless steel root canal instruments. *Int. Endod. J.* **2011**, *44*, 357–361. [CrossRef] [PubMed]
26. Pruett, J.P.; Clement, D.J.; Carnes, D.L. Cyclic fatigue testing of nickel-titanium endodontic instruments. *J. Endod.* **1997**, *23*, 77–85. [CrossRef]
27. Roda-Casanova, V.; Zubizarreta-Macho, A.; Sanchez-Marin, F.; Alonso Ezpeleta, O.; Albaladejo Martinez, A.; Galparsoro Catalan, A. Computerized Generation and Finite Element Stress Analysis of Endodontic Rotary Files. *Appl. Sci.* **2021**, *11*, 4329. [CrossRef]
28. Auricchio, F.; Petrini, L. A three-dimensional model describing stress-temperature induced solid phase transformations: Solution algorithm and boundary value problems. *Int. J. Numer. Methods Eng.* **2004**, *61*, 807–836. [CrossRef]

29. de Arruda Santos, L.; López, J.B.; de Las Casas, E.B.; de Azevedo Bahia, M.G.; Buono, V.T.L. Mechanical behavior of three nickel-titanium rotary files: A comparison of numerical simulation with bending and torsion tests. *Mater. Sci. Eng. C* **2014**, *37*, 258–263. [CrossRef]
30. Ha, J.H.; Cheung, G.S.; Versluis, A.; Lee, C.J.; Kwak, S.W.; Kim, H.C. 'Screw-in' tendency of rotary nickel-titanium files due to design geometry. *Int. Endod. J.* **2015**, *48*, 666–672. [CrossRef]
31. Karolczuk, A.; Macha, E. Selection of the critical plane orientation in two-parameter multiaxial fatigue failure criterion under combined bending and torsion. *Eng. Fract. Mech.* **2008**, *75*, 389–403. [CrossRef]
32. Kang, G.; Song, D. Review on structural fatigue of NiTi shape memory alloys: Pure mechanical and thermo-mechanical ones. *Theor. Appl. Mech. Lett.* **2015**, *5*, 245–254. [CrossRef]
33. Gavini, G.; dos Santos, M.; Caldeira, C.L.; Machado, M.E.d.L.; Freire, L.G.; Iglecias, E.F.; Peters, O.A.; Candeiro, G.T.d.M. Nickel-titanium instruments in endodontics: A concise review of the state of the art. *Braz. Oral Res.* **2018**, *32*, e67. [CrossRef] [PubMed]

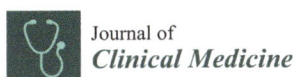

Article

The Effect of Ultrasonic Agitation on the Porosity Distribution in Apically Perforated Root Canals Filled with Different Bioceramic Materials and Techniques: A Micro-CT Assessment

Saulius Drukteinis [1,*], Goda Bilvinaite [1], Hagay Shemesh [2], Paulius Tusas [1] and Vytaute Peciuliene [1]

1. Institute of Dentistry, Faculty of Medicine, Vilnius University, Zalgirio 115, LT-08217 Vilnius, Lithuania; goda.bilvinaite@gmail.com (G.B.); paulius.tusas@gmail.com (P.T.); vytaute.peciuliene@mf.vu.lt (V.P.)
2. Academic Centre for Dentistry Amsterdam (ACTA), Gustav Mahlerlaan 3044, 1081 LA Amsterdam, The Netherlands; h.shemesh@acta.nl
* Correspondence: saulius.drukteinis@mf.vu.lt; Tel.: +370-610-41808

Abstract: The present study evaluated the effect of ultrasonic agitation on the porosity distribution of BioRoot RCS/single gutta-percha cone (BR/SC) and MTA Flow (MF) root canals fillings used as apical plugs in moderately curved and apically perforated roots. Eighty mesial root canals of mandibular first molars were enlarged up to ProTaper NEXT X5 rotary instrument 2 mm beyond the apical foramen, simulating apical perforations. Specimens were randomly divided into four experimental groups (20 canals per group) according to the material and technique used for root canal obturation: BR/SC, BR/SC with ultrasonic agitation (BR/SC-UA), MF and MF with ultrasonic agitation (MF-UA). The ultrasonic tip was passively inserted into the root canal after the injection of flowable cement and activated for 10 s. The specimens were scanned before and after obturation with a high-resolution micro-computed tomography scanner, and the porosity of the apical plugs was assessed. The differences between groups were analyzed using the Kruskal-Wallis and Mann-Whitney tests, with the significance level set at 5%. None of the obturation materials and techniques used in this study was able to provide a pore-free root canal filling in the apical 5 mm. Considerably higher percentages of open and closed pores were observed in the MF and MF-UA groups, with the highest porosity being in the MF-UA group ($p < 0.05$). No significant differences were observed between the BR/SC and BR/SC-UA groups, where the quantity of open and closed pores remained similar ($p > 0.05$).

Keywords: apical plug; BioRoot RCS; micro-computed tomography; MTA Flow; porosity; root perforation; single cone; ultrasonic

Citation: Drukteinis, S.; Bilvinaite, G.; Shemesh, H.; Tusas, P.; Peciuliene, V. The Effect of Ultrasonic Agitation on the Porosity Distribution in Apically Perforated Root Canals Filled with Different Bioceramic Materials and Techniques: A Micro-CT Assessment. *J. Clin. Med.* **2021**, *10*, 4977. https://doi.org/10.3390/jcm10214977

Academic Editors: Massimo Amato, Giuseppe Pantaleo and Alfredo Iandolo

Received: 4 October 2021
Accepted: 25 October 2021
Published: 27 October 2021

Publisher's Note: MDPI stays neutral with regard to jurisdictional claims in published maps and institutional affiliations.

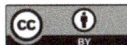

Copyright: © 2021 by the authors. Licensee MDPI, Basel, Switzerland. This article is an open access article distributed under the terms and conditions of the Creative Commons Attribution (CC BY) license (https:// creativecommons.org/licenses/by/ 4.0/).

1. Introduction

Root perforation is characterized as a communication between the root canal system and the surrounding periodontal tissues [1]. Perforations occurring due to dental caries or resorption are commonly defined as pathologic in nature [2], while iatrogenic perforations are usually related to inappropriate prosthodontic or endodontic treatment [3]. Up to 20% of endodontically treated teeth are diagnosed with root perforations, of which the majority are caused by various iatrogenic errors [4]. The most severe complication of root perforations is a persistent inflammation, breakdown of periodontal tissues and subsequent loss of bone attachment, ultimately leading to a tooth extraction [5]. Therefore, early diagnosis and appropriate perforation repair have a major influence on the long-term prognosis and survival of the affected tooth [4]. It is generally assumed that apical root perforation, which usually occurs because of endodontic instrumentation during the root canal preparation, has a good prognosis [6]. However, the management of apical root perforations frequently poses a challenge even for experienced endodontists, as visualization and direct access to the perforation site, especially in moderately or severely curved root canals, can be remarkably complicated, with a significant risk of collateral treatment mishaps, errors and complications [2].

The main goal of apical root perforation repair is to obtain a persistent bacteria-tight apical seal to prevent the percolation of fluids, microorganisms and their byproducts in the periapical tissues, allowing the healing and reorganization of damaged tissues [7]. Before the introduction of mineral trioxide aggregate (MTA), various dental materials, such as amalgam or glass ionomer cement, were used to repair root perforations. However, MTA instantly gained popularity due to its favorable biological, physical and chemical properties, which ensured an overall success rate of perforation repair of more than 80% [3,7]. Nevertheless, modifications of the original MTA formulation have been recently made to overcome its poor handling characteristics and long setting time [8]. MTA Flow (MF) (Ultradent Products Inc., South Jordan, UT, USA) is a relatively new MTA-based repair material, consisting of a di- and tri-calcium silicate grey powder and a water-soluble silicone-based gel [9]. MF was developed to give the clinician a variety of mixing options and consistencies, facilitating the manipulation and delivery of the material into the root canal [10]. Due to the extremely small particle size of less than 10μm, MF can be prepared in a thin consistency and delivered to the perforation site using a 29-G needle [11].

Although MTA-based materials have been widely used for root perforation repair since their first introduction [12], various investigations of hydraulic calcium silicate-based cements (HCSC) have shown that BioRoot RCS (Septodont, Saint-Maur-des-Fosses, France) could be effectively used as a filler and seal the apical root perforation as well [13]. BioRoot RCS possesses all the necessary antibacterial, biocompatible and bioactive properties, which promote the regeneration of periapical tissues and contribute to the recruitment of osteo-odontogenic stem cells within the apical environment [14]. Moreover, this material has the desirable dimensional stability and low solubility and provides high clinical success rates when used in conjunction with a single gutta-percha cone (SC) obturation technique [15–17]. In contrast to cold lateral compaction or various thermoplastic methods, the BioRoot RCS/single gutta-percha cone (BR/SC) obturation technique is clinically appealing due to its simplicity, as no superior clinical skills or any additional armamentarium and devices are needed [18]. However, the available data on the performance of the BR/SC technique used for an apical plug in apically perforated roots are still limited. There is only one study demonstrating the sealability of apical perforations using the BR/SC technique and porosity distribution in these fillings [19].

Ultrasonic devices have been successfully used in endodontics over the years for a wide range of clinical procedures, including root canal obturation [20,21]. It has been reported that ultrasonication of the sealers during the root canal filling procedure may increase their penetrability into the dentinal tubules and improve the interfacial adaptation between the filling material and the root canal wall [22,23]. Additionally, ultrasonic energy is capable of rearranging the material particles and removing the entrapped air and thus reducing the porosity [24,25]. Therefore, ultrasonic agitation has been recommended in order to improve the quality and homogeneity of root canal fillings [25,26]. However, most of the previous research has investigated the effect of ultrasonic agitation, applied to the sealers indirectly, and there are still no data available on the porosity distribution within the BR/SC and MF root canal fillings after the use of direct ultrasonication.

Micro-computed tomography (micro-CT) is a widely accepted non-destructive method to perform two-dimensional (2D) and three-dimensional (3D) assessments of root canal fillings using high-resolution images [27]. Micro-CT analysis, due to its high accuracy, can be used to determine the overall porosity of the fillings as well as to identify and quantify open and closed pores separately [28]. Therefore, the present study aimed to evaluate, by means of micro-CT analysis, the effect of direct ultrasonic agitation on the porosity distribution in BR/SC and MF root canal fillings used as apical plugs in artificially perforated and moderately curved roots of mandibular molars. The null hypothesis tested was that direct ultrasonic agitation significantly impacts the quality and homogeneity of BR/SC and MF apical plugs, decreasing their porosity.

2. Materials and Methods

2.1. Specimen Selection and Preparation

A total of 40 human mandibular first molars were selected for this study, under the approval of the local ethics committee (protocol no. EK-2). The minimum sample size was calculated using G*Power 3.1.9.7 software (Heinrich Heine, Iniversität Düsseldorf, Düsseldorf, Germany) followed by t-test family, α error probability of 0.05 and 1-β error probability of 0.95. Therefore, the requirement of 16 root canals per group was determined. Teeth were extracted for medical reasons unrelated to the present study and were stored in a saline solution at room temperature until use. Only molars with two separate mesial root canals, fully developed root apices and moderately curved roots (10°–20°) were selected. The root curvature was determined on preoperative radiographs using Shilder's method [29].

The orifices of root canals were accessed conventionally by preparing endodontic cavities with high-speed Endo Access burs (Dentsply Sirona, Ballaigues, Switzerland) under copious water-cooling. The presence of two separate mesial root canals was confirmed radiographically using the size 10 K-file (Dentsply Sirona, Ballaigues, Switzerland) inserted to the full working length (WL). The WL of both mesial canals was determined by inserting a size 10 K-file into the root canal until the tip approached the apical foramen and was visible under 10× magnification (OPMI Pico, Carl Zeiss, Oberkochen, Germany). Afterwards, the WL was increased by 2 mm to over-instrument the root canal and simulate apical perforation. All mesial canals were enlarged beyond the apical foramen. The glide path was created using size 15 and 20 K-Flexofiles (Dentsply Sirona, Ballaigues, Switzerland), and the root canal shaping was performed with ProTaper NEXT (Dentsply Sirona, Ballaigues, Switzerland) nickel-titanium rotary instruments at the established WL in the following sequence: X1 (17/0.04), X2 (25/0.06), X3 (30/0.07), X4 (40/0.06) and X5 (50/0.06). Instruments were driven using an X-Smart (Dentsply Sirona, Ballaigues, Switzerland) endodontic motor at the rotation speed of 300 rpm and the torque of 1 Ncm.

After the use of each instrument, root canals were repeatedly irrigated with 5 mL 3% sodium hypochlorite (Ultradent Products Inc., South Jordan, UT, USA), while 5 mL of 18% ethylenediaminetetraacetic acid (Ultradent Products Inc., South Jordan, UT, USA) followed by 5 mL of distilled water was used for the final flush at the end of instrumentation. The irrigants were delivered using 29-G NaviTip needles (Ultradent Products Inc., South Jordan, UT, USA) attached to disposable syringes. Afterwards, the root canals were dried with paper points.

The imitation of surrounding periodontal tissues and the alveolar bone was achieved using prefabricated A-silicone (3M ESPE, Seefeld, Germany) blocks. Specimens were fixed in these blocks up to the cement-enamel junction after the coverage of apices with a polytetrafluoroethylene tape (Tesa SE, Norderstedt, Germany).

2.2. Root Canal Obturation

A true randomness generator (www.random.org, accessed on 25 October 2021) was used for random allocation of the samples into four equal experimental groups (10 teeth/20 canals per group), according to the material and technique selected and used for root canal obturation:

- BR/SC group—the root canals were filled with BioRoot RCS sealer and single Pro-Taper NEXT size X5 gutta-percha point (Dentsply Sirona, Ballaigues, Switzerland). The apical 4 mm of the gutta-percha point was cut with a sterile scalpel to fit the gutta-percha with a tug-back effect at a length 2 mm shorter than the perforated apical foramen. The sealer was mixed according to the manufacturer's instructions, inserted into the Skini syringe (Ultradent Products Inc., South Jordan, UT, USA) and subsequently delivered into the root canal via attached plastic Capillary Tip cannula (Ultradent Products Inc., South Jordan, UT, USA). The tip was inserted approximately 2 mm shorter than the perforation site, and the plunger of the syringe was gently pressed while withdrawing the plastic cannula until reaching the orifice level. After the injection of BioRoot RCS, the pre-fitted gutta-percha point was coated with a thin amount of the sealer and gently inserted into the root canal 2 mm short of the perforated apex.

- BR/SC-UA group—the root canals were filled with BioRoot RCS sealer and single ProTaper NEXT size X5 gutta-percha point using ultrasonic agitation. The selection and adaptation of the gutta-percha point and the injection of the sealer were accomplished identically to the BR/SC group. After delivering the sealer into the root canal, an Ultrawave ET25 ultrasonic tip (Ultradent Products Inc., South Jordan, UT, USA) attached to an Ultrawave XS ultrasonic device (Ultradent Products Inc., South Jordan, UT, USA) was directly inserted into the root canal and BioRoot RCS sealer 2 mm short of the WL. The ultrasonic tip was activated for 10 s at the medium power using Reflex technology (Ultradent Products Inc.), capable of automatic real-time frequency adjustment of 28–36 kHz. The pre-fitted gutta-percha point was subsequently coated with a small amount of the sealer and slowly inserted into the root canal 2 mm shorter than the apical foramen.
- MF group—the root canals were filled with MTA Flow cement. A total of 0.19 g of powder and 3 drops of liquid were mixed according to the manufacturer's recommendations to get a thin consistency of the cement. The mixed material was inserted into the clear Skini syringe, and the flowability of the material was checked by extruding the small amount of the cement through the attached 29-G NaviTip needle. The filling material was delivered into the root canal by slowly pressing the plunger of the syringe and withdrawing the tip, which was inserted 2 mm short of the perforated apex.
- MF-UA group—the root canals were filled with MTA Flow cement using ultrasonic agitation. The filling material was prepared and injected into the root canal in the same manner as in the MF group. Afterwards, the Ultrawave ET25 ultrasonic tip was directly inserted into the root canal and MTA Flow cement 2 mm short of the perforation site and activated for 10 s at the 28–36 kHz frequency and the power described previously.

Postoperative radiographs were made immediately after the obturation of the root canals to evaluate the filling quality. The obturation procedure was repeated when a lack of homogeneity or inadequate filling length was observed. New radiographs were taken to confirm the quality of the root canal fillings afterwards. The heat carrier was used to cut the gutta-percha point at the orifice level in the BR/SC and BR/SC-UA groups. The endodontic access cavities of all specimens were sealed with temporary filling material Cavit™-W (3M ESPE, Seefeld, Germany), and the teeth were stored at 37 °C and 100% humidity for 7 days to allow the filling materials to set completely.

All specimens were prepared and obturated by a single operator: an experienced endodontist.

2.3. Micro-CT Analysis

Teeth were scanned before and after root canal obturation with a high-resolution micro-CT scanner SkyScan 1272 (Bruker, Kontich, Belgium). The scanning parameters were set at 100 kV source voltage, 100 µA beam current, 9.9 µm isotropic resolution, 0.11 mm copper filter, 1073 ms exposure time, 0.4° rotation step and 360° rotation angle. The obtained images were reconstructed using NRecon v.1.6.9.18 software (Bruker, Kontich, Belgium) under a beam hardening correction of 20% and a ring artefact reduction factor of 6.

The CTAn v.1.14.4.1 software (Bruker, Kontich, Belgium) was used to analyze the quality of root canal fillings in the apical 5 mm. All grayscale images from the selected region of interest were converted to binary images using a global threshold method in a density histogram. The original and segmented scans were thoroughly compared to confirm the segmentation accuracy before further analysis with a custom-processing tool. Images obtained from pre-obturation scans were used for quantification of the root canal volume (C_{Vol}), while post-obturation images were used to determine volumes of filling material (F_{Vol}) and closed pores (CP_{Vol}). The total volume of pores (V_{Vol}) and volume of open pores (OP_{Vol}) were calculated using the following formulas, respectively:

$$V_{Vol} = C_{Vol} - F_{Vol},$$

$$OP_{Vol} = V_{Vol} - CP_{Vol}.$$

Afterwards, the percentage volume of open (%OP_{Vol}) and closed (%CP_{Vol}) pores was determined as follows:

$$\%OP_{Vol} = OP_{Vol}/C_{Vol} \times 100,$$

$$\%CP_{Vol} = CP_{Vol}/C_{Vol} \times 100$$

The evaluation of micro-CT images was performed by a single person who was blinded to data regarding the root canal filling material and technique.

2.4. Statistical Analysis

The porosity distribution between experimental groups was compared using a non-parametric Kruskal-Wallis test followed by the Mann-Whitney test due to a non-normal distribution of the data and validated with the Shapiro-Wilk test. All comparisons were performed using SPSS 25.0 software (SPSS Inc., Chicago, USA), with the significance level set at $p < 0.05$.

3. Results

None of the techniques used was able to provide a pore-free root canal filling in the apical 5 mm pores; size and shape diversity were observed in all apical plugs, with open pores being the dominant type of porosity. The results of quantitative volumetric analysis of open and closed pores are summarized in Table 1. The micro-CT assessment revealed that volumes of prepared root canals had no considerable volumetric variances before the root obturation procedure ($p = 0.34$), indicating the initial equality among all experimental groups. However, the porosity distribution in root canal fillings was significantly different between all experimental groups evaluated ($p < 0.05$).

Table 1. Mean values (%) and standard deviations (SD) of open and closed pores in the respective groups.

Group	N	Open Pores	Closed Pores
BR/SC	20	3.374 ± 2.751 [A]	0.061 ± 0.080 [A]
BR/SC-UA	20	3.390 ± 3.428 [A]	0.066 ± 0.070 [A]
MF	20	18.832 ± 3.334 [B]	0.292 ± 0.226 [B]
MF-UA	20	29.075 ± 9.440 [C]	0.923 ± 0.684 [C]

Different superscript letters in the same column indicate significant differences between groups (pairwise Mann-Whitney test; $p < 0.05$).

A considerably higher quantity of open and closed pores was observed in both MF groups (with/without ultrasonic agitation), when compared to the fillings of BR/SC and BR/SC-UA ($p < 0.05$). The interaction between the MF and MF-UA groups was detected to be statistically significant ($p < 0.05$), with the highest porosity being in the MF-UA group (Figure 1).

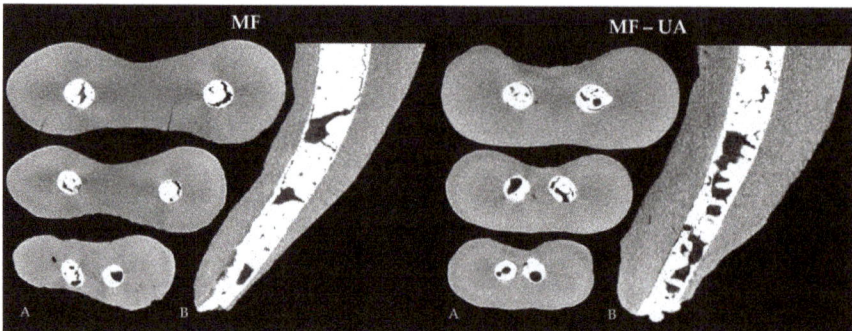

Figure 1. Representative cross-sections of random samples at the level of 5 mm, 3 mm and 1 mm from the apex (**A**) and longitudinal sections (**B**), demonstrating the porosity distribution within the fillings of MF (MTA Flow) and MF-UA (MTA Flow with ultrasonic agitation) groups.

However, no significant differences were observed between the specimens of the BR/SC and BR/SC-UA groups, where the quantity of open and closed pores within the fillings remained similar ($p = 0.82$ and $p = 0.57$, respectively) regardless of a lower mean porosity determined in the BR/SC group (Figure 2).

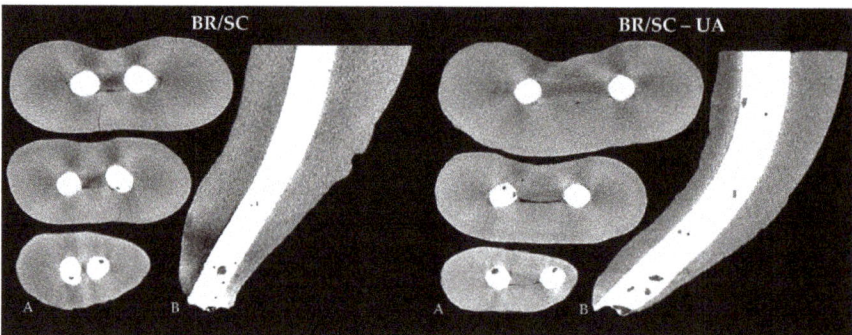

Figure 2. Cross-sectional images at the level of 5 mm, 3 mm and 1 mm from the apex (**A**) and longitudinal images (**B**), representing the quality and homogeneity of BR/SC (BioRoot RCS/single cone) and BR/SC-UA (BioRoot RCS/single cone with ultrasonic agitation) apical plugs.

4. Discussion

Root perforations are one of the most common complications observed in modern endodontology [4]. Regardless of recent advances in the field of endodontic instruments and devices, the mechanical preparation of curved root canals still remains a significant challenge, even for experienced clinicians [30]. It has been reported that the risk of root perforation occurring strongly correlates with the degree of root canal curvature, and the prevalence of apical root perforations is significantly higher in molars as compared to other teeth [2,31]. Therefore, mandibular first molars with a moderate curvature of mesial roots were selected in the present study to maximize its clinical relevance.

The management of root perforation is a time-dependent procedure, where hermetic physical seal is crucial to improve the prognosis and survival of the affected tooth [32]. It has been reported that up to 52–79% of the root canal may remain unprepared, regardless of the instruments or instrumentation technique used [33], and no currently available irrigation protocol is capable of completely disinfecting the entire root canal system [34]. Therefore, the obturation phase of the endodontic treatment has undeniable importance in order to create an unfavorable environment for the microorganisms left inside the root canal system after the preparation and to prevent their penetration into periapical tissues [4,35]. The homogeneity of root canal obturation highly depends on the porosity of the fillings [25], as open pores communicating with dentinal walls may create an excellent pathway for microleakage and eventually decrease the success rate and outcome of endodontic treatment [28,36]. Closed pores are considered to be less clinically relevant, as they represent empty spaces completely surrounded by filling material [37]. Nevertheless, it has been shown that this type of porosity may negatively affect the physical properties of the material, such as hardness and strength [36,38]. Therefore, the quantification of both open and closed pores is necessary to evaluate the quality of root canal fillings properly. Previously, various porosity and leakage measuring approaches, such as dye staining, glucose or radioactive isotope penetration, protein loss, scanning electron microscopy, mercury and capillary flow porometry, were applied to assess the sealing feature of the material used [39]. However, the significant limitations of these methods, e.g., the need to section the samples and hence the creation of artifacts, led to micro-CT being the technique of choice for accurate 3D evaluation of root canal fillings [20]. Therefore, micro-CT analysis was used in the present study to quantify and qualify the pores within the apical plugs. The isotropic resolution was set at 9.9 μm, as it has been shown that a voxel size of 11.2 μm or less is a reliable cutoff value to assess the filling porosity [36,40], even though there is always a risk of tiny pores left undetected due to a high radiopacity of the material used [18].

Techniques and materials applied for root perforation repair have not been standardized. However, MTA is generally assumed to be a benchmark for sealing various types of root perforations [32]. MF is one of the newest MTA-based repair materials, which surpasses traditional MTA in terms of clinical applicability due to its superior handling and delivery characteristics as well as faster setting time and thus increased washout resistance [10,19]. Moreover, MF retains all desirable biological properties of the original MTA, such as biocompatibility and bioactivity, which are the crucial requirements for perforation repair material exposed to periodontal tissues [41]. The biocompatibility and bioactivity are attributed mainly to the continuous calcium ion release and the formation of calcium phosphate apatite crystals, which induce the regeneration and remineralization of adjacent hard tissues while also reducing the porosity of filling material [28,41]. Nevertheless, a previous study has shown that, despite all the improvements and advantageous characteristics, MF results in highly porous apical plugs [19]. These results are in accordance with the present study, in which both MF groups (with/without ultrasonic agitation) exhibited a high porosity. The incidence of pores within MF fillings can be attributed to the increased water-to-cement ratio used during the mixing procedure to achieve a highly flowable consistency of the cement. It has been reported that excess water in the mixture eventually dries off and leaves pores that are not filled by hydration products [42]. Additionally, bismuth oxide, which is added to the MF composition as a radiopacifier, can negatively affect the sealing features by interfering with the hydration reaction and leaving more unreacted water within the filling [43]. Instead of bismuth oxide, some HCSC formulations, e.g., BioRoot RCS, contain zirconium oxide, which appears to have no impact on the material porosity [44]. These findings may correlate with the results of the present study, where significantly more homogeneous apical plugs were observed in both BR/SC groups than the MF groups.

Sealing apical root perforations with BioRoot RCS, together with a modified SC obturation technique, was proposed mainly due to the simplicity and effectiveness previously reported in in vitro and in vivo studies [16,17,19]. The concept of the SC obturation technique refers to the desirable physico-chemical properties of BioRoot RCS [14,15], which was designed as a biological filler [45], and to the tapered gutta-percha cone, acting as a piston on the flowable sealer [46]. As reported previously, the insertion of the tapered gutta-percha cone creates hydraulic pressure, which improves the material distribution throughout the root canal [47]. Therefore, the gutta-percha cone may be considered as the main factor leading to the significant differences between the BR/SC and MF groups. No porosity associated with gutta-percha cones was observed in the present study through micro-CT analysis. Therefore, the superior overall homogeneity of BR/SC apical plugs can be attributed to the use of solid gutta-percha cones.

Attempts to minimize the occurrence of pores within BR/SC and MF fillings by using ultrasonic agitation were made in our previous study, which demonstrated that neither of these techniques was able to produce pore-free apical plugs [19]. The effect of ultrasonic application mainly refers to the acoustic energy transmission and the formation of cavitation bubbles, which eventually implode, increasing the temperature and the pressure inside the root canal [21]. According to previous investigations, which have reported significantly better results in terms of porosity after the use of indirect ultrasonication, the increased pressure may remove the entrapped air, disperse agglomerated particles, reduce their surface friction and provide a more efficient incorporation of filler particles into the organic matrix, with no changes in particle size or material composition [23,25,48]. Additionally, the pressure generated during ultrasonic agitation may lead to superior interfacial adaptation between the filling material and the root canal wall, with better tubular penetration as well [21,22]. However, these advantageous effects of ultrasonic application did not provide more homogeneous apical plugs in the present study; the increased percentages of open and closed pores were observed in both BR/SC-UA and MF-UA groups. Therefore, the null hypothesis was rejected.

The lower overall homogeneity of ultrasonicated apical plugs could be attributed to the direct ultrasonic agitation, resulting in excessive vibratory forces. It has been reported that excessive ultrasonic energy potentially can lead to air incorporation into the filling material and thus contribute to the higher porosity [26,49]. However, the use of direct ultrasonic agitation should not be directly associated with less homogenous root canal fillings, since it has been reported that indirect ultrasonication may also increase the porosity [20]. Instead of ultrasonication type, more attention should be paid to the agitation time, which is potentially directly related to both the rearrangement of cement particles and the heat generation [20,50]. The ultrasonic agitation of 10 s was selected in the present study in accordance with Sisli et al. [8], who agitated 5 mm apical plugs for 10 s and afterwards reported a lower incidence of pores. It has been reported that a short agitation time may create a shock-like effect, and the duration of 5 to 10 s is necessary to rearrange the cement particles and decrease the porosity [20]. On the other hand, the prolonged agitation time may be responsible for the increase in temperature, ultimately leading to water loss from HCSC [22,49]. Even though the number of published studies evaluating the temperature changes in filling materials is still limited, there are few reports in the literature indicating that ultrasonic agitation is capable of raising the temperature inside the root canal by 2 °C [7], which can be sufficient to increase the water desorption occurring at temperatures as low as 20 °C [51]. The water loss may alter the rheological properties of the material and increase the porosity [7,51], which is considered the result of spaces between unhydrated cement particles [42]. Nevertheless, it can be speculated that indirect ultrasonic application is not prone to these adverse effects of temperature changes, as ultrasonic energy is transmitted to the material through the gutta-percha cone, plugger or another instrument. This would explain the contradictory findings in terms of porosity obtained between the present study and previous investigations [8,24], which also performed ultrasonic agitation for 10 s. However, it is difficult to directly compare the present study results with the available literature, as they differ in too many aspects, including the type and properties of filling material, the application technique, ultrasonication type and duration, assessment method, etc.

The present study suggests that all apical plugs, regardless of the obturation technique used, may potentially lead to microleakage, as none of the fillings was pore-free, and the percentages of open pores surpassed the closed porosity in all experimental groups. Nevertheless, MF apical plugs (with/without ultrasonic agitation) demonstrated significantly higher percentages of open and closed pores as compared to the BR/SC obturation technique. Therefore, reinforcing the findings of Benavides-García et al. [52], it can be concluded that MF prepared in a thin consistency should not be the material of choice for apical root perforation repair. Even though there is still no clear evidence what porosity level is critical, the significantly higher amount of pores observed in both MF groups may theoretically contribute to a worse outcome of endodontic treatment [27,28]. On the other hand, it has been shown that HCSC reduces their porosity with time in the presence of tissue fluids [42]. Therefore, the results of the present study should be evaluated with caution, as it is impossible to fully reproduce the clinical conditions using in vitro models. Further studies are needed to determine the clinical efficacy of BR/SC and MF obturation techniques in apically perforated and moderately curved roots and to confirm the adverse impact of direct ultrasonic agitation on the quality and homogeneity of root canal fillings.

5. Conclusions

Within the limitations of this in vitro study, it can be concluded that none of the obturation techniques was able to provide pore-free root canal fillings in the apical 5 mm. Significantly higher porosity was observed in the MF and MF-UA groups as compared to the BR/SC and BR/SC-UA groups. The direct ultrasonic agitation had no considerable impact on the porosity distribution in BR/SC fillings, while MF fillings demonstrated significantly higher overall porosity after ultrasonic agitation.

Author Contributions: Conceptualization, S.D. and H.S.; methodology, S.D.; software, P.T.; validation, S.D., G.B. and H.S.; formal analysis, V.P.; investigation, S.D. and G.B.; resources, H.S.; data curation, G.B.; writing—original draft preparation, G.B. and S.D.; writing—review and editing, P.T., H.S. and V.P.; visualization, S.D.; supervision, H.S.; project administration, S.D. All authors have read and agreed to the published version of the manuscript.

Funding: This research received no external funding.

Institutional Review Board Statement: The study was conducted according to the guidelines of the Declaration of Helsinki and approved by the Ethics Committee of Vilnius University Hospital Zalgirio Clinics (protocol no. EK-2, 2016 06 03).

Informed Consent Statement: Informed consent was obtained from all subjects involved in the study.

Data Availability Statement: Data is contained within the article.

Acknowledgments: The authors would like to thank Leo J. van Ruijven for his help in operating the SkyScan 1272 μCT scanner and Septodont and Ultradent Products Inc. for the donation of the materials.

Conflicts of Interest: The authors declare no conflict of interest. The sponsors had no role in the design of the study; in the collection, analyses, or interpretation of data; in the writing of the manuscript, and in the decision to publish the results.

References

1. Bueno, M.R.; Estrela, C.; De Figueiredo, J.A.; Azevedo, B.C. Map-reading strategy to diagnose root perforations near metallic intracanal posts by using cone beam computed tomography. *J. Endod.* **2011**, *37*, 85–90. [CrossRef]
2. Sarao, S.K.; Berlin-Broner, Y.; Levin, L. Occurrence and risk factors of dental root perforations: A systematic review. *Int. Dent. J.* **2021**, *71*, 96–105. [CrossRef] [PubMed]
3. Siew, K.; Lee, A.H.; Cheung, G.S. Treatment outcome of repaired root perforation: A systematic review and meta-analysis. *J. Endod.* **2015**, *41*, 1795–1804. [CrossRef]
4. Gorni, F.G.; Andreano, A.; Ambrogi, F.; Brambilla, E.; Gagliani, M. Patient and clinical characteristics associated with primary healing of iatrogenic perforations after root canal treatment: Results of a long-term Italian study. *J. Endod.* **2016**, *42*, 211–215. [CrossRef]
5. Estrela, C.; Decurcio, D.A.; Rossi-Fedele, G.; Silva, J.A.; Guedes, O.A.; Borges, Á.H. Root perforations: A review of diagnosis, prognosis and materials. *Braz. Oral. Res.* **2018**, *32*, e73. [CrossRef] [PubMed]
6. Tsesis, I.; Fuss, Z. Diagnosis and treatment of accidental root perforations. *Endod. Top.* **2006**, *13*, 95–107. [CrossRef]
7. Lopes, F.C.; Zangirolami, C.; Mazzi-Chaves, J.F.; Silva-Sousa, A.C.; Crozeta, B.M.; Silva-Sousa, Y.T.C.; Sousa-Neto, M.D. Effect of sonic and ultrasonic activation on physicochemical properties of root canal sealers. *J. Appl. Oral. Sci.* **2019**, *27*, e20180556. [CrossRef]

8. Sisli, S.N.; Ozbas, H. Comparative micro-computed tomographic evaluation of the sealing quality of ProRoot MTA and MTA Angelus apical plugs placed with various techniques. *J. Endod.* **2017**, *43*, 147–151. [CrossRef]
9. Mondelli, J.A.S.; Hoshino, R.A.; Weckwerth, P.H.; Cerri, P.S.; Leonardo, R.T.; Guerreiro-Tanomaru, J.M.; Tanomaru-Filho, M.; da Silva, G.F. Biocompatibility of mineral trioxide aggregate flow and biodentine. *Int. Endod. J.* **2019**, *52*, 193–200. [CrossRef] [PubMed]
10. Guimarães, B.M.; Vivan, R.R.; Piazza, B.; Alcalde, M.P.; Bramante, C.M.; Duarte, M.A.H. Chemical-physical properties and apatite-forming ability of mineral trioxide aggregate flow. *J. Endod.* **2017**, *43*, 1692–1696. [CrossRef]
11. Ultradent. Ultradent Products, Inc. Proudly Introduces MTA Flow™ Repair Cement. Available online: https://www.ultradent.com/company/newsroom/article/ultradent-products-inc-proudly-introduces-mta-flow-repair-cement (accessed on 25 October 2021).
12. Liu, M.; He, L.; Wang, H.; Su, W.; Li, H. Comparison of in vitro biocompatibility and antibacterial activity of two calcium silicate-based materials. *J. Mater. Sci. Mater. Med.* **2021**, *32*, 52. [CrossRef] [PubMed]
13. Drukteinis, S. Bioceramic Materials for Management of Endodontic Complications. In *Bioceramic Materials in Clinical Endodontics*, 1st ed.; Drukteinis, S., Camilleri, J., Eds.; Spinger: Cham, Germany, 2021; pp. 59–85.
14. Siboni, F.; Taddei, P.; Zamparini, F.; Prati, C.; Gandolfi, M.G. Properties of BioRoot RCS, a tricalcium silicate endodontic sealer modified with povidone and polycarboxylate. *Int. Endod. J.* **2017**, *50*, 120–136. [CrossRef]
15. Sfeir, G.; Zogheib, C.; Patel, S.; Giraud, T.; Nagendrababu, V.; Bukiet, F. Calcium silicate-based root canal sealers: A narrative review and clinical perspectives. *Materials* **2021**, *14*, 3965. [CrossRef] [PubMed]
16. Bardini, G.; Casula, L.; Ambu, E.; Musu, D.; Mercadè, M.; Cotti, E. A 12-month follow-up of primary and secondary root canal treatment in teeth obturated with a hydraulic sealer. *Clin. Oral Investig.* **2021**, *25*, 2757–2764. [CrossRef]
17. Zavattini, A.; Knight, A.; Foschi, F.; Mannocci, F. Outcome of root canal treatments using a new calcium silicate root canal sealer: A non-randomized clinical trial. *J. Clin. Med.* **2020**, *9*, 782. [CrossRef] [PubMed]
18. Drukteinis, S.; Bilvinaite, G.; Tusas, P.; Shemesh, H.; Peciuliene, V. Microcomputed tomographic assessment of the single cone root canal fillings performed by undergraduate student, postgraduate student and specialist endodontist. *J. Clin. Med.* **2021**, *10*, 1080. [CrossRef]
19. Drukteinis, S.; Peciuliene, V.; Shemesh, H.; Tusas, P.; Bendinskaite, R. Porosity distribution in apically perforated curved root canals filled with two different calcium silicate based materials and techniques: A micro-computed tomography study. *Materials* **2019**, *12*, 1729. [CrossRef]
20. El-Ma'aita, A.M.; Qualtrough, A.J.; Watts, D.C. A micro-computed tomography evaluation of mineral trioxide aggregate root canal fillings. *J. Endod.* **2012**, *38*, 670–672. [CrossRef]
21. da Silva Machado, A.P.; Câncio Couto de Souza, A.C.; Lima Gonçalves, T.; Franco Marques, A.A.; da Fonseca Roberti Garcia, L.; Antunes Bortoluzzi, E.; Acris de Carvalho, F.M. Does the ultrasonic activation of sealer hinder the root canal retreatment? *Clin. Oral Investig.* **2021**, *25*, 4401–4406. [CrossRef]
22. Aguiar, B.A.; Frota, L.M.A.; Taguatinga, D.T.; Vivan, R.R.; Camilleri, J.; Duarte, M.A.H.; de Vasconcelos, B.C. Influence of ultrasonic agitation on bond strength, marginal adaptation, and tooth discoloration provided by three coronary barrier endodontic materials. *Clin. Oral Investig.* **2019**, *23*, 4113–4122. [CrossRef]
23. Wiesse, P.E.B.; Silva-Sousa, Y.T.; Pereira, R.D.; Estrela, C.; Domingues, L.M.; Pécora, J.D.; Sousa-Neto, M.D. Effect of ultrasonic and sonic activation of root canal sealers on the push-out bond strength and interfacial adaptation to root canal dentine. *Int. Endod. J.* **2018**, *51*, 102–111. [CrossRef]
24. Dinçer, A.N.; Güneşer, M.B.; Sisli, S.N. Micro-CT analysis of the marginal adaptation and porosity associated with ultrasonic activation of coronally placed tricalcium silicate-based cements. *Aust. Endod. J.* **2020**, *46*, 323–329. [CrossRef]
25. Kim, J.A.; Hwang, Y.C.; Rosa, V.; Yu, M.K.; Lee, K.W.; Min, K.S. Root Canal Filling Quality of a Premixed Calcium Silicate Endodontic Sealer Applied Using Gutta-percha Cone-mediated Ultrasonic Activation. *J. Endod.* **2018**, *44*, 133–138. [CrossRef] [PubMed]
26. Kim, S.Y.; Jang, Y.E.; Kim, B.S.; Pang, E.K.; Shim, K.; Jin, H.R.; Son, M.K.; Kim, Y. Effects of ultrasonic activation on root canal filling quality of single-cone obturation with calcium silicate-based sealer. *Materials* **2021**, *14*, 1292. [CrossRef]
27. An, H.J.; Yoon, H.; Jung, H.I.; Shin, D.H.; Song, M. Comparison of obturation quality after MTA orthograde filling with various obturation techniques. *J. Clin. Med.* **2021**, *10*, 1719. [CrossRef] [PubMed]
28. Milanovic, I.; Milovanovic, P.; Antonijevic, D.; Dzeletovic, B.; Djuric, M.; Miletic, V. Immediate and long-term porosity of calcium silicate-based sealers. *J. Endod.* **2020**, *46*, 515–523. [CrossRef]
29. Schneider, S.W. A comparison of canal preparations in straight and curved root canals. *Oral Surg. Oral Med. Oral Pathol.* **1971**, *32*, 271–275. [CrossRef]
30. Ansari, I.; Maria, R. Managing curved canals. *Contemp Clin. Dent.* **2012**, *3*, 237–241. [CrossRef] [PubMed]
31. Schafer, E.; Dammaschke, T. Development and sequelae of canal transportation. *Endod. Top.* **2006**, *15*, 75–90. [CrossRef]
32. Abdelmotelb, M.A.; Gomaa, Y.F.; Khattab, N.M.A.; Elheeny, A.A.H. Premixed bioceramics versus mineral trioxide aggregate in furcal perforation repair of primary molars: In vitro and in vivo study. *Clin. Oral Investig.* **2021**, *25*, 4915–4925. [CrossRef] [PubMed]
33. Lopes, R.M.V.; Marins, F.C.; Belladonna, F.G.; Souza, E.M.; De-Deus, G.; Lopes, R.T.; Silva, E.J.N.L. Untouched canal areas and debris accumulation after root canal preparation with rotary and adaptive systems. *Aust. Endod. J.* **2018**, *44*, 260–266. [CrossRef]

34. Nagendrababu, V.; Jayaraman, J.; Suresh, A.; Kalyanasundaram, S.; Neelakantan, P. Effectiveness of ultrasonically activated irrigation on root canal disinfection: A systematic review of in vitro studies. *Clin. Oral Investig.* **2018**, *22*, 655–670. [CrossRef]
35. Selem, L.C.; Li, G.H.; Niu, L.N.; Bergeron, B.E.; Bortoluzzi, E.A.; Chen, J.H.; Pashley, D.H.; Tay, F.R. Quality of obturation achieved by a non-gutta-percha-based root filling system in single-rooted canals. *J. Endod.* **2014**, *40*, 2003–2008. [CrossRef]
36. Torres, F.F.E.; Guerreiro-Tanomaru, J.M.; Bosso-Martelo, R.; Espir, C.G.; Camilleri, J.; Tanomaru-Filho, M. Solubility, porosity, dimensional and volumetric change of endodontic sealers. *Braz. Dent. J.* **2019**, *30*, 368–373. [CrossRef] [PubMed]
37. Dioguardi, M.; Quarta, C.; Sovereto, D.; Troiano, G.; Zhurakivska, K.; Bizzoca, M.E.; Lo Muzio, L.; Lo Russo, L. Calcium silicate cements vs. epoxy resin based cements: Narrative review. *Oral* **2021**, *1*, 23–35. [CrossRef]
38. Antonijevic, D.; Zelic, K.; Djuric, M. Novel calcium silicate based dental material with the addition of biologically active soy compound. In Proceedings of the 2015 IEEE 15th International Conference on Bioinformatics and Bioengineering (BIBE), Belgrade, Serbia, 2–4 November 2015. [CrossRef]
39. Guerrero, F.; Berástegui, E. Porosity analysis of MTA and Biodentine cements for use in endodontics by using micro-computed tomography. *J. Clin. Exp. Dent.* **2018**, *10*, 237–240. [CrossRef] [PubMed]
40. Orhan, K.; Jacobs, R.; Celikten, B.; Huang, Y.; de Faria Vasconcelos, K.; Nicolielo, L.F.P.; Buyuksungur, A.; Van Dessel, J. Evaluation of threshold values for root canal filling voids in micro-CT and nano-CT images. *Scanning* **2018**, *2018*, 9437569. [CrossRef] [PubMed]
41. Bueno, C.R.E.; Vasques, A.M.V.; Cury, M.T.S.; Sivieri-Araújo, G.; Jacinto, R.C.; Gomes-Filho, J.E.; Cintra, L.T.A.; Dezan-Junior, E. Biocompatibility and biomineralization assessment of mineral trioxide aggregate flow. *Clin. Oral Investig.* **2019**, *23*, 169–177. [CrossRef] [PubMed]
42. Camilleri, J.; Grech, L.; Galea, K.; Keir, D.; Fenech, M.; Formosa, L.; Damidot, D.; Mallia, B. Porosity and root dentine to material interface assessment of calcium silicate-based root-end filling materials. *Clin. Oral Investig.* **2014**, *18*, 1437–1446. [CrossRef] [PubMed]
43. Coomaraswamy, K.S.; Lumley, P.J.; Hofmann, M.P. Effect of bismuth oxide radiopacifier content on the material properties of an endodontic Portland cement-based (MTA-like) system. *J. Endod.* **2007**, *33*, 295–298. [CrossRef]
44. Li, X.; Yoshihara, K.; De Munck, J.; Cokic, S.; Pongprueksa, P.; Putzeys, E.; Pedano, M.; Chen, Z.; Van Landuyt, K.; Van Meerbeek, B. Modified tricalcium silicate cement formulations with added zirconium oxide. *Clin. Oral Investig.* **2017**, *21*, 895–905. [CrossRef]
45. Camilleri, J. BioRoot RCS. Endo Sealer or Biological Filler? 2019. Available online: https://www.septodont.com.ru/sites/ru/files/2019-07/Septodont_BioRoot_Endo%20sealer%20or%20biological%20filler_JC.pdf (accessed on 25 October 2021).
46. Camilleri, J. Will bioceramics be the future root canal filling materials? *Curr. Oral Health Rep.* **2017**, *4*, 228–238. [CrossRef]
47. Kalantar Motamedi, M.R.; Mortaheb, A.; Zare Jahromi, M.; Gilbert, B.E. Micro-CT evaluation of four root canal obturation techniques. *Scanning* **2021**, *2021*, 6632822. [CrossRef] [PubMed]
48. Acris De Carvalho, F.M.; Silva-Sousa, Y.T.C.; Saraiva Miranda, C.E.; Miller Calderon, P.H.; Barbosa, A.F.S.; Domingues De Macedo, L.M.; Abi Rached-Junior, F.J. Influence of ultrasonic activation on the physicochemical properties of calcium silicate-based cements. *Int. J. Dent.* **2021**, *2021*, 6697988. [CrossRef]
49. Yeung, P.; Liewehr, F.R.; Moon, P.C. A quantitative comparison of the fill density of MTA produced by two placement techniques. *J. Endod.* **2006**, *32*, 456–459. [CrossRef] [PubMed]
50. Pérez-Alfayate, R.; Algar-Pinilla, J.; Mercade, M.; Foschi, F. Sonic activation improves bioceramic sealer's penetration into the tubular dentin of curved root canals: A confocal laser scanning microscopy investigation. *Appl. Sci.* **2021**, *11*, 3902. [CrossRef]
51. Atmeh, A.R.; AlShwaimi, E. The effect of heating time and temperature on epoxy resin and calcium silicate-based endodontic sealers. *J. Endod.* **2017**, *43*, 2112–2118. [CrossRef]
52. Benavides-García, M.; Hernández-Meza, E.; Reyes-Carmona, J. Ex vivo analysis of MTA FLOW® biomineralization and push-out strength: A pilot study. *Int. J. Dent. Sci.* **2021**, *23*, 76–90. [CrossRef]

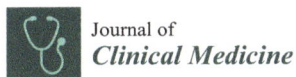

Article

Influence of the Geometrical Cross-Section Design on the Dynamic Cyclic Fatigue Resistance of NiTi Endodontic Rotary Files—An In Vitro Study

Vicente Faus-Llácer [1], Nirmine Hamoud-Kharrat [1], María Teresa Marhuenda Ramos [1], Ignacio Faus-Matoses [1], Álvaro Zubizarreta-Macho [2,3,*], Celia Ruiz Sánchez [1] and Vicente Faus-Matoses [1]

[1] Department of Stomatology, Faculty of Medicine and Dentistry, University of Valencia, 46010 Valencia, Spain; fausvj@uv.es (V.F.-L.); nirhak@alumni.uv.es (N.H.-K.); marhuen3@uv.es (M.T.M.R.); ignacio.faus@uv.es (I.F.-M.); celia.ruiz@uv.es (C.R.S.); vicente.faus@uv.es (V.F.-M.)
[2] Department of Endodontics, Faculty of Health Sciences, Alfonso X el Sabio University, 28691 Madrid, Spain
[3] Department of Surgery, Faculty of Medicine and Dentistry, University of Salamanca, 37008 Salamanca, Spain
* Correspondence: amacho@uax.es or alvaro.zubizarreta@usal.es

Citation: Faus-Llácer, V.; Hamoud-Kharrat, N.; Marhuenda Ramos, M.T.; Faus-Matoses, I.; Zubizarreta-Macho, Á.; Ruiz Sánchez, C.; Faus-Matoses, V. Influence of the Geometrical Cross-Section Design on the Dynamic Cyclic Fatigue Resistance of NiTi Endodontic Rotary Files—An In Vitro Study. *J. Clin. Med.* **2021**, *10*, 4713. https://doi.org/10.3390/jcm10204713

Academic Editors: Massimo Amato, Giuseppe Pantaleo and Alfredo Iandolo

Received: 6 September 2021
Accepted: 11 October 2021
Published: 14 October 2021

Publisher's Note: MDPI stays neutral with regard to jurisdictional claims in published maps and institutional affiliations.

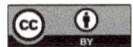

Copyright: © 2021 by the authors. Licensee MDPI, Basel, Switzerland. This article is an open access article distributed under the terms and conditions of the Creative Commons Attribution (CC BY) license (https://creativecommons.org/licenses/by/4.0/).

Abstract: The aim of this study was to analyze and compare the influence of the geometrical cross-section design on the dynamic cyclic fatigue resistance of NiTi endodontic rotary files. Materials and Methods: Forty sterile endodontic rotary files were selected and distributed into the following study groups: A: 25.06 double S-shaped cross-section NiTi alloy endodontic rotary files (Mtwo) ($n = 10$); B: 20.04 rectangular cross-section NiTi alloy endodontic rotary files (T Pro E1) ($n = 10$); C: 25.04 convex triangular cross-section NiTi alloy endodontic rotary files (T Pro E2) ($n = 10$); and D: 25.06 triangular cross-section NiTi alloy endodontic rotary files (T Pro E4) ($n = 10$). A cyclic fatigue device was used to conduct the static cyclic fatigue tests with stainless steel artificial root canal systems with 200 μm and 250 μm apical diameter, 60° curvature angle, 3 mm radius of curvature, 20 mm length, and 4% and 8% taper. The results were analyzed using the ANOVA test and Weibull statistical analysis. Results: All the pairwise comparisons presented statistically significant differences between the time to failure and number of cycles to failure for the cross-section design study groups ($p < 0.001$). Conclusions: the double S-shaped cross-section of Mtwo NiTi endodontic files shows higher cyclic fatigue resistance than the rectangular cross-section of T Pro E1 NiTi endodontic files, the convex triangular cross-section of T Pro E2 NiTi endodontic files, and the triangular cross-section of T Pro E4 NiTi endodontic files.

Keywords: endodontics; cyclic fatigue; cross-section design; NiTi; continuous rotation; energy-dispersive X-ray

1. Introduction

The introduction of nickel–titanium alloy (NiTi) in the manufacturing of root canal instruments entailed a great revolution in the field of endodontics, as these endodontic files decreased the iatrogenic complications [1,2]. However, the failure of endodontic rotary files is still a concern, despite the continuous mechanical and chemical improvements in the NiTi alloy endodontic rotary instruments made by manufacturers to reduce the incidence of complications during root canal treatment [3]. Nevertheless, the incidence of fracture of NiTi endodontic rotary files ranges from 0.09% to 5% [4,5]. The failure of NiTi endodontic rotary files occurs when fatigue resistance is overcome by torsional stress, flexural bending (cyclic) stress, or a combination of the two [6]. Specifically, torsional fatigue occurs when the tip of the endodontic file becomes blocked in the root canal while the instrument continues rotating [7], and flexural bending fatigue occurs by the alternating application of compressive and tensile stress cycles on a curved root canal, leading to overcoming plastic deformation and the subsequent failure of the endodontic rotary instrument [6,8].

In addition, the unexpected failure of the NiTi alloy endodontic rotary instruments might condition the outcome of the root canal treatment by blocking the advancement of disinfecting agents beyond the fractured instrument [9–11], which may lead to subsequent pulp necrosis and the formation of periapical lesions [12] or decrease the success rate of root canal treatment of teeth with periapical pathology [13]. Therefore, several reports have been conducted to analyze the influence of both the NiTi alloy and the geometrical parameters on the torsional and flexural bending resistance of endodontic rotary instruments to prevent the incidence of failure of endodontic rotary instruments. Both the chemical composition and crystalline structure of the NiTi alloy have been widely found to highly influence the fatigue resistance of endodontic rotary files, in particular, the endodontic rotary systems, composed of a higher concentration of the martensitic phase and manufactured by electropolishing, ion implantation, cryogenic treatment, and heat treatments, improve the mechanical behavior of NiTi endodontic rotary files, increasing their cyclic fatigue resistance [14]. However, some geometrical factors have also been reported to influence the instrument's performance, including the taper and apical diameter [15], cross-section design [16,17], flute length, helix angle, and pitch [18]. Unfortunately, the independent assessment of each factor associated with flexural bending fatigue may be difficult in a clinical setting due to the heterogeneous anatomy of the root canal system; thus, controlled experimental studies have been conducted to independently analyze each variable using custom-made cyclic fatigue devices [15].

The aim of this study was to analyze and compare the influence of the geometrical cross-section design on the dynamic cyclic fatigue resistance of NiTi endodontic rotary files, with a null hypothesis (H_0) stating that the geometry of the cross-section design would not affect the resistance of NiTi endodontic rotary files to dynamic cyclic fatigue.

2. Materials and Methods

2.1. Study Design

Forty (40) sterile and non-used NiTi alloy endodontic rotary instruments were used in this in vitro study. A controlled experimental trial was performed at the Department of Stomatology of the Faculty of Medicine and Dentistry at the University of Valencia (Valencia, Spain), between March and July 2021. The NiTi endodontic rotary files were selected and categorized into the following study groups: A: double S-shaped cross-section with 250 µm apical diameter and 6% taper conventional NiTi alloy endodontic rotary files mainly consisting of austenite phase at body temperature [19] (Ref.: 0236 025 025, Mtwo, VDW, Munich, Germany) ($n = 10$) (Mtwo); B: rectangular cross-section with 200 µm apical diameter and 4% taper austenite phase NiTi alloy endodontic rotary files (Ref.: 20010103, T Pro E1, Perfect Endo, Shenzhen Perfect Medical Instruments, Shanwei City, China) ($n = 10$) (T Pro E1); C: convex triangular cross-section with 250 µm apical diameter and 4% taper austenite phase NiTi alloy endodontic rotary file (Ref.: 20010103, T Pro E2, Perfect Endo, Shenzhen Perfect Medical Instruments, Shanwei City, China) ($n = 10$) (T Pro E2); and D: triangular cross-section with 250 µm apical diameter and 6% taper austenite phase NiTi alloy endodontic rotary file (Ref.: 20010103, T Pro E4, Perfect Endo, Shenzhen Perfect Medical Instruments, Shanwei City, China) ($n = 10$) (T Pro E4). All endodontic rotary files were manufactured in austenitic phase with an austenite finish (A_f), and the temperatures of the Mtwo, T Pro E1, T Pro E2, and T Pro E4 were approximately 15 °C [19], 15 °C, 20 °C, and 20 °C, respectively. The A_f temperatures of T Pro E1, T Pro E2, and T Pro E4 were provided by the manufacturer.

2.2. Scanning Electron Microscopy Analysis

All NiTi endodontic rotary files were initially analyzed under scanning electron microscopy (SEM) (HITACHI S-4800, Fukuoka, Japan) at ×30 and ×600 in the Central Support Service for Experimental Research of the University of Valencia (Burjassot, Spain) under the following exposure parameters: acceleration voltage: 20 kV, magnification from 100× to 6500×, and a resolution between −1.0 nm at 15 kV and 2.0 nm at 1 kV, to perform a surface characterization to discard further surface defects in its manufacture and analyze and compare the geometrical design of the NiTi endodontic rotary files (Figure 1).

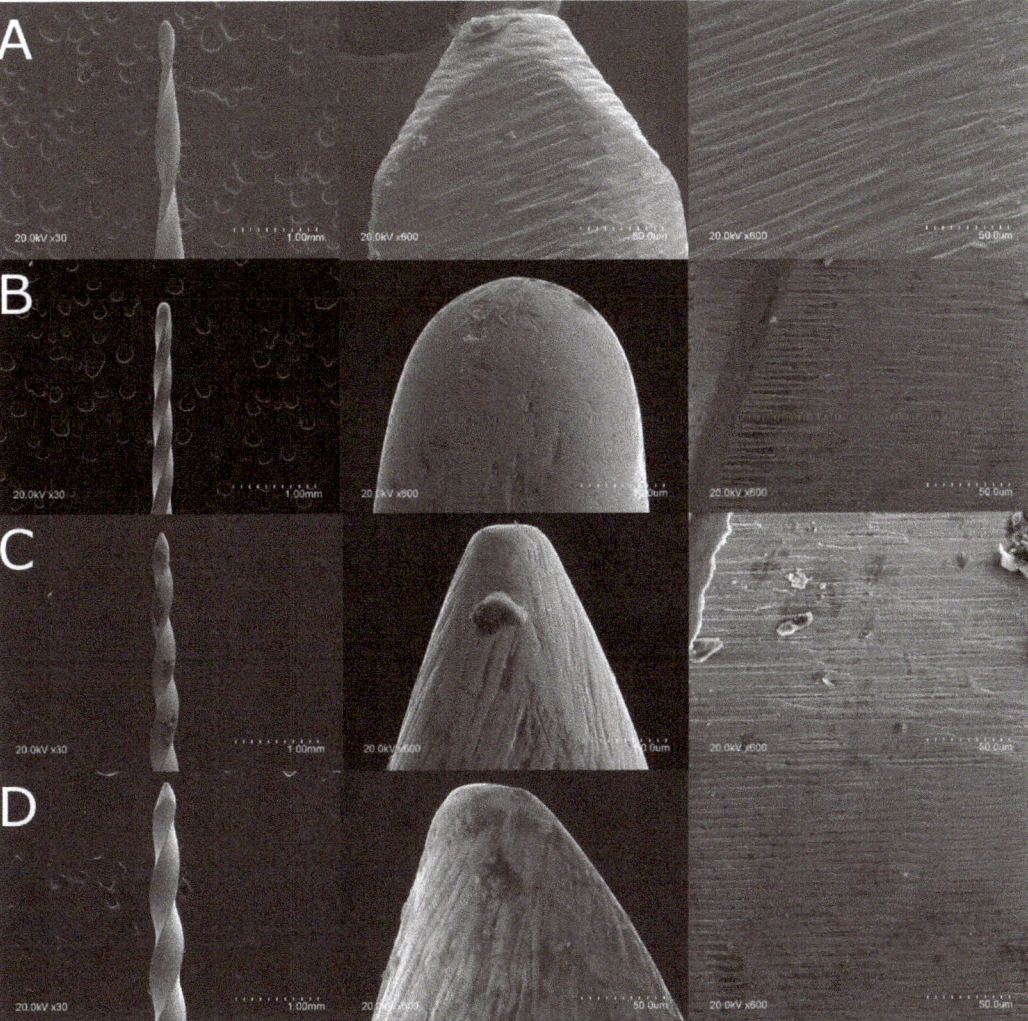

Figure 1. (**A**) SEM analysis of the Mtwo NiTi alloy endodontic rotary file, (**B**) T Pro E1 Gold-Wire NiTi alloy endodontic rotary file, (**C**) T Pro E2 Gold-Wire NiTi alloy endodontic rotary file, and (**D**) T Pro E4 Gold-Wire NiTi alloy endodontic rotary file.

2.3. Energy-Dispersive X-ray Spectroscopy Analysis

Additionally, an energy-dispersive X-ray spectroscopy (EDX) analysis was performed on all NiTi endodontic rotary files in the Central Support Service for Experimental Research of the University of Valencia (Burjassot, Spain) under the following exposure parameters: acceleration voltage: 20 kV; magnification: from 100× to 6500×; and a resolution between −1.0 nm at 15 kV and 2.0 nm at 1 kV, in order to analyze the elemental composition of the chemical elements of the NiTi endodontic rotary files used in the static fatigue tests, by means of the atomic weight percent measurement, at three randomized locations (Figure 2).

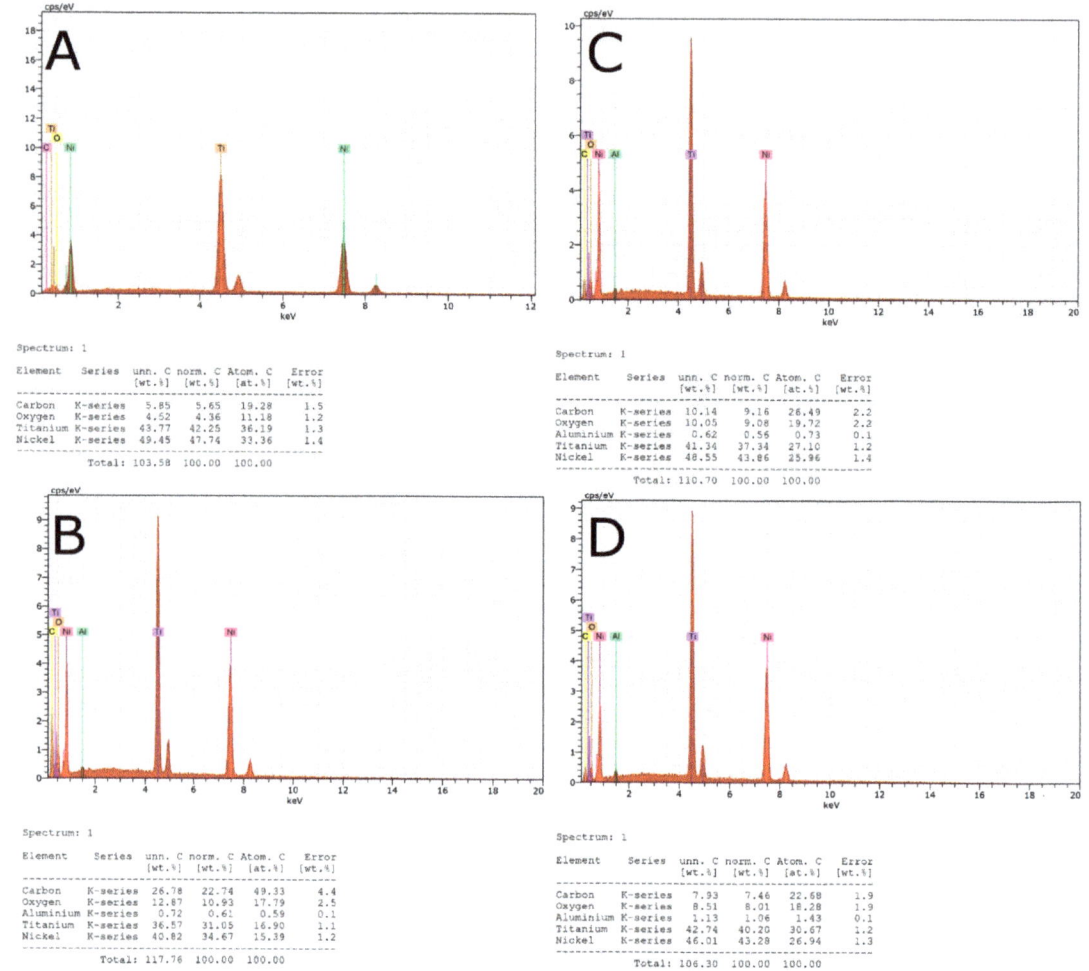

Figure 2. (**A**) EDX micro-analysis of the Mtwo NiTi alloy endodontic rotary file, (**B**) T Pro E1 austenite phase NiTi alloy endodontic rotary file, (**C**) T Pro E2 austenite phase NiTi alloy endodontic rotary file, and (**D**) T Pro E4 austenite phase NiTi alloy endodontic rotary file.

2.4. Experimental Cyclic Fatigue Model

Dynamic cyclic fatigue tests were performed using the previously described custom-made device (utility model patent number ES1219520) [20]. The structure of the dynamic cyclic fatigue test device was designed by computer aided design/computer aided engineering (CAD/CAE) 2D/3D software (Midas FX+®, Brunleys, Milton Keynes, UK) and created using 3D printing (ProJet® 6000 3D Systems©, Rock Hill, SC, USA) (Figure 3).

The custom-made artificial root canals were performed with a 60° curvature according to Schneider's measuring technique [21] and 3 mm radius of curvature using CAD/CAE 2D/3D software for inverse engineering technology. The artificial root canal was created from stainless steel using electrical discharge machining (EDM) molybdenum wire-cut technology (Cocchiola S.A., Buenos Aires, Argentina). This process ensured intimate contact between the NiTi endodontic reciprocating files and the artificial root canal walls. The artificial root canal was positioned on its support, and failure of the endodontic rotary instrument was detected using a Light-Dependent Resistor (LDR) sensor (Ref.: C000025, Arduino LLC®, Ivrea, Italy) located at the apex of the artificial root canal. The LDR sensor quantifies the continuous light source emitted by a high-brightness white Light-Emitting Diode (LED) (20000 mcd) (Ref.: 12.675/5/b/c/20k, Batuled, Coslada, Spain), which is located opposite the artificial root canal. The light signals emitted by the LED sensor were detected by the LDR (Ref.: C000025, Arduino LLC®) sensor with a frequency of 50 ms to accurately identify the precise time of failure.

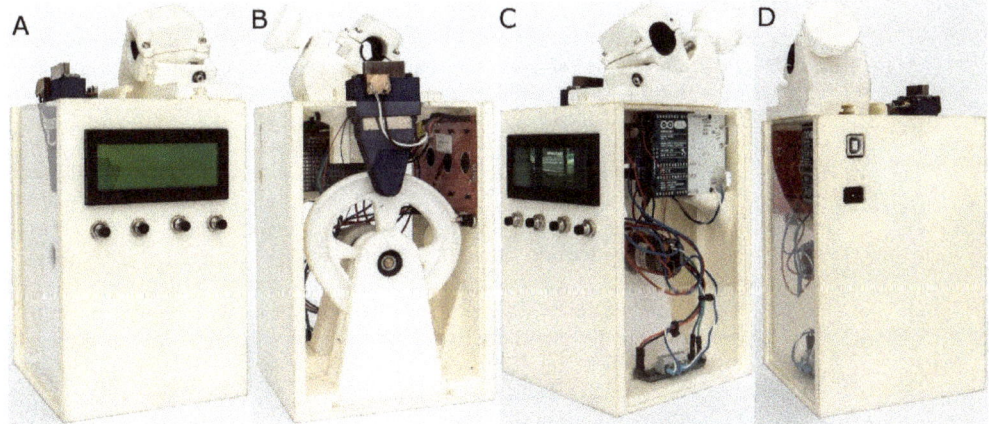

Figure 3. (**A**) Front, (**B**) back, (**C**) right, and (**D**) left surfaces of the dynamic cyclic fatigue device.

The direction and speed of the movement generated by the brushed DC gear motor (Ref.: 1589, Pololu® Corporation, Las Vegas, NV, USA) and controlled by the driver (Ref.: DRV8835, Pololu® Corporation, Las Vegas, NV, USA) were transferred to the artificial root canal support through a roller bearing system (Ref.: MR104ZZ, FAG, Schaeffler Herzogenaurach, Germany). The artificial root canal support moved in a pure axial motion using a lineal guide (Ref.: HGH35C 10249-1 001 MA, HIWIN Technologies Corp. Taichung, Taiwan). All the NiTi endodontic rotary files were used with a 6:1 reduction handpiece (X-Smart plus, Dentsply Maillefer, Baillagues, Switzerland) and torque-controlled motor. Mtwo NiTi alloy endodontic rotary files (Ref.: 0236 025 025, Mtwo, VDW, Munich, Germany) were used at 250 rpm and 2.3 N/cm torque, T Pro E1 austenite phase NiTi alloy endodontic rotary files (Ref.: 20010103, T Pro E1, Perfect Endo, Shenzhen Perfect Medical Instruments, Shanwei City, China) were used at 250 rpm and 2 N/cm torque, T Pro E2 austenite phase NiTi alloy endodontic rotary files (Ref.: 20010103, T Pro E1, Perfect Endo, Shenzhen Perfect Medical Instruments, Shanwei City, China) were used at 250 rpm and 2 N/cm torque, and T Pro E4 austenite phase NiTi alloy endodontic rotary files (Ref.: 20010103, T Pro E1, Perfect Endo, Shenzhen Perfect Medical Instruments, Shanwei City, China) were used at 250 rpm and 2 N/cm torque, according to the manufacturer's instructions.

All NiTi endodontic files were used in the dynamic cyclic fatigue device at a frequency of 60 pecking movements/min according to a previous study [20]. To reduce the friction between the rotating files and the artificial canal walls, special high-flow synthetic oil designed for the lubrication of mechanical parts (Singer All-Purpose Oil; Singer Corp., Barcelona, Spain) was applied.

All NiTi endodontic rotary files were used until fracture occurred. The time to failure and the number of cycles to failure were measured and recorded.

2.5. Statistical Tests

Statistical analysis of all the variables was carried out using SAS 9.4 (SAS Institute Inc., Cary, NC, USA). Descriptive statistics are expressed as the mean and standard deviation

(SD) for quantitative variables. Comparative analysis was performed by comparing the time to failure (in seconds) and the number of cycles to failure using the ANOVA test. For the comparisons, the p-values were adjusted using the Tukey method to correct the type I error. In addition, Weibull characteristic strength and Weibull modulus were calculated. The statistical significance was set at $p < 0.05$.

3. Results

SEM analysis of the T Pro E2 NiTi endodontic rotary files (Ref.: 20010103, T Pro E1, Perfect Endo, Shenzhen Perfect Medical Instruments, Shanwei City, China) showed accumulation of organic matter, but none of the NiTi endodontic rotary files showed relevant structural alterations. Moreover, manufacturing lines were distributed perpendicularly to the longitudinal axis in all of the endodontic rotary files and also parallel to each other due to the manufacturing process by laser machining. The width and spacing of the manufacturing lines and tubular porosity correspond to the precision and intensity of the laser machining process. In addition, the macroscopically geometrical design of the double S-shaped cross-section of Mtwo NiTi alloy endodontic rotary files (Ref.: 0236025025, Mtwo, VDW, Munich, Germany) showed a higher pitch than the rectangular cross-section of T Pro E1 NiTi endodontic files (Ref.: 20010103, T Pro E1, Perfect Endo, Shenzhen Perfect Medical Instruments, Shanwei City, China), the convex triangular cross-section of T Pro E2 NiTi endodontic files (Ref.: 20010103, T Pro E1, Perfect Endo, Shenzhen Perfect Medical Instruments, Shanwei City, China), and the triangular cross-section of T Pro E4 NiTi endodontic files (Ref.: 20010103, T Pro E1, Perfect Endo, Shenzhen Perfect Medical Instruments, Shanwei City, China).

EDX micro-analysis of the double S-shaped cross-section of Mtwo NiTi alloy endodontic rotary files (Ref.: 0236025025, Mtwo, VDW, Munich, Germany), the rectangular cross-section of T Pro E1 NiTi endodontic files (Ref.: 20010103, T Pro E1, Perfect Endo, Shenzhen Perfect Medical Instruments, Shanwei City, China), the convex triangular cross-section of T Pro E2 NiTi endodontic files (Ref.: 20010103, T Pro E1, Perfect Endo, Shenzhen Perfect Medical Instruments, Shanwei City, China), and the triangular cross-section of T Pro E4 NiTi endodontic files (Ref.: 20010103, T Pro E1, Perfect Endo, Shenzhen Perfect Medical Instruments, Shanwei City, China) was performed at 20 kV as this allowed a deeper analysis of the NiTi endodontic rotary files surface. In summary, the double S-shaped cross-section of Mtwo NiTi alloy endodontic rotary files (Ref.: 0236025025, Mtwo, VDW, Munich, Germany) differs in the chemical elements present in the metal alloy, in accordance with the rectangular cross-section of T Pro E1 NiTi endodontic files (Ref.: 20010103, T Pro E1, Perfect Endo, Shenzhen Perfect Medical Instruments, Shanwei City, China), the convex triangular cross-section of T Pro E2 NiTi endodontic files (Ref.: 20010103, T Pro E1, Perfect Endo, Shenzhen Perfect Medical Instruments, Shanwei City, China), and the triangular cross-section of T Pro E4 NiTi endodontic files (Ref.: 20010103, T Pro E1, Perfect Endo, Shenzhen Perfect Medical Instruments, Shanwei City, China), which include aluminum in the chemical composition of the metal alloy (Table 1).

Table 1. Mean atomic weight percent (%) of Mtwo NiTi alloy endodontic rotary files, T Pro E1 austenite phase NiTi alloy endodontic rotary files, T Pro E2 austenite phase NiTi alloy endodontic rotary files, and T Pro E4 austenite phase NiTi alloy endodontic rotary files.

Spectrum	C	O	Al	Ti	Ni
Mtwo 20 kV (1–3)	20.92	10.89	-	37.60	30.58
T Pro E1 20 kV (1–3)	42.51	21.15	0.52	19.48	16.34
T Pro E2 20 kV (1–3)	26.49	19.72	0.73	27.10	25.96
T Pro E4 20 kV (1–3)	39.52	19.25	2.43	20.58	18.23

The mean and SD values for the time to failure (in seconds) for each of the study groups are displayed in Table 2 and Figure 4.

Table 2. Descriptive statistics of the time to failure of Mtwo NiTi alloy endodontic rotary files, T Pro E1 austenite phase NiTi alloy endodontic rotary files, T Pro E2 austenite phase NiTi alloy endodontic rotary files, and T Pro E4 austenite phase NiTi alloy endodontic rotary files.

Study Group	n	Mean	SD	Minimum	Maximum
Mtwo	10	500.06 [a]	9.22	484.90	512.90
T Pro E1	10	256.05 [b]	7.96	242.90	269.20
T Pro E2	10	349.29 [c]	7.02	339.00	358.20
T Pro E14	10	400.64 [d]	8.72	387.10	411.60

[a,b,c,d] Statistically significant differences between groups ($p < 0.05$).

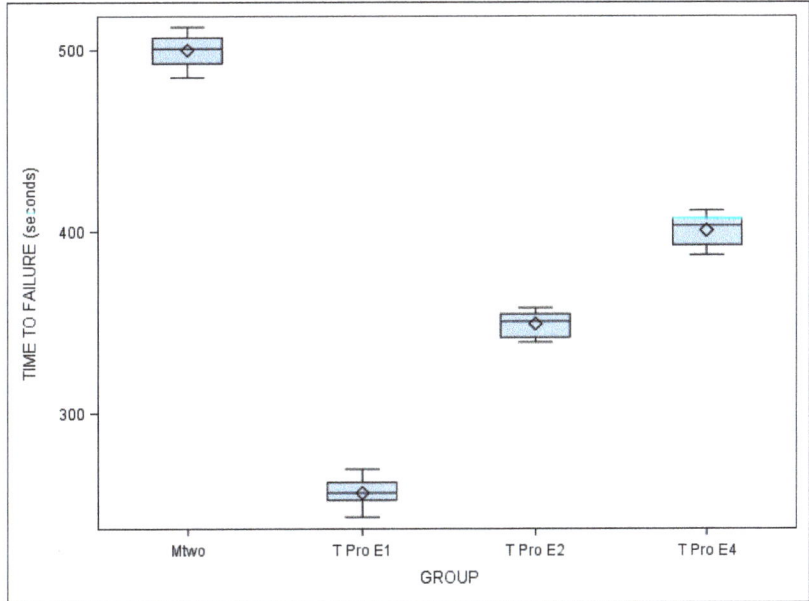

Figure 4. Box plot of the time to failure of Mtwo NiTi alloy endodontic rotary files, T Pro E1 austenite phase NiTi alloy endodontic rotary files, T Pro E2 austenite phase NiTi alloy endodontic rotary files, and T Pro E4 austenite phase NiTi alloy endodontic rotary files.

The ANOVA test showed statistically significant differences between the time to failure of all NiTi endodontic rotary files ($p < 0.001$) (Figure 4). The results related to the number of cycles to failure are similar as the dynamic cyclic fatigue device had a frequency of 60 pecking movements/min.

The scale distribution parameter (η) of the Weibull statistical analysis found statistically significant differences between the time to failure of all NiTi endodontic rotary files ($p < 0.001$) (Table 3, Figure 5). However, the shape distribution parameter (β) of the Weibull analysis found no statistically significant differences between the time to failure of any of the NiTi endodontic rotary files ($p > 0.05$). The results related to the number of cycles to failure are similar as the dynamic cyclic fatigue device had a frequency of 60 pecking movements/min (Table 3, Figure 5).

Table 3. Weibull statistics of time to failure of replica-like and original brand NiTi endodontic rotary files study groups.

Study Group	Weibull Shape (β)				Weibull Scale (η)			
	Estimate	St Error	Lower	Upper	Estimate	St Error	Lower	Upper
Mtwo	67.0256	16.7296	41.0943	109.3202	504.2430	2.5132	499.3413	509.1928
T Pro E1	37.0114	8.8527	23.1599	59.1472	259.6936	2.3498	255.1287	264.3402
T Pro E2	64.0224	16.4767	38.6606	106.0220	352.4523	1.8358	348.8725	356.0689
T Pro E14	59.2617	15.1900	35.8586	97.9388	404.5474	2.2760	400.1110	409.0329

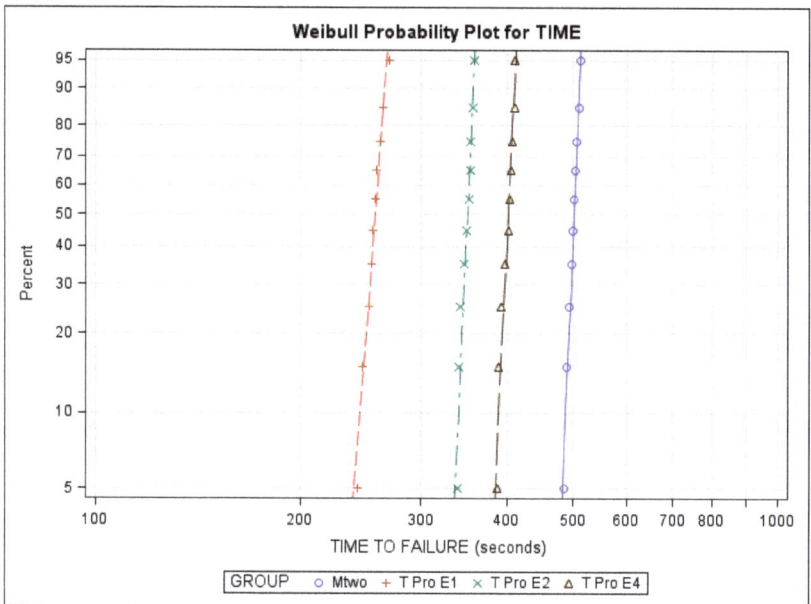

Figure 5. Weibull probability plot of time to failure of Mtwo NiTi alloy endodontic rotary files, T Pro E1 austenite phase NiTi alloy endodontic rotary files, T Pro E2 austenite phase NiTi alloy endodontic rotary files, and T Pro E4 austenite phase NiTi alloy endodontic rotary files.

4. Discussion

The results obtained in the present study reject the null hypothesis (H_0) that stated that the geometry of the cross-section design would not affect the resistance of NiTi endodontic rotary files to dynamic cyclic fatigue.

The results derived in the present study reported that Mtwo NiTi alloy endodontic rotary files with double S-shaped cross-section showed higher resistance to dynamic cyclic fatigue than T Pro E1 austenite phase NiTi alloy endodontic rotary files with rectangular cross-sections, T Pro E2 austenite phase NiTi alloy endodontic rotary files with convex triangular cross-sections, and T Pro E4 austenite phase NiTi alloy endodontic rotary files with triangular cross-sections. The results can be summarized in that with the increase in the mass and the contact points between the instrument surface and the dentin walls of the root canal, the cyclic fatigue resistance of the NiTi endodontic rotary files decreases. This can also influence the flexibility of the NiTi endodontic rotary files and lead the instrument to cause excessive root canal dentine removal, apical transportation [22], root perforations, and fractures [4,23,24].

The persistent bacterial load present in the root canal system after endodontic therapy has been highlighted as a relevant etiologic factor in the endodontic failure and secondary endodontic infections [25]; moreover, Sjögren established a relationship between the bacterial load reduction during the root canal treatment and the prognosis of the endodontic therapy, and reported that negative microbiological cultures obtained from the root canal system led to an endodontic success rate close to 94%, whereas positive cultures reduced the success rate to 68% [26]. This is the reason that the cyclic fatigue resistance of NiTi endodontic rotary files has been widely analyzed.

The design of the anatomical-based artificial root canal used in the present study was based on the method described by Schneider [21], selecting a 5 mm radius and 60° curvature angle and adapting the geometry to the NiTi endodontic rotary files included in this study. Previous studies have shown that the fatigue resistance of endodontic rotary files decreases as the angle of curvature increases and the radius of curvature decreases [10,27,28], since the stress accumulation on the endodontic rotary file is inversely proportional to the radius of curvature of the canal. As a result, in more abrupt root canals, there is an augmentation of the torsion and flexural bending fatigue that ultimately results in instrument fracture [10,21]. Moreover, clinical or even ex vivo experimental studies would be desirable to reproduce clinical conditions and extrapolate the cyclic fatigue results to the clinical setting; however, the difficulty to homogenize the radius, curvature angle, apical diameter, hardness, and cross-section of the root canals can bias the study by introducing more variables [28]. Therefore, custom-made static and dynamic cyclic fatigue devices have been developed to independently analyze the influence of the variable under study; unfortunately, there is neither a norm that regulates the characteristics of the custom-made cyclic fatigue devices nor an international standard for testing the cyclic fatigue behavior of NiTi endodontic rotary instruments with taper higher than 2% [29].

Static and dynamic testing devices have been used to analyze the cyclic fatigue. In the static cyclic fatigue testing models, the NiTi endodontic files are rotated until fracture occurs and the tension–compression cycles are concentrated in the maximum curvature angle of the root canal, resulting in microstructural alterations in the file and subsequent failure. Therefore, dynamic cyclic fatigue testing devices are preferable to better reproduce the clinical conditions, especially the pecking motion of the NiTi endodontic rotary files. Thus, this study used a dynamic cyclic fatigue testing model, an anatomical-based artificial root canal and an automatic detection system to objectively and accurately identify failures of endodontic rotary files [28,30,31].

Previous studies have analyzed the influence of cross-section design on the mechanical behavior of the NiTi endodontic rotary files. Sekar et al. analyzed the role of the cross-section on the cyclic fatigue resistance of NiTi endodontic rotary files under continuous and reciprocation motion and reported that the 25.06 Mtwo rotary files were significantly more resistant to failure than Revo-S SU and One Shape files in both continuous ($p < 0.001$) and reciprocating motion ($p < 0.001$) [17]. These findings are consistent with the results of our study, which concluded that the double S-shaped cross-section of Mtwo NiTi endodontic files showed higher cyclic fatigue resistance than the rectangular cross-section of T Pro E1 NiTi endodontic files, the convex triangular cross-section of T Pro E2 NiTi endodontic files, and the triangular cross-section of T Pro E4 NiTi endodontic files. In addition, de Menezes et al. reported that ProDesign endodontic rotary files with a modified double S-shaped cross-section design presented a significantly higher ($p < 0.05$) number of cycles to failure (910.37 ± 472.10) than Wave One Gold endodontic reciprocating files with a parallelogram cross-section design (264.76 ± 305.42) in artificial root canals with a 60° curvature and 5 mm radius of curvature [32]. Moreover, Adiguzel et al. showed that XP-endo Shaper endodontic rotary files with triangular cross-sections design presented a significantly higher ($p < 0.05$) number of cycles to failure (3064.0 ± 248.1) than HyFlex CM endodontic rotary files with a variable cross-section design (from triangular to trapezoidal and quadratic) (1120.5 ± 106.1) in artificial root canals with a 60° curvature and 3 mm radius of curvature [33]; however, Uygun et al. showed that HyFlex EDM endodontic rotary files with a variable cross-section design (from triangular to trapezoidal and quadratic) presented a significantly higher ($p < 0.05$) number of cycles to failure (1710.42 ± 114.89) than Vortex Blue endodontic rotary files with a convex triangular cross-section design

(548.39 ± 77.64), ProTaper Gold endodontic rotary files with a convex triangular cross-section design (600.83 ± 66.49), and One Curve endodontic rotary files with a variable cross-section design (from double S-shaped to triangular) (959.58 ± 61.18) in artificial root canals with a 60° curvature and 3 mm radius of curvature [34].

Unfortunately, the limitations of the present study prevented the analysis of more cross-section designs to standardize the NiTi alloy, apical diameter, pitch, helix angle, manufacturing process, speed, and taper. In addition, the study was not developed in a clinical environment due to the difficulty in standardizing the sample.

5. Conclusions

The conclusion derived from the present study is that the double S-shaped cross-section of Mtwo NiTi endodontic files shows higher cyclic fatigue resistance than the rectangular cross-section of T Pro E1 NiTi endodontic files, the convex triangular cross-section of T Pro E2 NiTi endodontic files, and the triangular cross-section of T Pro E4 NiTi endodontic files.

Author Contributions: Conceptualization, V.F.-L., N.H.-K. and Á.Z.-M.; design, I.F.-M.; data acquisition, C.R.S.; formal analysis, V.F.-M.; statistical analyses, Á.Z.-M. and V.F.-L.; review and editing, N.H.-K. and M.T.M.R. All authors have read and agreed to the published version of the manuscript.

Funding: This research received no external funding.

Institutional Review Board Statement: Not applicable.

Informed Consent Statement: Not applicable.

Data Availability Statement: Data are available on request due to restrictions, e.g., privacy or ethical.

Conflicts of Interest: The authors declare no conflict of interest.

References

1. Walia, H.; Brantley, W.A.; Gerstein, H. An initial investigation of the bending and torsional properties of nitinol root canal files. *J. Endod.* **1988**, *14*, 346–351. [CrossRef]
2. Esposito, P.T.; Cunningham, C.J. A comparison of canal preparation with nickel-titanium and stainless steel instruments. *J. Endod.* **1995**, *21*, 173–176. [CrossRef]
3. Bergmans, L.; Van Cleynenbreugel, J.; Wevers, M.; Lambrechts, P. Mechanical root canal preparation with NiTi rotary instruments: Rationale, performance and safety. Status report for the American Journal of Dentistry. *Am. J. Dent.* **2001**, *14*, 324–333. [PubMed]
4. Parashos, P.; Gordon, I.; Messer, H.H. Factors Influencing Defects of Rotary Nickel-Titanium Endodontic Instruments After Clinical Use. *J. Endod.* **2004**, *30*, 722–725. [CrossRef] [PubMed]
5. Spili, P.; Parashos, P.; Messer, H.H. The Impact of Instrument Fracture on Outcome of Endodontic Treatment. *J. Endod.* **2005**, *31*, 845–850. [CrossRef] [PubMed]
6. Sattapan, B.; Nervo, G.J.; Palamara, J.E.; Messer, H.H. Defects in Rotary Nickel-Titanium Files After Clinical Use. *J. Endod.* **2000**, *26*, 161–165. [CrossRef] [PubMed]
7. Peters, O.; Barbakow, F. Dynamic torque and apical forces of ProFile .04 rotary instruments during preparation of curved canals. *Int. Endod. J.* **2002**, *35*, 379–389. [CrossRef]
8. Kuhn, G.; Tavernier, B.; Jordan, L. Influence of Structure on Nickel-Titanium Endodontic Instruments Failure. *J. Endod.* **2001**, *27*, 516–520. [CrossRef] [PubMed]
9. Pruett, J.P.; Clement, D.J.; Carnes, D.L., Jr. Cyclic fatigue testing of nickel-titanium endodontic instruments. *J. Endod.* **1997**, *23*, 77–85. [CrossRef]
10. Parashos, P.; Messer, H.H. Rotary NiTi Instrument Fracture and its Consequences. *J. Endod.* **2006**, *32*, 1031–1043. [CrossRef]
11. Topçuoğlu, H.S.; Topçuoğlu, G. Cyclic Fatigue Resistance of Reciproc Blue and Reciproc Files in an S-shaped Canal. *J. Endod.* **2017**, *43*, 1679–1682. [CrossRef]
12. Siqueira, J.F., Jr.; Rôças, I.N. Polymerase chain reaction–based analysis of microorganisms associated with failed endodontic treatment. *Oral. Surg. Oral. Med. Oral. Pathol. Oral. Radiol. Endod.* **2014**, *97*, 85–94. [CrossRef]
13. Strindberg, L. The Dependence of the Results of Pulp Therapy on Certain Factors: An Analytic Study Based on Radiographic and Clinical Follow-up Examinations. *Acta Odontol. Scand.* **1956**, *14*, 1–175.
14. Zupanc, J.; Vahdat-Pajouh, N.; Schäfer, E. New thermomechanically treated NiTi alloys—A review. *Int. Endod. J.* **2018**, *51*, 1088–1103. [CrossRef] [PubMed]

15. Faus-Llácer, V.; Kharrat, N.H.; Ruiz-Sánchez, C.; Faus-Matoses, I.; Zubizarreta-Macho, Á.; Faus-Matoses, V. The Effect of Taper and Apical Diameter on the Cyclic Fatigue Resistance of Rotary Endodontic Files Using an Experimental Electronic Device. *Appl. Sci.* **2021**, *11*, 863. [CrossRef]
16. Turpin, Y.L.; Chagneau, F.; Vulcain, J.M. Impact of Two Theoretical Cross-Sections on Torsional and Bending Stresses of Nickel-Titanium Root Canal Instrument Models. *J. Endod.* **2000**, *26*, 414–417. [CrossRef] [PubMed]
17. Sekar, V.; Kumar, R.; Nandini, S.; Ballal, S.; Velmurugan, N. Assessment of the role of cross section on fatigue resistance of rotary files when used in reciprocation. *Eur. J. Dent.* **2016**, *10*, 541–545. [CrossRef] [PubMed]
18. Kwak, S.W.; Ha, J.-H.; Lee, C.-J.; El Abed, R.; Abu-Tahun, I.H.; Kim, H.-C. Effects of Pitch Length and Heat Treatment on the Mechanical Properties of the Glide Path Preparation Instruments. *J. Endod.* **2016**, *42*, 788–792. [CrossRef] [PubMed]
19. Keskin, C.; Yilmaz, Ö.S.; Keleş, A.; Inan, U. Comparison of cyclic fatigue resistance of Rotate instrument with reciprocating and continuous rotary nickel–titanium instruments at body temperature in relation to their transformation temperatures. *Clin. Oral Investig.* **2021**, *25*, 151–157. [CrossRef] [PubMed]
20. Zubizarreta-Macho, Á.; Álvarez, J.M.; Martínez, A.A.; Segura-Egea, J.J.; Bruchelli, J.C.; Agustín-Panadero, R.; Píriz, R.L.; Alonso-Ezpeleta, Ó. Influence of the Pecking Motion Frequency on the Cyclic Fatigue Resistance of Endodontic Rotary Files. *J. Clin. Med.* **2019**, *9*, 45. [CrossRef] [PubMed]
21. Schneider, S.W. A comparison of canal preparations in straight and curved root canals. *Oral Surg. Oral Med. Oral Pathol.* **1971**, *32*, 271–275. [CrossRef]
22. Freire, L.G.; Gavini, G.; Cunha, R.S.; Dos Santos, M. Assessing apical transportation in curved canals: Comparison between cross-sections and micro-computed tomography. *Braz. Oral Res.* **2012**, *26*, 222–227. [CrossRef] [PubMed]
23. Ounsi, H.F.; Salameh, Z.; Al-Shalan, T.; Ferrari, M.; Grandini, S.; Pashley, D.H.; Tay, F.R. Effect of Clinical Use on the Cyclic Fatigue Resistance of ProTaper Nickel-Titanium Rotary Instruments. *J. Endod.* **2007**, *33*, 737–741. [CrossRef] [PubMed]
24. Grande, N.M.; Plotino, G.; Pecci, R.; Bedini, R.; Malagnino, V.A.; Somma, F. Cyclic fatigue resistance and three-dimensional analysis of instruments from two nickel–titanium rotary systems. *Int. Endod. J.* **2006**, *39*, 755–763. [CrossRef] [PubMed]
25. Siqueira, J.F., Jr. Aetiology of root canal treatment failure: Why well-treated teeth can fail. *Int. Endod. J.* **2001**, *34*, 1–10. [CrossRef]
26. Sjögren, T.; Figdor, D.; Persson, S.; Sundqvist, G. Influence of infection at the time of root filling on the outcome of endodontic treatment of teeth with apical periodontitis. *Int. Endod. J.* **1997**, *30*, 297–306. [CrossRef]
27. Azimi, S.; Delvari, P.; Hajarian, H.C.; Saghiri, M.A.; Karamifar, K.; Lotfi, M. Cyclic Fatigue Resistance and Fractographic Analysis of Race and Protaper Rotary NiTi Instruments. *Iran. Endod. J.* **2011**, *6*, 80–86.
28. Haïkel, Y.; Serfaty, R.; Bateman, G.; Senger, B.; Allemann, C. Dynamic and cyclic fatigue of engine-driven rotary nickel-titanium endodontic instruments. *J. Endod.* **1999**, *25*, 434–440. [CrossRef]
29. ISO. *Dentistry—Root Canal Instruments—Part 1: General Requirements and Test Methods*; ISO 3630–3631; ISO; Geneva, Switzerland, 2008.
30. Whipple, S.J.; Kirkpatrick, T.C.; Rutledge, R.E. Cyclic Fatigue Resistance of Two Variable-taper Rotary File Systems: ProTaper Universal and V-Taper. *J. Endod.* **2009**, *35*, 555–558. [CrossRef]
31. Gambarini, G. Cyclic Fatigue of Nickel-Titanium Rotary Instruments after Clinical Use with Low-and High-Torque Endodontic Motors. *J. Endod.* **2001**, *27*, 772–774. [CrossRef]
32. De Menezes, S.E.A.C.; Batista, S.M.; Lira, J.O.P.; de Melo Monteiro, G.Q. Cyclic Fatigue Resistance of WaveOne Gold, ProDesign R and ProDesign Logic Files in Curved Canals In Vitro. *Iran Endod. J.* **2017**, *12*, 468–473. [PubMed]
33. Adiguzel, M.; Isken, I.; Pamukcu, I.I. Comparison of cyclic fatigue resistance of XP-endo Shaper, HyFlex CM, FlexMaster and Race instruments. *J. Dent. Res. Dent. Clin. Dent. Prospect.* **2018**, *12*, 208–212. [CrossRef] [PubMed]
34. Uygun, A.D.; Unal, M.; Falakaloglu, S.; Guven, Y. Comparison of the cyclic fatigue resistance of hyflex EDM, vortex blue, protaper gold, and onecurve nickel-Titanium instruments. *Niger J. Clin. Pract.* **2020**, *23*, 41–45. [PubMed]

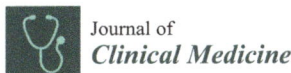

Journal of
Clinical Medicine

Review

Influence of Guided Tissue Regeneration Techniques on the Success Rate of Healing of Surgical Endodontic Treatment: A Systematic Review and Network Meta-Analysis

Álvaro Zubizarreta-Macho [1,2,3,*], Roberta Tosin [1], Fabio Tosin [1], Pilar Velasco Bohórquez [1], Lara San Hipólito Marín [1], José María Montiel-Company [4], Jesús Mena-Álvarez [3] and Sofía Hernández Montero [1]

1. Department of Implant Surgery, Faculty of Health Sciences, Alfonso X El Sabio University, 28691 Madrid, Spain; rtosi@myuax.com (R.T.); ftosi@myuax.com (F.T.); mvelaboh@uax.es (P.V.B.); lsanhmar@uax.es (L.S.H.M.); shernmon@uax.es (S.H.M.)
2. Department of Surgery, Faculty of Medicine and Dentistry, University of Salamanca, 37008 Salamanca, Spain
3. Department of Endodontics, Faculty of Health Sciences, Alfonso X El Sabio University, 28691 Madrid, Spain; jmenaalv@uax.es
4. Department of Stomatology, Faculty of Medicine and Dentistry, University of Valencia, 46010 Valencia, Spain; jose.maria.montiel@uv.es
* Correspondence: amacho@uax.es

Abstract: Several regeneration techniques and materials have been proposed for the healing of bone defects after surgical endodontic treatment; however, the existing literature does not provide evidence on the most recommended techniques or materials. The aim of the present systematic review and network meta-analysis (NMA) is to summarize the clinical evidence on the efficacy of guided tissue regeneration techniques (GRTs). The PRISMA recommendations were followed. Four databases were searched up to December 2021. Randomized clinical trials (RCTs) with a minimum follow-up of 6 months were included. The risk of bias was assessed using the Cochrane Collaboration tool. A fixed effects model and frequentist approach were used in the NMA. Direct GRT technique comparisons were combined to estimate indirect comparisons, and the estimated effect size of the comparisons was analyzed using the odds ratio (OR). Inconsistency was assessed with the Q test, with a significance level of $p < 0.01$, and a net heat plot. A total of 274 articles was identified, and 11 RCTs (6 direct comparisons of 15 techniques) were included in the NMA, which examined 6 GRT techniques: control, Os, PL, MB, MB + Os, and MB + PL. The MB + Os group compared to the control (OR = 3.67, 95% CI: 1.36–9.90) and to the MB group (OR = 3.47, 95% CI: 1.07–11.3) showed statistically significant ORs ($p < 0.05$). The MB + Os group presented the highest degree of certainly (P-score = 0.93).

Keywords: endodontic surgery; periapical lesion; guided tissue regeneration; bone graft; membrane; platelet rich fibrin

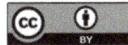

1. Introduction

Bacterial infection plays an important role in establishing pulp tissue inflammation, which may lead to subsequent pulp necrosis and the formation of periapical lesions [1]. The complete removal of, or at least significant reduction in, the bacterial load during non-surgical endodontic treatment is an important factor determining the final prognosis of root canal treatment. However, the development of apical periodontitis was reported in 44.9% of studied cases [2], mainly related to persistent or secondary endodontic infections [3].

Endodontic surgery is recommended after unsuccessful retreatment, when retreatment is impossible, or when there is an unfavorable prognosis [4]. Surgical endodontic procedures include removing necrotic and infected periapical tissues, resecting the apical part of the tooth (apicoectomy), and preparing the root-end cavity for the insertion of retrograde filling material [5]. Conventional endodontic surgery has been reported to result in a complete periapical tissue healing rate of 90% [6].

Recently, guided tissue regeneration (GTR) techniques have been widely used in medicine, including in dentistry, to improve tissue healing. Furthermore, GTR techniques have been recommended as an adjunct to endodontic surgery to promote periapical tissue healing and improve the treatment outcome [7].

Complete periapical healing involves the regeneration of alveolar bone, periodontal ligament cells, and cementum [8]. However, the surrounding connective tissues may grow into the osseous defect, preventing bone healing [6]. GTR techniques have been proposed as an adjunct to endodontic surgery approaches to promote bone healing and prevent the collapse of connective tissues [9].

Numerous studies reported the clinical effectiveness of GTR techniques to promote healing and improve the outcome of surgical endodontic treatments [10,11]. However, the wide range of available biomaterials, the treatment protocols, and the lack of standardization in assessment criteria lead to inconsistent and confusing results. Therefore, an evidence-based review and meta-analysis of the available literature regarding the influence of GTR techniques on the outcome of surgical endodontic treatment is necessary to help clinicians select the most predictable tissue regeneration technique for surgical endodontic treatment success.

Network meta-analysis (NMA) extends the principles of meta-analysis to the evaluation of several treatments in a single analysis, comparing multiple treatments simultaneously by combining direct and indirect evidence within an array of randomized controlled trials [12]. It is the best tool to examine the success rates of different procedures, such as GTR techniques in endodontic surgery.

The aim of the present study is to conduct a systematic review and NMA to analyze the influence of GTR techniques on the success rate of surgical endodontic treatment. The null hypothesis (H0) was that GTR techniques do not influence the success rate of surgical endodontic treatment.

2. Materials and Methods

2.1. Study Design and Registration

This systematic review and NMA was conducted following the Preferred Reporting Items for Systemic Reviews and Meta-Analyses (PRISMA, http://www.prisma-statement.org, accessed on 30 July 2020) guidelines. The review also fulfilled the PRISMA 2009 Checklist [13]. The registration number is CRD42020203447 (PROSPERO).

2.2. Literature Search Process

The search strategy was based on the following population, intervention, comparison, outcome (PICO) question: in adult patients undergoing endodontic surgery (P), does the use of regeneration techniques (I) compared to not applying regeneration techniques (C) influence the success rate (O)? An electronic search was conducted in the PubMed, Scopus, EMBASE, and Web of Science databases. The search covered all of the literature published internationally up to December 2021. The search included the following medical subject heading (MeSH) terms: "apicoectomy", "periapical surgery", "endodontic surgery", "periapical lesion", "surgical endodontic treatment", "root-end surgery", "root-end resection", "periradicular surgery", "guided tissue regeneration", "bone graft", "bone regeneration", and "membrane". The Boolean operators applied were OR and AND. The search terms were structured as follows: ((("apicoectomy") OR ("periapical surgery") OR ("endodontic surgery") OR ("periapical lesion") OR ("surgical endodontic treatment") OR ("root-end surgery") OR ("root-end resection") OR ("periradicular surgery")) AND ((("guided tissue regeneration") OR ("bone graft") OR ("bone regeneration")) AND (("membrane")). Two researchers (R.T. and A.Z.M.) independently conducted the database searches in duplicate. Titles and abstracts were selected by applying the inclusion and exclusion criteria. One researcher (R.T.) extracted data for the relevant variables. The systematic review was carried out by R.T., and two researchers not involved in the selection process (A.Z.M. and J.M.C.) performed the subsequent meta-analysis.

2.3. Inclusion and Exclusion Criteria

The inclusion criteria for the selected studies were as follows: randomized clinical trials (RCTs) that had a minimum follow-up period of at least 6 months; studies that analyzed GTR techniques (bone graft, membrane, membrane plus bone graft, platelet-rich plasma, or membrane plus platelet-rich plasma) or compared GTR techniques with a control treatment; patients that were 18 years old or older; and endodontic surgery procedures that were used to treat apical and/or apical-marginal lesions. No restrictions were placed on the year of publication or language.

The exclusion criteria for the selected studies were as follows: systematic or bibliographic reviews, clinical cases, case series, retrospective studies, and editorials and studies, including patients younger than 18 years.

2.4. Data Extraction

The following data were extracted from each study by independent reviewers (S.H.M. and J.M.A.): author and year of publication, title, journal in which the article was published, sample size (n), follow-up time, measurement procedure, type of GTR technique, success rate, periapical reduction, and bone density. The success of healing was analyzed according to the radiographic criteria established by Rud et al. [14] and Molven et al. [15], with complete healing defined as the reformation of periodontal space (intact lamina dura) with one cavity filled with bone (which can be of different radiopacity) and complete bone repair, but no discernable PDL around the apex. A third reviewer (P.V.B.) was consulted if the independent reviewers did not agree.

2.5. Risk of Bias

The risk of bias in the selected studies was assessed using the Cochrane Collaboration tool for methodological quality assessment of clinical trials [16]. This tool consists of 7 items that evaluate sequence generation, allocation concealment, participant blinding, assessment blinding, incomplete data, free selective reporting, and other sources of bias (Table 1 and Figure 1).

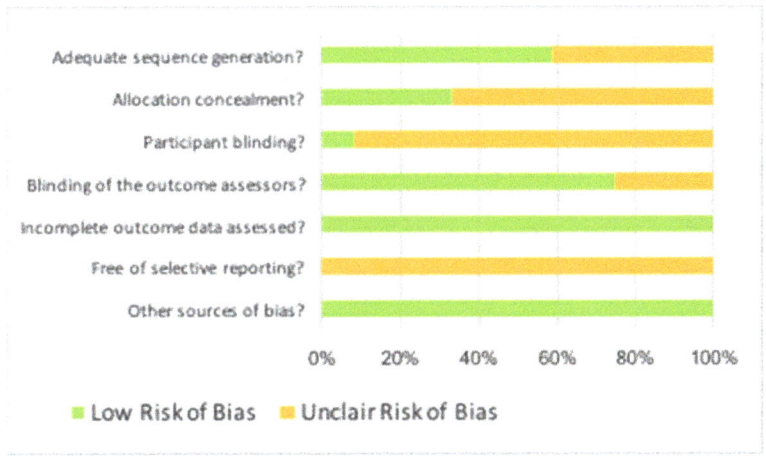

Figure 1. Risk of bias. Green color means "low risk of bias", and yellow color means "unclair risk of bias".

Table 1. Cochrane Collaboration tool for assessing risk of bias.

Author, Year	Adequate Sequence Generation?	Allocation Concealment?	Participant Blinding?	Blinding of Outcome Assessors?	Incomplete Outcome Data Assessed?	Free of Selective Reporting?	Other Sources of Bias?
Dhamija, 2020	Low	Low	Unclear	Low	Low	Unclear	Low
Dhiamn, 2015	Unclear	Low	Unclear	Low	Low	Unclear	Low
Goyal, 2011	Low	Low	Unclear	Low	Low	Unclear	Low
Marin Botero, 2006	Low	Low	Unclear	Low	Low	Unclear	Low
Parmar, 2019	Low	Unclear	Low	Low	Low	Unclear	Low
Pecora, 2002	Low	Low	Unclear	Low	Low	Unclear	Low
Stassen, 1994	Unclear	Unclear	Unclear	Low	Low	Unclear	Low
Taschieri, 2007a	Low	Unclear	Unclear	Low	Low	Unclear	Low
Taschieri, 2007b	Low	Unclear	Unclear	Low	Low	Unclear	Low
Taschieri, 2008	Low	Unclear	Unclear	Low	Low	Unclear	Low
Tobon, 2002	Unclear	Unclear	Unclear	Unclear	Low	Unclear	Low

2.6. Data Synthesis and Statistical Analysis

The meta-analysis was carried out using a random effects model to estimate the success rate of endodontic surgery with and without GTR techniques, along with the confidence intervals. Heterogeneity among the combined studies for each treatment group was assessed using the I^2 statistical index [17], which describes the percentage of total variation of studies due to heterogeneity and is not random. The effect of heterogeneity was quantified as being between 0 and 100% (low 0–25%, mild 25–50%, moderate 50–75%, high > 75%) [17]. The results of the meta-analysis are represented by forest plots.

Direct treatment comparisons were combined with a fixed effects model in a frequentist NMA to estimate indirect comparisons. The estimated effect size of the comparisons was analyzed by the OR. The inconsistency of studies included in the NMA was assessed with the Q test [18], with a significance level of $p < 0.01$, and a net heat plot [19].

Direct comparisons were performed using a NETWORK graph, and treatments were ranked on a scale of 0 to 1 using a P-score measuring the degree of certainty and indicating whether one treatment was superior to another [20].

Publication bias was analyzed using the trim and fill adjustment method for funnel plot asymmetry. In this analysis, each study was represented by a point, and the effect size and standard error were represented on the X-axis (logit transformed proportion). If there were no significant differences between the initial and adjusted estimates, the publication bias was considered to be low. R software was used with the Metaprop and Netmetaprop statistical packages to perform the meta-analysis.

3. Results

3.1. Results of the Search Process

The systematic electronic search identified 159 articles in PubMed, 40 in Web of Science, 64 in EMBASE, 12 in Scopus, and 1 in the gray literature, which was found in the bibliography of a previous review [21]. Of the 276 articles, 56 were discarded as duplicates using RefWorks (https://refworks.proquest.com/reference/upload/recent/, accessed on 14 August 2020). After reading the titles and abstracts, an additional 130 articles were eliminated, leaving 90 articles; a further 55 articles were rejected because they did not fulfil the inclusion criteria: they did not include complete success rate data, did not use in vivo patient data, or presented a minimum follow-up time of less than 6 months. Finally, 11 articles were included in the qualitative and quantitative synthesis because they included all of the required data and variables (Figure 2).

3.2. Qualitative Analysis

All 11 articles that were included were randomized clinical trials [22–32]. Among them, 7 studies analyzed both clinical and radiographic parameters [23,24,26–28,30,31], and 4 studies analyzed radiographic parameters, such as bone density and periapical defect volume [22,25,27,32]. Most of the studies presented a sample size of approximately

25–30 patients, although the sample size ranged from 25 [30] to 101 [23], with subject ages ranging from 18 to 70 years and a follow-up time from 12 to 24 months. The results are presented in Table 2.

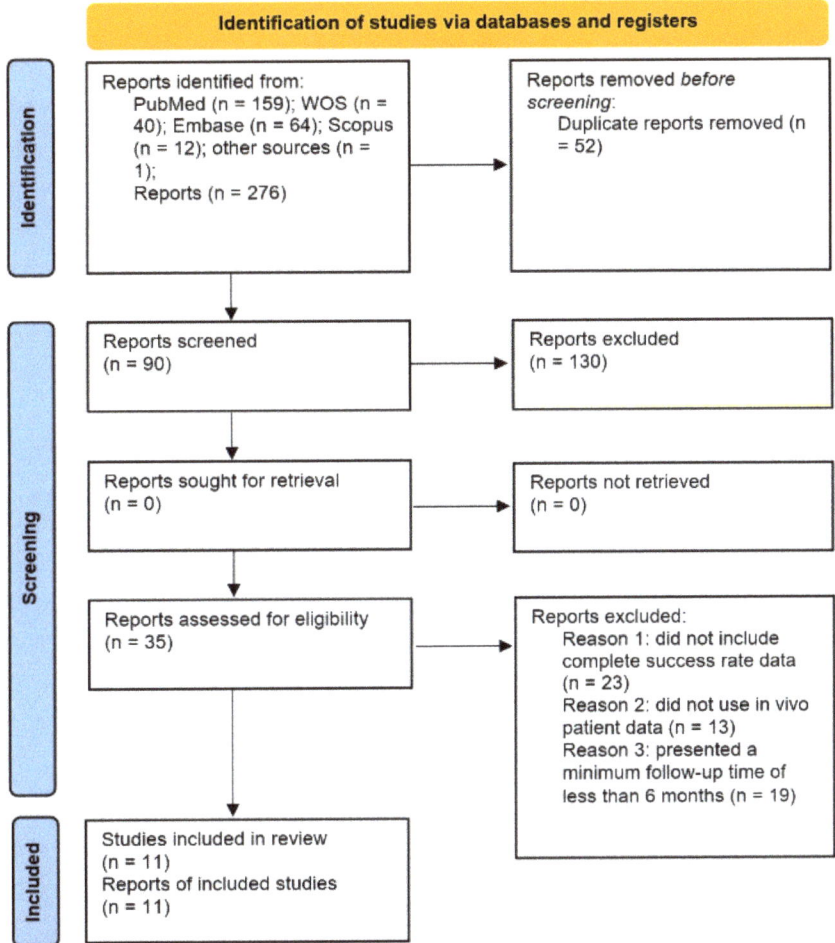

Figure 2. Preferred Reporting Items for Systematic Reviews and Meta-Analyses (PRISMA) flow diagram.

3.3. Assessment of Risk of Bias

The methodological quality results were assessed using the Cochrane Collaboration tool and are shown in Table 1. All selected studies showed a low risk of bias related to incomplete data outcome assessment and other sources of bias. Moreover, most studies showed a low risk of bias related to sequence generation assessment and blinding of outcome assessors; however, most studies also showed an unclear risk of bias related to allocation concealment and participant blinding, and all studies showed an unclear risk of bias related to free selective reporting.

Table 2. Qualitative analysis of articles included in systematic review.

Author/Year	Study Type	Sample (n)	Follow-Up Time (Months)	Measurement Procedure	GTR Technique	Complete Healing Rate	Periapical Healing Results
Dhiamn, 2015	RCT	26	12	Clinical and radiographic	Control PL	8/11 8/15	Control: 53.3% complete healing PL: 53.33% complete healing
Goyal, 2011	RCT	25	3	Clinical and radiographic	MB PL PL + MB	NAv NAv NAv	MB: 38.7 ± 22.3% periapical size reduction PL: 39.2 ± 11.7% periapical size reduction PL + MB: 45.6 ± 14.2% periapical size reduction
		25	6		MB PL PL + MB	NAv NAv NAv	MB: 67.9 ± 16.3% periapical size reduction PL: 84.9 ± 10.4% periapical size reduction PL + MB: 75.9 ± 12.2% periapical size reduction
		25	9		MB PL PL + MB	NAv NAv NAv	MB: 88.6 ± 10.1% periapical size reduction PL: 93.3 ± 3.0% periapical size reduction PL + MB: 90.3 ± 6.9% periapical size reduction
		25	12		MB PL PL + MB	7/10 5/6 7/9	MB: 97.0 ± 3.2 periapical size reduction PL: 96.3 ± 3.0% periapical size reduction PL + MB: 97.3 ± 3.3% periapical size reduction
Marin Botero, 2006	RCT	30	12	Clinical and radiographic	Control Mb Os	9/15 6/15 50/68	Control: 91.1 ± 18.1% periapical size reduction MB: 87.0 ± 18.6% periapical size reduction
Parmar, 2019	RCT	30	12	Radiographic 2D	Control MB	12/15 11/15	Control: 12 ± 21mm^2 (92 ± 12% reduction) MB: 31 ± 30 mm^2 (86 ± 14% reduction)
		30	12	Radiographic 3D	Control MB	9/15 8/15	Control: 174 ± 264 mm^3 (85 ± 19% reduction) MB: 324 ± 364 mm^3 (82 ± 13% reduction)
Pecora, 2002	RCT	20	6	Clinical and radiographic	Control Os	3/10 8/10	Significant reduction in periapical defects ($p < 0.05$)
		18	12		Control Os	3/9 7/9	
Dhamija, 2020	RTC	32	12	Clinical and radiographic	PL Control	9/16 5/16	Significant reduction in periapical defects ($p < 0.05$)

Table 2. Cont.

Author/Year	Study Type	Sample (n)	Follow-Up Time (Months)	Measurement Procedure	GTR Technique	Complete Healing Rate	Periapical Healing Results
Stassen, 1994	RTC	101	24	Clinical and radiographic	Control Os	50/56 29/45	No significant reduction in periapical defects ($p = 0.057$)
Taschieri, 2007	RTC	59	12	Radiographic 4-wall defects	Control MB + Os	18/22 14/16	Control: 80.0–83.3% complete healing MB + Os: 81.8–100% complete healing
		59	12	Radiographic through-and-through	Control MB + Os	8/13 6/8	Control: 55.6–75.0% complete healing MB + Os: 75.0% complete healing
Taschieri, 2008	RTC	31	12	Clinical and radiographic	Control MB + Os	8/14 15/17	Control: 57.1% complete healing Os: 88.2% complete healing
Taschieri, 2008	RTC	69	12	Clinical and radiographic 2-wall defects	Control MB + Os	9/14 15/17	Statistically significant differences ($p = 0.02$)
				Clinical and radiographic 4-wall defects	Control MB + Os	18/22 14/16	No statistically significant differences ($p = 0.21$).
Tobon, 2002	RTC	26	12	Radiographic	Control MB MB + Os	4/9 6/9 8/8	Control: 44.4% complete healing MB: 66.6% complete healing MB + Os: 100% complete healing

RCT, randomized controlled trial; CT, controlled trial; CS, case series; NAv, not available; PL, platelet enriched plasma; Os, bone graft; MB, membrane.

3.4. Quantitative Analysis Results

Odds ratios among regeneration techniques for the success of healing after endodontic surgery (meta-analysis):

Six meta-analyses of direct comparisons between GRT techniques (PL vs. control, MB vs. PL, MB + PL vs. MB, MB vs. control, Os vs. control, MB + Os vs. control) were carried out with the data obtained from the eleven selected RCTs. The meta-analysis of combined studies comparing MB-Os versus control (fixed effects model with the absence of heterogeneity; $I^2 = 0\%$) estimated a significant OR of 3.53 with a 95% confidence interval between 1.33 and 9.33. The remaining comparisons do not produce a significant OR (Figure 3).

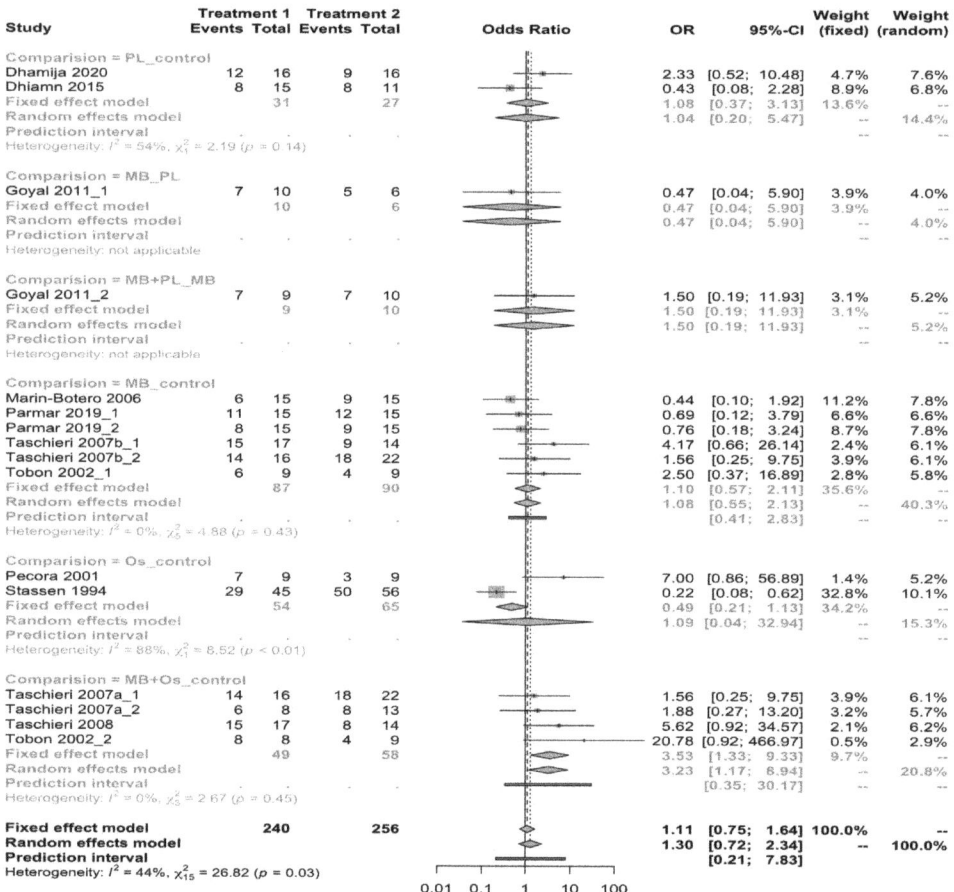

Figure 3. Forest plot of ORs among guided tissue regeneration techniques for healing success after endodontic surgery. Column 1 lists the articles included in the meta-analysis. Columns 2 and 3 show us the results of the articles in the form of a proportion. Column 3 is the forest plot itself, the graphic part of the representation. It plots the effect measures for each study on both sides of the null effect line, which is the one for the odds ratio. In the lower part of the graph, the global result of the meta-analysis is represented. Column 4 describes the estimated weight of each study in percentage, and column 5 presents the estimates of the weighted effect of each one. Diamonds indicate the mean and confidence interval of combined effect, and squares indicate the mean and confidence interval of each study. Red lines represent the prediction interval.

Odds ratios were among the regeneration techniques for the success of healing after endodontic surgery (net meta-analysis).

Eleven RCTs (sixteen pairs of comparisons) were included in a frequentist NMA examining six GRT techniques (control, Os, PL, MB, MB + Os, and MB + PL) to analyze their influence on the success of healing after endodontic surgery. The data were combined with a fixed effects model (Mantel–Haenszel method). The nodes represent treatments, and the lines connecting the nodes are the six direct comparisons included in the NMA (Figure 4).

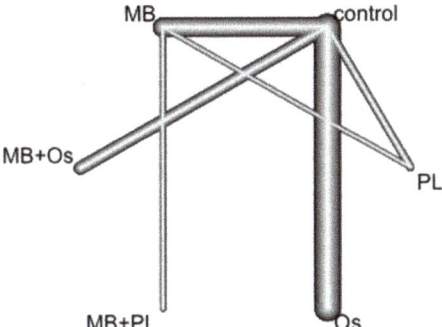

Figure 4. NETWORK plot of GTR techniques. Node size is proportional to the number of participants randomized to that technique, and the edge width is proportional to number of trials comparing two techniques.

The outcome of GTR techniques was estimated in terms of OR and 95% confidence interval. OR > 1 indicated that the treatment in the first column on the left was superior to the comparator, while OR < 1 indicated the opposite. Statistically significant ORs are shown in bold ($p < 0.05$). Direct comparisons (6/15) are highlighted in gray, and indirect comparisons are uncolored. Only two statistically significant ORs were found (in bold) ($p < 0.05$). The probability of obtaining a successful result was 3.67 times greater in the MB + Os group than in the control group ($p < 0.05$). The success of healing was 3.47 times greater in the MB + Os group than in the MB group ($p < 0.05$). The remaining comparisons among the groups do not show significance ($p > 0.05$) (Table 3 and Figure 5).

The ranking of the GTR techniques was performed according to the P-score, which measures the degree of certainty and indicates whether one alternative is superior to the others. The P-score is measured on a scale of 0 to 1. The MB + Os group presents the highest P-score (0.93), followed by MB + PL (0.60) and PL (0.53) (Figure 6).

Table 3. Comparison between GTR techniques using OR and 95% confidence intervals estimated in Netmeta. * $p < 0.05$.

	Control	MB	MB + Os	MB + PL	Os	PL
Control	1	0.95 0.50; 1.78	0.27 * 0.10; 0.73	0.63 0.07; 5.52	2.04 0.88; 4.66	0.82 0.31; 2.21
MB	1.06 0.56; 1.99	1	0.29 * 0.09; 0.94	0.66 0.08; 5.30	2.14 0.76; 6.11	0.87 0.29; 2.68
MB + Os	3.67 * 1.36; 9.90	3.47 * 1.07; 11.3	1	2.31 0.21; 25.1	7.46 2.04; 27.2	3.04 0.75; 12.3
MB + PL	1.58 0.18; 13.9	1.50 0.19; 11.9	0.43 0.04; 4.69	1	3.22 0.32; 32.9	1.31 0.12; 13.8
Os	0.49 0.21; 1.13	0.47 0.16; 1.32	0.13 0.04; 0.49	0.31 0.03; 3.16	1	0.41 0.11; 1.47
PL	1.21 0.45; 3.23	1.14 0.37; 3.49	0.33 0.08; 1.33	0.76 0.07; 8.04	2.46 0.68; 8.32	1

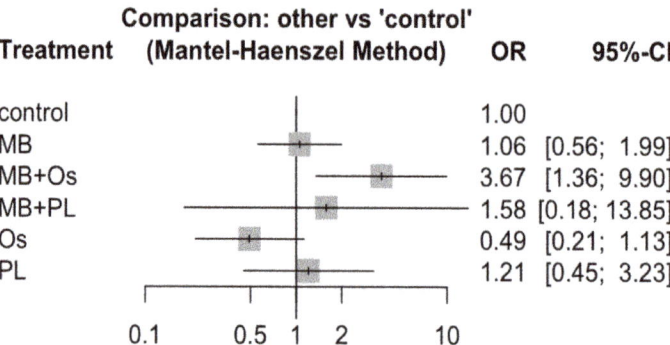

Figure 5. Forest plot of healing success using GTR techniques (odds ratio) compared to control group.

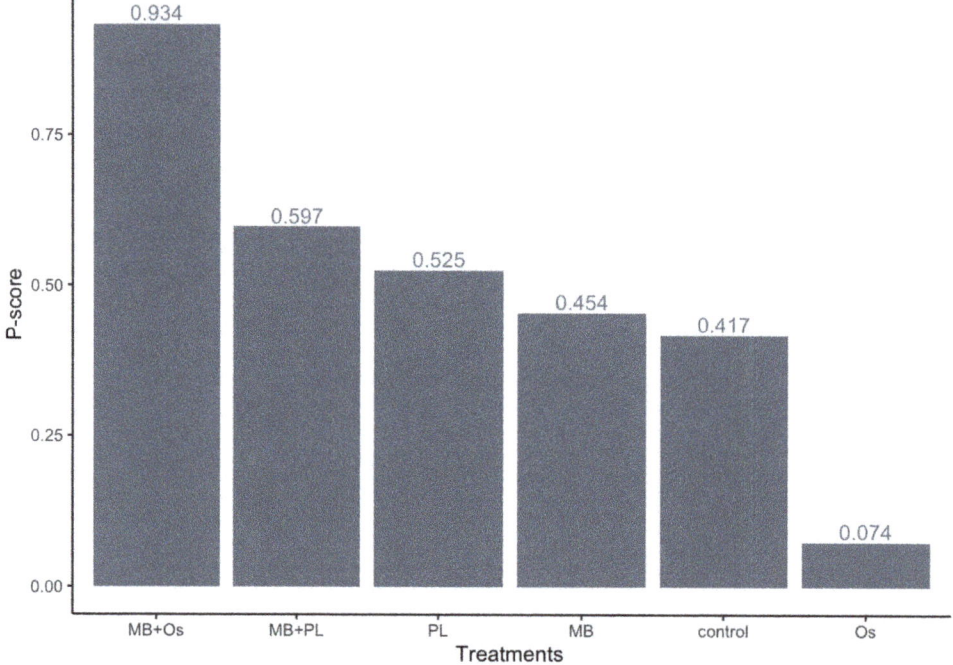

Figure 6. Ranking of GTR techniques by P-score.

No heterogeneity or inconsistency was found in the NMA (test of heterogeneity/inconsistency Q = 0.29; p = 0.589). The net heat plot (Figure 7), which provides a detailed assessment of inconsistency, detected a very slight inconsistency between direct and indirect estimations, which was not significant.

3.5. Publication Bias

Six new studies were incorporated using the trim and fill method to adjust for funnel plot asymmetry, and a new OR for the six direct comparisons analyzed was estimated. No statistically significant differences were found with respect to the initially estimated OR (Figure 8).

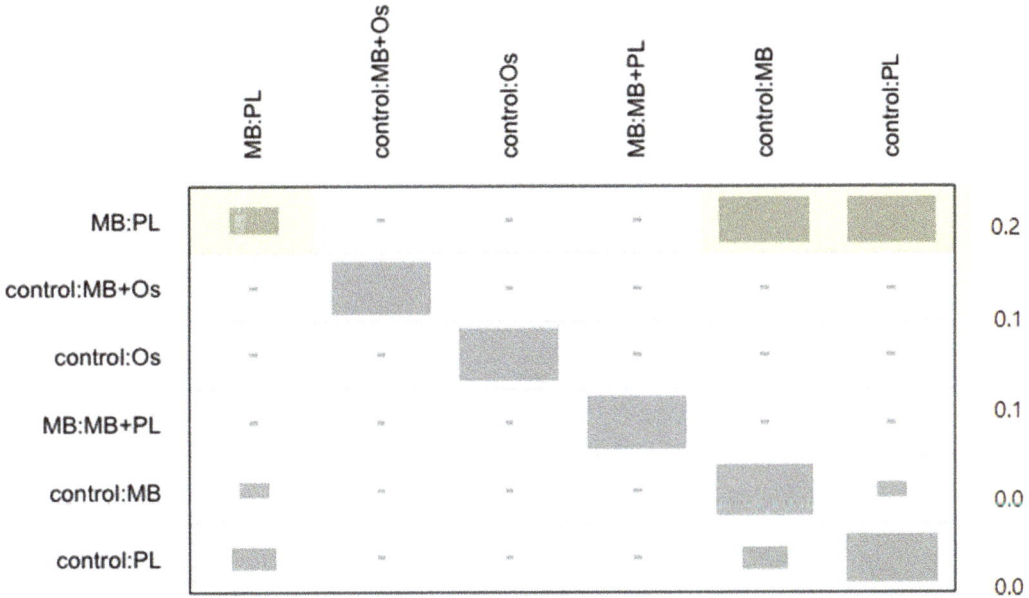

Figure 7. Net heat plot. Gray boxes signify the importance of one treatment comparison to the estimation of another treatment comparison. Larger boxes indicate more important comparisons. Color background, ranging from blue to red, signifies the inconsistency of comparison (row) attributable to design (column).

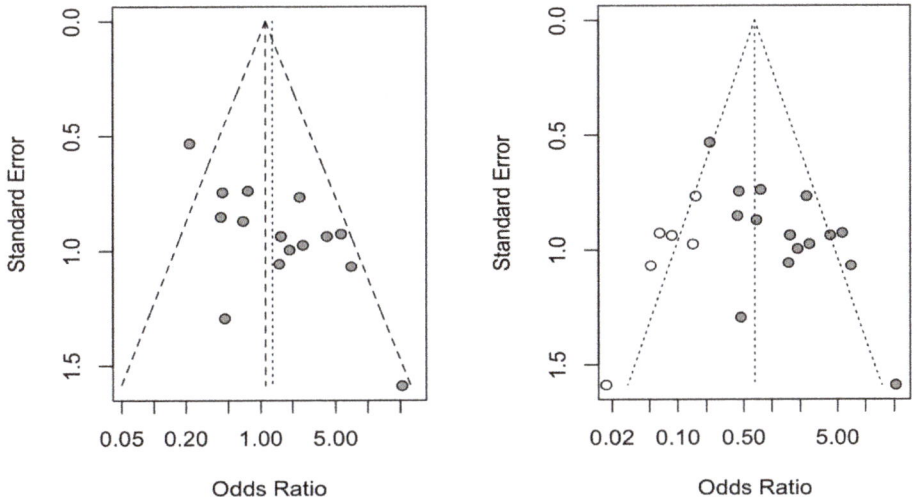

Figure 8. Initial funnel plot after trim and fill adjustment of OR of periapical healing among guided tissue regeneration techniques.

4. Discussion

The objective of this systematic review and NMA was to investigate the influence of different GTR techniques used as adjuncts to endodontic surgery and analyze their efficacy, assessed in terms of success rates. The results of the NMA show that the success rate of endodontic surgery can be improved using GTR techniques as adjuncts, and combined therapy with bone grafts plus membranes results in a higher success rate.

Since the NMA did not show heterogeneity or inconsistency (Q = 1.16; p = 0.2821), the present NMA satisfied the assumption of transitivity, indicating that there were no systematic differences among the compared techniques other than the GTR techniques being compared [33]. Evaluating the transitivity assumption is critical, because the existence of intransitivity will bias treatment effect estimates [12]. Therefore, the calculated OR (3.6; p < 0.05) for the comparison between membrane plus bone grafting and endodontic surgery alone indicates that the success rate of this combination was almost four times higher than that of surgery without an adjunct GTR technique.

Most authors highlighted the relevance of membranes to promoting the healing of bone defects and preventing adjacent soft tissue ingrowth. The use of a membrane alone, without a bone graft, was 1.02 times more effective than endodontic surgery without a GTR technique (control), and more effective than platelet-rich plasma techniques. However, the membrane plus bone graft combination was 3.6 times more successful than membrane only.

The success rate of the combined membrane plus bone graft was 3.7 times higher than that of endodontic surgery alone (control). Parmar et al. (2019) reported a nonsignificant radiographic reduction in periapical bone defects regenerated using a resorbable collagen membrane. Complete periapical healing was observed in the control group, with rates of 60 to 80% and 53.3 to 73.3% of those of the membrane group, depending on the radiodiagnostic technique [32].

Marin-Botero et al. (2006) also reported that polyglactin-910 resorbable membranes had little influence on the complete healing of periapical bone defects after endodontic surgery (40%) compared with the control treatment (60%) [26]. Garret et al. (2002) reported that resorbable membranes did not show a statistically significant (p > 0.05) radiographic reduction in periapical bone defects after endodontic surgery. Additionally, they did not recommend the use of resorbable membranes for bone defects with four walls that are confined to the apical region [34]. Santamaria Zuazua et al. (1998) analyzed the bone density and radiographic reduction in periapical bone defects after endodontic surgery using resorbable and non-resorbable membranes, and found no statistically significant difference (p > 0.05) in bone density at 6 months after surgery between the two types of membranes.

These results suggest that GTR techniques using membranes do not contribute to increased periapical bone regeneration regardless of the membrane type [35]. However, Taschieri et al. (2011) retrospectively analyzed clinical and radiographic periapical bone healing after endodontic surgery procedures using a collagen resorbable membrane and recommended its application for through-and-through lesions [36]. Goyal et al. (2011) analyzed the impact of membranes and platelet-rich plasma on the complete periapical healing of periapical bone defects after endodontic surgery. They found no statistically significant differences (p > 0.05) among the membrane alone, platelet-rich plasma alone, and the two combined [30]. Dhiman et al. (2015) reported no statistically significant difference (p > 0.05) in the clinical and radiographic reduction in periapical bone defects after endodontic surgery using platelet-rich plasma techniques with respect to the control group [32].

Most authors reported that bone grafts stimulate bone defect healing and prevent adjacent soft tissue collapse [4,23,37–39]. Kattimani et al. (2014) highlighted the use of bovine-derived and synthetic hydroxyapatite bone grafts for the radiographic reduction in periapical bone defects after endodontic surgery. They found no statistically significant difference (p > 0.05) in radiographic reduction between the two bone graft materials [38]. Kattimani et al. (2016) also compared the clinical and radiographic outcomes of bovine-derived and synthetic hydroxyapatite bone grafts after endodontic surgery. They found no statistically significant (p > 0.05) difference between the two bone graft materials at 6-month follow-up [39]. Stassen et al. (1994) also analyzed the clinical and radiographic effects of bovine-derived hydroxyapatite bone grafts and did not recommend their use as adjuncts in endodontic surgery [23]. However, Sreedevi (2011) reported complete clinical and radiographic periapical bone healing after endodontic surgery using hydroxyapatite bone graft material with respect to the control group [4].

Other bone graft materials have been used as adjuncts to GTR techniques in endodontic surgery. Pantchev et al. (2009) retrospectively analyzed the clinical and radiographic outcomes of a synthetic bioactive glass material used as a bone graft after endodontic surgery. They found a statistically significant difference ($p < 0.05$) at short-term follow-up (9–24 months), but no statistically significant difference ($p > 0.05$) at long-term follow-up (33–48 months) [37]. It is more difficult to apply endodontic surgery using a GTR technique to 4-wall defects and through-and-through lesions because of the higher risk of soft tissue collapse and decreased stability of the bone regeneration material. Pecora et al. (2001) demonstrated that the addition of calcium sulfate as a bone graft material in GTR techniques for the treatment of through-and-through lesions improves the clinical outcome [24]. However, Taschieri et al. (2007, 2008) showed no statistically significant difference ($p > 0.05$) after endodontic surgery when using resorbable collagen membrane and bovine-derived hydroxyapatite bone graft material for through-and-through lesions [27] and four-wall defects [29]. Tobon et al. (2002) reported that the simultaneous use of nonresorbable membrane and bovine-derived hydroxyapatite bone graft material produced complete clinical and radiographic periapical bone healing after endodontic surgery [25].

In addition, the wound healing scales and indices used in oral surgery do not capture the relationships between outcome parameters; therefore, Hamzani et al. (2018) proposed a novel scale that allows the assessment of wound healing phases [40]. Recently, Haj Yahya et al. (2020) described a novel procedure for measuring the healing process after surgical extraction based on an inflammatory proliferative remodeling scale that could also be used in further studies for the assessment of wound healing following endodontic surgery [41].

A limitation of this systematic review and meta-analysis is the possibility that not all articles related to the selection criteria were identified, although the risk was decreased because three databases were searched. In addition, most of the studies were of poor quality, according to the Cochrane Collaboration tool [16]. Furthermore, the most effective GTR technique (MB + Os) was only included in a single study. Therefore, further, better designed clinical studies with higher quality are necessary.

5. Conclusions

Within the limitations of this study, it was found that GTR techniques increased the success rate of endodontic surgery. The use of bone grafts plus membranes as an adjunct to surgical endodontic treatment promoted complete periapical bone healing, with a higher success rate, and improved the prognosis of endodontic surgery. Therefore, we recommend the use of bone grafts plus membranes as a GTR technique in endodontic surgery.

Author Contributions: Conceptualization, Á.Z.-M., R.T. and F.T.; data acquisition, P.V.B.; design, L.S.H.M.; review and editing, J.M.-Á. and S.H.M.; all statistical analyses, J.M.M.-C. All authors have read and agreed to the published version of the manuscript.

Funding: This research received no external funding.

Institutional Review Board Statement: Not applicable.

Informed Consent Statement: Not applicable.

Data Availability Statement: Information is available upon request in accordance with relevant restrictions (e.g., privacy or ethical).

Conflicts of Interest: The authors have no conflict of interest.

References

1. Siqueira, J.F., Jr.; Rôças, I.N. The microbiota of acute apical abscesses. *J. Dent. Res.* **2009**, *88*, 61–65. [CrossRef] [PubMed]
2. Kielbassa, A.M.; Frank, W.; Madaus, T. Radiologic assessment of quality of root canal fillings and periapical status in an Austrian subpopulation—An observational study. *PLoS ONE* **2017**, *12*, e0176724. [CrossRef] [PubMed]
3. Siqueira, J.F., Jr. Aetiology of root canal treatment failure: Why well-treated teeth can fail. *Int. Endod. J.* **2001**, *34*, 1–10. [CrossRef] [PubMed]
4. Sreedevi, P.; Varghese, N.; Varugheese, J.M. Prognosis of periapical surgery using bonegrafts: A clinical study. *J. Conserv. Dent.* **2011**, *14*, 68–72. [CrossRef]
5. Chong, B.S.; Rhodes, J.S. Endodontic surgery. *Br. Dent. J.* **2014**, *216*, 281–290. [CrossRef]
6. Tsesis, I.; Rosen, E.; Taschieri, S.; Telishevsky Strauss, Y.; Ceresoli, V.; Del Fabbro, M. Outcomes of surgical endodontic treatment performed by a modern technique: An updated meta-analysis of the literature. *J. Endod.* **2013**, *39*, 332–339. [CrossRef]
7. Mastromihalis, N.; Goldstein, S.; Greenberg, M.; Friedman, S. Applications for guided bone regeneration in endodontic surgery. *N. Y. State Dent. J.* **1999**, *65*, 30–32.
8. Kim, S.; Kratchman, S. Modern endodontic surgery concepts and practice: A review. *J. Endod.* **2006**, *32*, 601–623. [CrossRef]
9. Corbella, S.; Taschieri, S.; Elkabbany, A.; Del Fabbro, M.; von Arx, T. Guided Tissue Regeneration Using a Barrier Membrane in Endodontic Surgery. *Swiss Dent. J.* **2016**, *126*, 13–25.
10. Von Arx, T.; Cochran, D.L. Rationale for the application of the GTR principle using a barrier membrane in endodontic surgery: A proposal of classification and literature review. *Int. J. Periodontics Restor. Dent.* **2001**, *21*, 127–139.
11. Tsesis, I.; Rosen, E.; Tamse, A.; Taschieri, S.; Del Fabbro, M. Effect of guided tissue regeneration on the outcome of surgical endodontic treatment: A systematic review and meta-analysis. *J. Endod.* **2011**, *37*, 1039–1045. [CrossRef] [PubMed]
12. Rouse, B.; Chaimani, A.; Li, T. Network meta-analysis: An introduction for clinicians. *Intern. Emerg. Med.* **2017**, *12*, 103–111. [CrossRef] [PubMed]
13. Banzi, R.; Moja, L.; Liberati, A.; Gensini, G.F.; Gusinu, R.; Conti, A.A. Measuring the impact of evidence: The Cochrane systematic review of organised stroke care. *Intern. Emerg. Med.* **2009**, *4*, 507–510. [CrossRef] [PubMed]
14. Rud, J.; Andreasen, J.O.; Jensen, J.E. Radiographic criteria for the assessment of healing after endodontic surgery. *Int. J. Oral Surg.* **1972**, *1*, 195–214. [CrossRef]
15. Molven, O.; Halse, A.; Grung, B. Observer strategy and the radiographic classification of healing after endodontic surgery. *Int. J. Oral Maxillofac. Surg.* **1987**, *16*, 432–439. [CrossRef]
16. Higgins, J.P.T.; Green, S. (Eds.) *Cochrane Handbook for Systematic Reviews of Interventions Version 5.1.0*; The Cochrane Collaboration: London, UK, 2011.
17. Higgins, J.P.; Thompson, S.G.; Deeks, J.J.; Altman, D.G. Measuring inconsistency in meta-analyses. *BMJ* **2003**, *327*, 557–560. [CrossRef]
18. Dias, S.; Welton, N.J.; Caldwell, D.M.; Ades, A.E. Checking consistency in mixed treatment comparison meta-analysis. *Stat. Med.* **2010**, *29*, 932–944. [CrossRef]
19. Freeman, S.C.; Fisher, D.; White, I.R.; Auperin, A.; Carpenter, J.R. Identifying inconsistency in network meta-analysis: Is the net heat plot a reliable method? *Stat. Med.* **2019**, *38*, 5547–5564. [CrossRef]
20. Rücker, G.; Schwarzer, G. Ranking treatments in frequentist network meta-analysis works without resampling methods. *BMC Med. Res. Methodol.* **2015**, *15*, 58. [CrossRef]
21. Liu, T.J.; Zhou, J.N.; Guo, L.H. Impact of different regenerative techniques and materials on the healing outcome of endodontic surgery: A systematic review and meta-analysis. *Int. Endod. J.* **2021**, *54*, 536–555. [CrossRef]
22. Dhamija, R.; Tewari, S.; Sangwan, P.; Duhan, J.; Mittal, S. Impact of Platelet-rich Plasma in the Healing of Through-and-through Periapical Lesions Using 2-dimensional and 3-dimensional Evaluation: A Randomized Controlled Trial. *J. Endod.* **2020**, *46*, 1167–1184. [CrossRef] [PubMed]
23. Stassen, L.F.; Hislop, W.S.; Still, D.M.; Moos, K.F. Use of anorganic bone in periapical defects following apical surgery—a prospective trial. *Br. J. Oral Maxillofac. Surg.* **1994**, *32*, 83–85. [CrossRef]
24. Pecora, G.; De Leonardis, D.; Ibrahim, N.; Bovi, M.; Cornelini, R. The use of calcium sulphate in the surgical treatment of a 'through and through' periradicular lesion. *Int. Endod. J.* **2001**, *34*, 189–197. [CrossRef] [PubMed]
25. Tobón, S.I.; Arismendi, J.A.; Marín, M.L.; Mesa, A.L.; Valencia, J.A. Comparison between a conventional technique and two bone regeneration techniques in periradicular surgery. *Int. Endod. J.* **2002**, *35*, 635–641. [CrossRef]
26. Marín-Botero, M.L.; Domínguez-Mejía, J.S.; Arismendi-Echavarría, J.A.; Mesa-Jaramillo, A.L.; Flórez-Moreno, G.A.; Tobón-Arroyave, S.I. Healing response of apicomarginal defects to two guided tissue regeneration techniques in periradicular surgery: A double-blind, randomized-clinical trial. *Int. Endod. J.* **2006**, *39*, 368–377. [CrossRef] [PubMed]
27. Taschieri, S.; Del Fabbro, M.; Testori, T.; Weinstein, R. Efficacy of xenogeneic bone grafting with guided tissue regeneration in the management of bone defects after surgical endodontics. *J. Oral Maxillofac. Surg.* **2007**, *65*, 1121–1127. [CrossRef] [PubMed]
28. Taschieri, S.; Del Fabbro, M.; Testori, T.; Saita, M.; Weinstein, R. Efficacy of guided tissue regeneration in the management of through-and-through lesions following surgical endodontics: A preliminary study. *Int. J. Periodontics Restor. Dent.* **2008**, *28*, 265–271.
29. Taschieri, S.; Testori, T.; Azzola, F.; Del Fabbro, M.; Valentini, P. Régénération tissulaire guidée en chirurgie endodontique [Guided-tissue regeneration in endodontic surgery]. *Rev. Stomatol. Chir. Maxillofac.* **2008**, *109*, 213–217. [CrossRef]

30. Goyal, B.; Tewari, S.; Duhan, J.; Sehgal, P.K. Comparative evaluation of platelet-rich plasma and guided tissue regeneration membrane in the healing of apicomarginal defects: A clinical study. *J. Endod.* **2011**, *37*, 773–780. [CrossRef]
31. Dhiman, M.; Kumar, S.; Duhan, J.; Sangwan, P.; Tewari, S. Effect of Platelet-rich Fibrin on Healing of Apicomarginal Defects: A Randomized Controlled Trial. *J. Endod.* **2015**, *41*, 985–991. [CrossRef]
32. Parmar, P.D.; Dhamija, R.; Tewari, S.; Sangwan, P.; Gupta, A.; Duhan, J.; Mittal, S. 2D and 3D radiographic outcome assessment of the effect of guided tissue regeneration using resorbable collagen membrane in the healing of through-and-through periapical lesions—A randomized controlled trial. *Int. Endod. J.* **2019**, *52*, 935–948. [CrossRef] [PubMed]
33. Salanti, G. Indirect and mixed-treatment comparison, network, or multiple-treatments meta-analysis: Many names, many benefits, many concerns for the next generation evidence synthesis tool. *Res. Synth. Methods.* **2012**, *3*, 80–97. [CrossRef]
34. Garrett, K.; Kerr, M.; Hartwell, G.; O'Sullivan, S.; Mayer, P. The effect of a bioresorbable matrix barrier in endodontic surgery on the rate of periapical healing: An in vivo study. *J. Endod.* **2002**, *28*, 503–506. [CrossRef] [PubMed]
35. Santamaría, J.; García, A.M.; de Vicente, J.C.; Landa, S.; López-Arranz, J.S. Bone regeneration after radicular cyst removal with and without guided bone regeneration. *Int. J. Oral Maxillofac. Surg.* **1998**, *27*, 118–120. [CrossRef]
36. Taschieri, S.; Corbella, S.; Tsesis, I.; Bortolin, M.; Del Fabbro, M. Effect of guided tissue regeneration on the outcome of surgical endodontic treatment of through-and-through lesions: A retrospective study at 4-year follow-up. *Oral Maxillofac. Surg.* **2011**, *15*, 153–159. [CrossRef]
37. Pantchev, A.; Nohlert, E.; Tegelberg, A. Endodontic surgery with and without inserts of bioactive glass PerioGlas—A clinical and radiographic follow-up. *Oral Maxillofac. Surg.* **2009**, *13*, 21–26. [CrossRef]
38. Kattimani, V.S.; Chakravarthi, S.P.; Neelima Devi, K.N.; Sridhar, M.S.; Prasad, L.K. Comparative evaluation of bovine derived hydroxyapatite and synthetic hydroxyapatite graft in bone regeneration of human maxillary cystic defects: A clinico-radiological study. *Indian J. Dent. Res.* **2014**, *25*, 594–601. [CrossRef]
39. Kattimani, V.; Lingamaneni, K.P.; Chakravarthi, P.S.; Kumar, T.S.; Siddharthan, A. Eggshell-Derived Hydroxyapatite: A New Era in Bone Regeneration. *J. Craniofac. Surg.* **2016**, *27*, 112–117. [CrossRef]
40. Hamzani, Y.; Chaushu, G. Evaluation of early wound healing scales/indexes in oral surgery: A literature review. *Clin. Implant. Dent. Relat. Res.* **2018**, *20*, 1030–1035. [CrossRef]
41. Haj Yahya, B.; Chaushu, G.; Hamzani, Y. Evaluation of wound healing following surgical extractions using the IPR Scale. *Int. Dent. J.* **2020**, *71*, 133–139. [CrossRef]

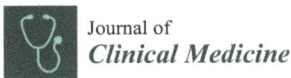

Review

Vital and Nonvital Pulp Therapy in Primary Dentition: An Umbrella Review

Luísa Bandeira Lopes [1,2,*], Catarina Calvão [1,2], Filipa Salema Vieira [1,2], João Albernaz Neves [2,3], José João Mendes [2,4], Vanessa Machado [2,4] and João Botelho [2,4]

1. Dental Pediatrics Department, Egas Moniz—Cooperativa de Ensino Superior, 2829-511 Almada, Portugal; catarinacalvao@hotmail.com (C.C.); filipasalemavieira@gmail.com (F.S.V.)
2. Clinical Research Unit (CRU), Centro de Investigação Interdisciplinar Egas Moniz (CiiEM), Egas Moniz—Cooperativa de Ensino Superior, 2829-511 Almada, Portugal; jalbernazneves@gmail.com (J.A.N.); jmendes@egasmoniz.edu.pt (J.J.M.); vmachado@egasmoniz.edu.pt (V.M.); jbotelho@egasmoniz.edu.pt (J.B.)
3. Endodontics Department, Egas Moniz—Cooperativa de Ensino Superior, 2829-511 Almada, Portugal
4. Evidenced-Based Hub, Centro de Investigação Interdisciplinar Egas Moniz, Egas Moniz—Cooperativa de Ensino Superior, 2829-511 Almada, Portugal
* Correspondence: luisabpmlopes@gmail.com

Abstract: Dental caries is the most common non-communicable disease in children with significant aesthetic, functional, and quality of life deterioration. Depending on the depth, two approaches may be considered in primary dentition: vital pulp therapy (VPT) or non-vital therapy (NPT). This umbrella review aimed to critically assess the available systematic reviews (SRs) on VPT and NPT. An electronic database search was conducted (PubMed, Embase, Scopus, Cochrane, Web of Science, and LILACS) until June 2021. The Risk of Bias (RoB) of SRs was analyzed using the Measurement Tool to Assess SRs criteria 2 (AMSTAR2). From 272 entries, 33 SRs were included. Regarding the methodological quality, three studies were critically low, nine low, seventeen moderate, and six were rated as high quality. The quality of evidence produced by the available SRs was moderate. Future high standard SRs and well-designed clinical trials are warranted to better elucidate the clinical protocols and outcomes of VPT and NPT.

Keywords: endodontics; pediatric dentistry; oral health; dental medicine; systematic review; umbrella review

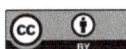

1. Introduction

Dental caries is the most common non-communicable disease in children with significant aesthetic, functional and quality of life deterioration [1]. Caries lesions can jeopardize the teeth vitality, as its progression cause infection, pain, and even early tooth loss [1,2]. Thus, a timely intervention is key to avoid unpleasant consequences for the child. Depending on the depth of caries (which may have pulp involvement), two approaches may be considered in the primary dentition: vital pulp therapy (VPT) or non-vital therapy (NPT) [1,3].

When the pulp is still recuperable, VPT may be an option and three options are available: indirect pulp treatment (IPT), direct pulp cap (DPC), and pulpotomy [1–5]. When the caries lesion progresses to the point where pulp necrotizes, then an NPT is performed, such as pulpectomy [3].

The efficacy of VPT and NPT has been widely researched [2–5]. However, the variability of designs, techniques, and material contributes to high heterogeneity regarding the evidence produced. IPT is a technique that leaves at the bottom of the cavity some deep caries to avoid pulp exposure, being covered with a biocompatible material to produce a biological seal [2,4,5]. DPC is a procedure in which there is a pulp exposure, being covered with a biocompatible material. There is a controversy about this method since it has shown limited success [2–5]. Pulpotomy is an approach applied when there is a carious pulp exposure and where the entire coronal pulp is removed, hemostasis of the radicular pulp is accomplished, and the remaining radicular pulp is treated with a medicament [3,6]. In contrast, pulpectomy is a nonvital treatment (NVT), being a root canal treatment with irreversibly inflamed or necrotic pulp resulting from caries or trauma [1,3,5,6]. Due to the clinical interest of these procedures in endodontics, several systematic reviews (SRs) have been published. Thus, appraising all the available evidence-based information would be of great interest.

Therefore, this umbrella review aimed to appraise the existing evidence on VPT and NVT in primary teeth. Our main focus was to ascertain the overall clinical efficacy of each procedure and its quality of evidence.

2. Materials and Methods

We followed the Preferred Reporting Items for Systematic Reviews and Meta-Analyses (PRISMA) guideline updated in 2020 [7] (Supplementary Table S1) and the guide for systematic reviews of systematic review [8]. The review protocol was approved a priori by all authors.

The Review question was: "How effective are VPT and NPT for treating deep carious lesion on primary dentition?".

The following PECO statements were set: Population (P)—Patients with deep caries on primary dentition; Exposure (E)—Clinical management; Comparison (C)—VPT (IPT, DPC and pulpotomy) and NPT (pulpectomy); Outcome (O)—Diagnosis and a variety of dental treatment types.

2.1. Eligibility Criteria

The inclusion criteria were as follows: (1) systematic review (with or without meta-analysis); (2) retrieving data from human studies; (3) addressing VPT and NPT on primary teeth. No restrictions to publication year or language were applied. Grey literature was searched through three appropriate databases (opensigle.inist.fr, https://www.ntis.gov/, https://www.apa.org/pubs/databases/psycextra, all accessed in June 2021).

2.2. Information Sources Search

Electronic data search was performed in seven electronic databases: PubMed (via Medline), Scopus, Cochrane Database of Systematic Reviews, Scielo (Scientific Electronic Library Online), EMBASE (The Excerpta Medica Database), LILACS (Latin-American scientific literature in health sciences), and TRIP (Turning Research Into Practise) up to June 2021. We merged keywords and subject headings in accordance with the thesaurus of each database and applied exploded subject headings, with the following syntax "(Primary teeth [MeSH] OR Pulp therapy [MeSH] OR Tooth [MeSH]) AND (Pulpotomy OR Pulpectomy OR Vital pulp therapy OR Deciduous teeth) AND (Systematic Review OR Meta-analysis)".

2.3. Study Selection

Two researchers (FV and CC) independently screened titles and abstracts. The agreement between the reviewers was assessed by Kappa statistics. Any paper classified as potentially eligible by either reviewer was ordered as a full-text and independently screened by the reviewers. All disagreements were resolved through discussion with a third reviewer (LBL).

2.4. Data Extraction Process and Data Items

Two researchers (FV and CC) independently extracted: authors and year of publication, objective/focused question, databases searched, number of studies included, type of studies included, main results and main conclusions. All disagreements were resolved through discussion with a third reviewer (LBL).

2.5. Risk of Bias Assessment

Two researchers (FV and CC) employed the MeaSurement Tool to Assess Systematic Reviews (AMSTAR 2) to determine the methodological quality of the included reviews [8]. AMSTAR 2 is a comprehensive 16-item tool that rates the overall confidence of the results of the review. According to the AMSTAR guidelines, the quality of the systematic reviews was considered as follows: High means 'Zero or one non-critical weakness'; Moderate means 'More than one non-critical weakness'; Low means 'One critical flaw with or without non-critical weaknesses'; and Critically low means 'More than one critical flaw with or without non-critical weaknesses. The estimation of the AMSTAR quality rate for each study was calculated through the AMSTAR 2 online tool (https://amstar.ca/Amstar_Checklist.php).

3. Results

3.1. Study Selection

Electronic searches retrieved a total of 272 titles through the database search. After manual assessment of title/abstract and removal of duplicates, 60 potentially eligible full-texts were screened (Figure 1). Full-text screening excluded thirteen studies with reasons (Supplementary Table S2), resulting in thirty-five systematic reviews that fulfilled the inclusion criteria. Inter-examiner reliability at the full-text screening was recorded as high (kappa score = 1.00).

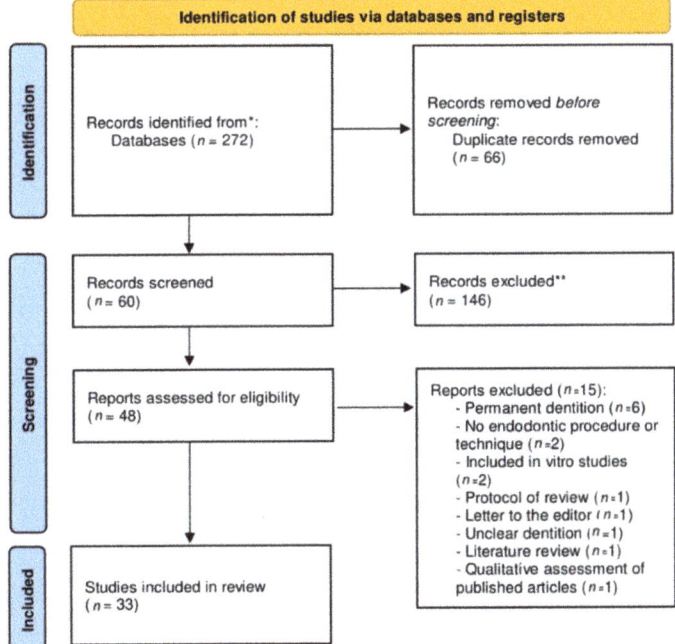

Figure 1. PRISMA flowchart of included studies.

3.2. Study Characteristics

In total, 33 systematic reviews [1–6,9–35] were included in the present umbrella review (Table 1). All SRs covered a defined timeframe; however, one did not mention such information [33]. Three systematics reviews failed to report a language restriction [2,10,11], seventeen restricted their search to studies in English [12–25], one restricted to English and Persia [26], and the remaining had no language restrictions [1,3–6,9,27–35].

Table 1. Characteristics of included studies.

Authors (Year)	N	Search Period	Interventions	Quality Assessment Tool	Sample	Method of Analysis	Outcomes	AMSTAR2 Score *	Funding
Ansari et al. (2018) [12]	17	Up to November 2017	Laser vs. FC in pulpotomy	None	15 NRSI and 2 case reports	SR & MA	Success rate (clinical and radiographic)	Critically Low	NI
Asgary et al. (2014) [13]	4	Up to June 2013	MTA vs. FS in pulpotomy	Modified van Tulder list [1]	4 RCTs	SR & MA	Success rate (clinical)	Moderate	NI
Barcelos et al. (2011) [14]	2	Up to May 2017	ZOE vs. No ZOE pulpectomy	Jadad's scale [2]	2 RCTs	SR	Success rate (clinical and radiographic)	Moderate	NI
Bossu et al. (2020) [15]	41	Up to October 2019	MTA vs. Biodentine vs. FS vs. FC in pulpotomy	Cochrane Collaboration Tool	NI	SR	Success rate (clinical and radiographic)	Low	Self-funded
Chandran et al. (2020) [16]	14	Unclear (up to 2020)	Laser pulpotomy vs. conventional pulpotomy	Cochrane Collaboration Tool	14 RCTs	SR & MA	Success rate (clinical and radiographic)	High	NI
Chugh et al. (2020) [17]	11	Up to March 2020	Rotary vs. hand root canal instrumentation	ROB 2.0 [3]	11 RCTs	SR & MA	Success rate (clinical)	High	NI
Coll et al. (2017) [4]	87	Since 1990	Indirect Pulp Therapy vs Direct pulp capping Vs Pulpotomy	ROB	-	SR & MA	Success rate (clinical and radiographic)	High	NR
Coll et al. (2020) [1]	-	Unclear (up to 2020)	Pulpotomy rate success in teeth with and without root resorption.	ROB	-	SR & MA	Success rate (clinical and radiographic)	High	NR
De Coster et al. (2013) [27]	7	Unclear (up to 2012)	Laser vs. conventional pulpotomy procedures	Dutch Cochrane Collaboration tool	5 RCTs and 2 Case series	SR	Success rate (clinical)	Critically Low	NI
Duarte et al. (2020) [9]	6	Up to December 2019	Lesion sterilization and tissue repair (LSTR) pulpotomy vs. pulpectomy	Cochrane Collaboration Tool	6 RCTs	SR & MA	Success rate (clinical and radiographic)	Moderate	Research Grant
Gadallah et al. (2018) [2]	4	Up to March 2018	Pulpotomy Vs pulpectomy	Cochrane Collaboration Tool	4 RCTs	SR & MA	Success rate (clinical and radiographic)	Low	Self-funded
Garrocho Rangel et al. (2019) [18]	12	Up to December 2019	Direct pulp capping with no carious or small carious exposure of pulp	Criteria developed by the authors	12 RCTs	SR	Success rate (clinical and radiographic)	Moderate	Partially by Research Grant
Ghajari et al. (2008) [26]	8	Up to March 2008	MTA vs. FC in pulpotomy	Jadad's scale [2]	8 RCTs	SR & MA	Success rate (clinical and radiographic)	Moderate	NI
Junior et al. (2019) [11]	9	Up to August 2017	Biodentine vs. MTA in pulpotomy	Cochrane Collaboration Tool	7 RCTs and 2 NRSI	SR & MA	Success rate (clinical and radiographic)	High	NI
Lin et al. (2014) [28]	37	Up to December 2012	MTA vs. Biodentine vs. FS vs. FC vs. Laser in pulpotomy	Criteria developed by the authors	37 RCTs	SR and Network MA	Success rate (clinical and radiographic)	Moderate	Research Grant
Manchanda et al. (2020) [19]	13	Up to January 2019	Rotary vs. hand root canal instrumentation	ROB 2.0 [3]	13 RCTs	SR & MA	Success rate (clinical and radiographic)	Low	NI
Marghalani et al. (2014) [29]	20	Up to May 2013	MTA vs. FC in pulpotomy	Cochrane Collaboration Tool	20 RCTs	SR & MA	Success rate (clinical and radiographic)	Moderate	NI
Nagendrababu et al. (2018) [20]	8	Up to October 2017	MTA vs. Biodentine in pulpotomy	ROB 2.0 [3]	8 RCTs	SR & MA	Success rate (clinical and radiographic)	Moderate	NI
Najjar et al. (2019) [30]	15	Up to January 2018	CH/iodoform vs ZOE in pulpectomy	CONSORT [4]	15 RCTs	SR & MA	Success rate (clinical and radiographic)	Moderate	Self-funded
Nematollahi et al. (2019) [31]	12	Up to September 2017	Laser vs no laser pulpotomy	Jadad's scale [2]	12 RCTs	SR & MA	Success rate (clinical and radiographic)	Low	Self-funded

Table 1. Cont.

Authors (Year)	N	Search Period	Interventions	Quality Assessment Tool	Sample	Method of Analysis	Outcomes	AMSTAR2 Score *	Funding
Nuvvula et al. (2018) [21]	20	Up to January 2017	FS vs. other agents in pulpotomy	Fuks and Papagiannoulis criteria [5]	NI	SR	Success rate (clinical and radiographic)	Low	Self-funded
Peng et al. (2007) [10]	11	Up to May 2006	FC vs. FS in pulpotomy	Jadad's scale [2]	4 RCTs, 4 CCTs, 3 retrospective studies	SR & MA	Success rate (clinical and radiographic)	Moderate	NI
Pintor et al. (2016) [32]	2	Up to May 2013	Smear layer removal vs non removal	Cochrane Collaboration Tool	2 RCTs	SR	Success rate (clinical and radiographic)	Moderate	NI
Pozos-Guillen et al. (2016) [33]	7	NI	Clinical efficacy of intracanal irrigants in pulpectomy	Criteria developed by the authors	7 RCTs	SR & MA	Success rate (clinical)	Moderate	Research Grant
da Rosa et al. (2019) [22]	17	Up to February 2018	CH vs. no-CH as pulp capping	Cochrane Collaboration Tool	14 RCTs and 1 retrospective study on primary teeth	SR & MA	Success rate (clinical)	Moderate	Research Grant
Schwendicke et al. (2016) [34]	11	Up to April 2015	Comparing direct pulp capping materials	Cochrane Collaboration Tool	11 RCTs	SR & MA	Success rate (clinical and radiographic)	Moderate	Self-funded
Shafaee et al. (2019) [35]	10	Up to July 2018	MTA vs. Biodentine vs. FS vs. FC in pulpotomy	Cochrane Collaboration Tool	10 RCTs	SR & MA	Success rate (clinical and radiographic)	Low	NI
Shirvani et al. (2014 a) [23]	19	Up to March 2013	MTA vs. FC in pulpotomy	Modified van Tulder list [1]	19 RCTs	SR & MA	Success rate (clinical)	Moderate	Self-funded
Shirvani et al. (2014 b) [24]	4	Up to March 2013	MTA vs. CH in pulpotomy	Modified van Tulder list [1]	4 RCTs	SR & MA	Success rate (clinical and radiographic)	Moderate	NI
Smail-Faugeron et al. (2016) [6]		Up to February 2015	Indirect pulp capping Vs Pulpotomy	Cochrane Collaboration Tool	8 Survey of dental prattise, 1 non-randomized study, 2 protocols of ongoing randomized trials	SR	Success rate (clinical and radiographic)	Low	NR
Smail-Faugeron et al. (2018) [3]	87	Up to August 2017	MTA vs. Biodentine vs. FS vs. FC vs. Laser in pulpotomy	Cochrane Collaboration Tool	87 RCTs	SR & MA	Success rate (clinical and radiographic)	High	NR
Subramanyam et al. (2017) [25]	8	Up to May 2017	Herbal medicines vs. standard pulpotomy	Criteria developed by the authors	8 RCTs	SR	Success rate (clinical and radiographic)	Low	Self-funded
Tedesco et al. (2021) [5]	9	Up to May 2020	Best approach for deep caries lesion	Cochrane Collaboration Tool	9 RCTs	SR & MA	Success rate (clinical)	Moderate	Self-funded

CCTs—controlled clinical trials; CH—calcium hydroxide; FC—formocresol; FS—Ferric Sulfate; MA—Meta-Analysis; MTA—mineral trioxide aggregate; N—number of included studies; NRSI—Nonrandomized study of intervention; RCTs—randomized-clinical trials; SR—Systematic Review; ZOE—zinc oxide eugenol; NI—no information; NR—not reported. * Detailed information regarding the methodological quality assessment is present in Table 2.

3.3. Methodological Quality

Regarding the methodological quality of SRs, three studies were assessed as of critically low quality [12,27], nine as of low quality [2,6,15,19,21,25,31,35], seventeen studies as of moderate quality [5,9,10,13,14,18,20,22–24,26,28–30,32–34], and six as of high quality [1,3,4,11,16,17] (detailed in Table 2). None of the included SR fully complied with the AMSTAR2 checklist. Overall, SRs mostly failed on: reporting on the sources of funding for the studies included in the review (93.9%, $n = 31$); providing a satisfactory explanation for, and discussion of, any heterogeneity observed in the results (27.3%, $n = 9$); reporting any potential sources of conflict of interest, including funding sources (27.3%, $n = 9$); explaining their selection literature search strategy (20.0%, $n = 7$).

Table 2. Results of the methodological quality assessment via AMSTAR2.

First Author	1	2	3	4	5	6	7	8	9	10	11	12	13	14	15	16	Review Quality
Ansari 2018 [12]	Y	N	Y	PY	Y	Y	Y	PY	N/N	N	N/0	N	N	N	N	Y	Critically Low
Asgary 2014 [13]	Y	Y	Y	PY	Y	Y	N	Y	PY/0	N	Y/0	Y	Y	Y	Y	N	Moderate
Barcelos 2011 [14]	Y	PY	Y	PY	Y	Y	PY	PY	PY/0	N	0/0	0	Y	N	0	N	Moderate
Bossù 2020 [15]	Y	PY	Y	N	Y	Y	Y	PY	PY/PY	N	0/0	0	Y	Y	0	Y	Low
Chandran 2020 [16]	Y	PY	Y	PY	Y	Y	Y	PY	PY/0	N	Y/0	Y	Y	Y	Y	Y	High
Chugh 2020 [17]	Y	PY	Y	PY	Y	Y	Y	PY	PY/0	N	Y/0	Y	Y	Y	Y	Y	High
Coll 2017 [4]	Y	PY	Y	PY	Y	Y	PY	PY	PY/0	N	Y/0	Y	Y	Y	Y	Y	High
Coll 2020 [1]	Y	PY	Y	PY	Y	Y	PY	PY	PY/PY	Y	Y/Y	Y	Y	Y	Y	N	High
De Coster 2013 [27]	Y	PY	N	PY	Y	Y	PY	PY	N/N	N	0/0	0	N	Y	0	N	Critically Low
Duarte 2020 [9]	Y	PY	N	PY	Y	Y	Y	PY	PY/0	N	Y/0	Y	Y	Y	Y	Y	Moderate
Gadallah 2018 [2]	Y	PY	N	PY	Y	Y	PY	PY	PY/0	N	Y/0	Y	Y	Y	Y	Y	Low
Garrocho Rangel 2019 [18]	Y	PY	N	PY	Y	Y	PY	N	PY/0	N	0/0	0	Y	N	0	Y	Moderate
Ghajari 2008 [26]	Y	PY	Y	PY	Y	Y	N	N	PY/0	N	Y/0	Y	Y	Y	Y	Y	Moderate
Junior 2018 [11]	Y	Y	Y	PY	Y	Y	PY	PY	PY/0	N	Y/0	Y	Y	Y	Y	Y	High
Lin 2014 [16]	Y	N	Y	PY	Y	Y	PY	N	PY/0	N	Y/0	Y	Y	Y	Y	Y	Moderate
Manchanda 2020 [19]	Y	PY	Y	PY	Y	Y	Y	PY	PY/0	N	N/0	Y	Y	N	Y	Y	Low
Marghalani 2014 [29]	Y	PY	Y	PY	Y	Y	N	Y	PY/0	N	Y/0	Y	Y	Y	N	Y	Moderate
Nagendrababu 2018 [20]	Y	PY	Y	PY	Y	Y	Y	PY	PY/0	N	Y/0	Y	Y	Y	Y	N	Moderate
Najjar 2019 [30]	Y	PY	Y	PY	Y	Y	N	Y	PY/PY	N	Y/Y	Y	Y	Y	Y	Y	Moderate
Nematollahi 2019 [31]	Y	PY	N	PY	Y	Y	N	N	PY/N	N	Y/Y	Y	Y	Y	N	Y	Low
Nuvvula 2018 [21]	Y	PY	Y	PY	Y	Y	N	PY	N/0	N	0/0	0	N	N	0	Y	Low
Peng 2007 [10]	N	PY	Y	PY	Y	Y	N	N	PY/PY	N	Y/Y	Y	Y	Y	N	N	Moderate
Pintor 2016 [32]	Y	PY	Y	PY	Y	Y	N	Y	Y/0	N	0/0	0	Y	N	0	N	Moderate
Pozos-Guillen 2016 [33]	Y	Y	Y	Y	Y	Y	N	Y	Y/0	N	Y/0	Y	Y	Y	Y	Y	Moderate
Da Rosa 2019 [22]	N	PY	Y	PY	Y	Y	N	PY	Y/0	N	Y/0	Y	Y	Y	Y	Y	Moderate
Schwendicke 2016 [34]	N	Y	N	Y	Y	Y	N	Y	Y/Y	N	Y/Y	Y	Y	Y	Y	Y	Moderate
Shafaee 2019 [35]	N	N	Y	N	Y	Y	N	Y	Y/0	N	Y/0	N	Y	Y	Y	Y	Low
Shirvani 2014 [23]	N	PY	Y	PY	Y	Y	N	Y	PY/0	N	Y/0	N	Y	N	Y	Y	Moderate
Shirvani 2014 (2) [24]	Y	PY	Y	PY	Y	Y	N	PY	Y/0	N	Y/0	Y	Y	Y	Y	Y	Moderate
Smaïl-Faugeron 2016 [6]	N	N	Y	N	Y	Y	N	N	PY/PY	N	0/0	0	Y	N	0	N	Low
Smaïl-Faugeron 2018 [3]	Y	Y	Y	Y	Y	Y	Y	Y	Y/0	Y	Y/0	Y	Y	Y	Y	Y	High
Subramanyam 2017 [25]	Y	Y	Y	PY	N	N	N	Y	Y/0	N	0/0	0	N	N	0	N	Low
Tedesco 2021 [5]	Y	Y	Y	Y	Y	Y	N	Y	PY/0	N	Y/0	Y	Y	Y	Y	Y	Moderate

0—No meta-analysis conducted, N—No, Y—Yes, PY—Partial Yes. 1. Research questions and inclusion criteria? 2. Review methods established a priori? 3. Explanation of their selection literature search strategy? 4. Did the review authors use a comprehensive literature search strategy? 5. Study selection performed in duplicate? 6. Data selection performed in duplicate? 7. List of excluded studies and exclusions justified? 8. Description of the included studies in adequate detail? 9. Satisfactory technique for assessing the risk of bias (RoB)? 10. Report on the sources of funding for the studies included in the review? 11. If meta-analysis was performed, did the review authors use appropriate methods for statistical combination of results? 12. If meta-analysis was performed, did the review authors assess the potential impact of RoB? 13. RoB accounted when interpreting/discussing the results of the review? 14. Did the review authors provide a satisfactory explanation for, and discussion of, any heterogeneity observed in the results of the review? 15. If they performed quantitative synthesis, was publication bias performed? 16. Did the review authors report any potential sources of conflict of interest, including funding sources?.

3.4. Synthesis of Results

3.4.1. Vital Pulp Therapy

Indirect Pulp Treatment (IPT)

In an IPT approach, the caries lesion is not fully removed during instrumentation to avoid pulp exposure, and the remaining affected dentin is then covered with a biocompatible material as a biological seal [4].

Dentin coverage with a liner provides no benefit to the IPT clinical success either using calcium hydroxide (CH) or inert materials (adhesive system or glass-ionomer cement

[GIC] [4,22], and with a certain level of confidence as they are based on SRs of high [4] and moderate methodological quality [22].

Also, IPT demonstrates higher clinical success rate than pulpotomy, with low confidence [6]. The Hall technique (an adapted IPT approach) showed 78% success versus a 76% success of pulpectomy, with moderate confidence [5].

Direct Pulp Capping (DPC)

In the DPC approach, the pulp is exposed during caries removal and covered with a biocompatible material [3–5].

A high-quality SR concluded that DPC presents an 88.8%, success rate regardless of the applied material (CH, dentin bonding agents, MTA and FC) (Coll 2017). These results are corroborated by a moderate quality SR [18] and a high quality Cochrane SR [3]. MTA or enamel matrix proteins do not present uppermost efficacy than CH, and bonding agent directly upon the exposed pulp without previous etching had no significantly different efficacy when compared to CH, MTA or calcium-enriched cement [34].

Also, DPC was shown to present lower clinical success than pulpotomy with moderate confidence [5].

Pulpotomy

A pulpotomy is delivered to exposed pulps during deep caries lesions removal with previously confirmed pulp vitality [4]. Clinically, this approach comprises: total coronal pulp removal; successful hemostasis; and coverage of the remaining radicular pulp with a biocompatible material.

A systematic review and meta-analyses with low quality stated no statistically significant difference in the clinical success rate between pulpotomy and pulpectomies in primary incisors [2].

Regarding the materials required in pulpotomy, the studies were diverse. One systematic review from Cochrane library with high quality stated that the evidence suggests MTA may be the most efficacious medicament to heal the root pulp after pulpotomy [3]. Considering MTA and Biodentine, no significant difference was found in clinical and radiographic success with a moderate quality review [20] and a high-quality review [11]. Already in turn, MTA showed superior long-term treatment outcome than ferric sulfate (FS) with moderate quality review [13], and in three meta-analyses with moderate quality, better rates of clinical and radiographic success than formocresol (FC) [23,26,29] were also mentioned, as well as CH, also with moderate quality review, with good quality of the RCT and homogeneity among the studies [24]. Another meta-analyses with moderate quality that addressed FC and FS demonstrated no significant difference in terms of clinical and radiographic outcomes [10]. Two studies with low quality that compared MTA, Biodentin, FC, and SF agreed that there was no significant difference between those materials, but MTA was considered a better option [15,35], the quality of evidence on the included studies being in one a systematic review regarding the comparisons of Biodentine and formocresol, as well as Biodentine and ferric sulfate, low and very low, respectively [35]. On the other hand, a systematic review with low quality referred MTA as the material of choice, and CH with the worst clinical performance [15]. Another systematic review with low quality compared the previously stated materials with herbal medicines (allium satvum, ankaferd blood stopper, elaegnus angustifolia, propolis), which found similar clinical and radiographic success rates when compared to the usual pulpotomy materials, the overall quality of research in the clinical success of herbal medicine as a pulpotomy medicament not being adequate [25]. One other systematic review with low quality assessed the effectiveness of FS, which reported a high success rate, but the studies included in the review were with limited evidence of high-quality studies [21]. A meta-analysis with moderate quality presented by Lin et al. (2014) showed MTA had the best performance, followed by FC and CH, and CH had more failures than FC and FS [28].

Seven systematic reviews also investigated the effect of lasers as well as the materials mentioned above. Several types of lasers were considered, such as diode, Er:YAG, Nd:YAG, He-Ne, CO2, and low level laser. One meta-analysis with low methodological quality showed no statistically significant difference in clinical and radiographic outcomes between laser pulpotomy and conventional pulpotomy [16]. Another meta-analysis with critically low quality revealed that laser had superior clinical results at a 36-month follow-up period [12]. On the contrary, two studies reported that laser had inferior success than conventional pulpotomy techniques, one being of critically low quality [27], and the other with moderate quality [28]. Finally, another systematic review with low quality showed no significant differences in clinical and radiographic pulpotomy outcomes with laser compared with other techniques [31]. One other meta-analysis with high quality compared different materials, referring that MTA and FC success rates were the highest of all pulpotomy types, including laser, were not significantly different [4]. A recent systematic review from the Cochane Library with high quality stated that the evidence shows MTA may be the best material for pulpotomy of primary teeth. However, other materials should be considered as alternatives like Biodentine, enamel matrix derivative, laser treatment or Ankaferd Blood Stopper. When these materials are not available, application of sodium hypochlorite is the safest option [3].

Note that several studies with different quality, but most with moderate quality mentioned that FC, because of its constitution that presents formaldehyde, presents a concern due its potential carcinogenicity, mutagenicity, and cytotoxicity effect [3,4,10,12,13, 15,16,18,21,23,26,28,29,31,34,35].

3.4.2. Non-Vital Pulp Therapy (NPT)

Among the NVT techniques, pulpectomy of primary teeth is indicated when irreversible pulpitis or necrotic pulp occurs [1].

As far as obturation concerns, resorbable materials are mandatory. Zinc oxide eugenol (ZOE) pulpectomies yielded similar outcome than Vitapex and Sealapex, with moderate methodological confidence [14]. A systematic review from Cochrane with high quality mentioned no conclusive evidence that one medicament or technique is superior to another. Therefore, the choice of medicament remains at the clinician's discretion, since comparison between Metapex and (ZOE) paste was inconclusive, as well as Endoflas and ZOE, and finally suggested ZOE paste may be better than Vitapex [3]. In pulpectomy on primary teeth nearing exfoliation, $Ca(OH)_2$/iodoform the best filling material to be used for pulpectomy in primary teeth nearing exfoliation, being moderate risk [30]. One other study considered zinc oxide eugenol/iodoform/calcium hydroxide or ZOE fillers perform better than iodoform filler, where the risk of bias was high despite heterogeneity between the studies [1]. Regarding lesion sterilization and tissue repair (LSTR) technique and pulpectomy, two meta-analyses showed a nonsignificant difference, one being with moderate quality [9], and another one with high quality [1].

Concerning smear layer, there is no consensus, with one study considering studies at a moderate risk of bias [5,32], despite one systematic review only having taken into account two studies [32]. The root canal irrigation has several products despite the controversy on their performance, as the study exhibited moderate risk of bias [33].

Regarding rotary instrumentation, there are similar clinical and radiographic success rate, but with a better-quality treatment in less time [1,19], despite the evidence showing low quality [19] and high quality, although there was heterogeneity among the studies [1]. On the contrary, another study referred there were not enough studies to assess whether rotary versus manual instrumentation affects clinical and radiological success, with a publication bias low [17].

4. Discussion

This umbrella review clearly summarizes the evidence sourced in VPT and NPT in primary teeth. The methodological quality of the included SRs ranged from very low to high quality, and therefore current evidence is of moderate confidence.

A correct diagnosis of the pulp status is crucial for correct treatment options and therefore for prognosis. In this regard and attending that the preservation of pulp vitality is fundamental, VPT treatment approaches must be considered. IPT allows selective tissue removal when compared to DPC and pulpotomy. IPT does not expose or damage the pulp and allows it to recover and heal by itself; this way selective caries removal are recommended [4–6,22]. However, the hall technique should be considered since it showed a superior success rate compared to non-selective and selective caries removal [5]. On the contrary, DPC is controversial, since there is not sufficient support to recommend it [4,5,33,34,36], due to its great occurrence of complications like mobility, percussion sensitivity, swelling, parulis, or presence of fistulous tract [5]. It is considered that DPC can succeed in case of vital pulp or reversible pulpitis without evidence of radicular pathology [5,36] and appropriate sealing of the cavity [5,34,36]. Already, although considering the pulpotomy is an acceptable and common procedure in case of deep caries, its success depends on several factors such as removing caries prior pulp exposure to avoid pulp contamination, rubber dam isolation application of different medicaments, and experience of the professional [4,11].

Regarding medicaments, the studies sometimes compare only two or several medicaments, MTA, Biodentine, FC, SF, and sodium hypochlorite being considered suitable despite the heterogeneity of the studies [2–4,10,11,13,15,20,21,23,26,29,35]; however, there is an agreement that CH is considered to have a less success rate [4,15,23]. In this sense, more well-designed studies with longer follow-up periods and superior methodology are required in order to obtain high evidence [2,4,10,11,15,29,35]. One systematic review highlighted the clinical and radiographic success rates of herbal medicine being suitable replacements to standard pulpotomy medicaments, but due to the heterogeneity of the studies and commercial availability, more studies are necessary to achieve alternatives to the standard medication [25]. Another option has been considered—the laser pulpotomy—which has been described as controversial in its results. Several factors must be determined such as pulp diagnosis, longer observation times, control group, and evaluation of different types of lasers [12,16,27,28,31]. It is also necessary to take into account that there is a learning curve for laser application [27] and there are some advantages of the laser on children like less chair time, painless treatment, and no high-speed rotors [16]; thus, more well-designed randomized clinical trials are required.

The lifecycle of primary teeth are fundamental to a normal growth and development of arch length and occlusal balance [33]. Therefore, sometimes, pulpectomy is necessary to keep the tooth in the arch. However, this procedure is a challenge because of the characteristics of the root canal system like side channels and accessories at the apex and furcation regions, as well as the root anatomy itself and the proximity of the apex to the germs of the permanent tooth [9,32]. Thus, it is of the utmost importance to consider several aspects of the clinical procedure, such as initial pulp condition, type of teeth, manual versus mechanical instrumentation, irrigants used, number of visits, root canal filling material, and type of restoration [14,32]. Therefore, further studies are important with a bigger sample, higher methodological quality, and particularly with longer follow-up, given the controversy between the studies.

Strengths and Limitations

The present umbrella review benefits from its comprehensive review of the available SRs using a transparent methodology. However, one limitation does need to be accounted for when interpreting the results. In each SR, the individual studies included were not explored. Thus, the conclusions of this review are based on the interpretation of the authors.

5. Conclusions

Both VPT and NPT present high clinical efficacy in primary teeth. The results should be interpreted with caution, as the quality of SRs included is overall moderate. Well-designed clinical trials and high standard systematic reviews are necessary to verify the efficacy of treatment options, clinical outcome efficacy, and material suitability.

Supplementary Materials: The following are available online at https://www.mdpi.com/article/10.3390/jcm11010085/s1, Table S1: PRISMA 2020 Checklist, Table S2: Detailed list of excluded articles with reasons.

Author Contributions: Conceptualization, L.B.L., C.C. and F.S.V.; methodology, J.B. and V.M.; validation, L.B.L., J.A.N. and J.B.; formal analysis, J.B. and V.M.; investigation, C.C. and F.S.V.; resources, J.J.M.; writing—original draft preparation, L.B.L. and J.A.N.; writing—review and editing, V.M., J.B. and J.J.M.; supervision, L.B.L.; project administration, J.J.M.; funding acquisition, J.J.M. All authors have read and agreed to the published version of the manuscript.

Funding: This work is financed by national funds through the FCT—Foundation for Science and Technology, I.P., under project UIDB/04585/2020.

Institutional Review Board Statement: Not applicable.

Informed Consent Statement: Not applicable.

Data Availability Statement: Data is available in the manuscript. Any further information is available upon request on the corresponding author.

Conflicts of Interest: The authors declare no conflict of interest.

References

1. Coll, J.A.; Vargas, K.; Marghalani, A.A.; Chen, C.Y.; AlShamali, S.; Dhar, V.; Crystal, Y.O. A Systematic Review and Meta-Analysis of Nonvital Pulp Therapy for Primary Teeth. *Pediatric Dent.* **2020**, *42*, 256–461.
2. Gadallah, L.; Hamdy, M.; El Bardissy, A.; Abou El Yazeed, M. Pulpotomy versus Pulpectomy in the Treatment of Vital Pulp Exposure in Primary Incisors. A Systematic Review and Meta-Analysis. *F1000Research* **2018**, *7*, 1560. [CrossRef]
3. Smaïl-Faugeron, V.; Glenny, A.M.; Courson, F.; Durieux, P.; Muller-Bolla, M.; Fron Chabouis, H. Pulp Treatment for Extensive Decay in Primary Teeth. *Cochrane Database Syst. Rev.* **2018**, *2018*. [CrossRef]
4. Coll, J.A.; Seale, N.S.; Vargas, K.; Marghalani, A.A.; Al Shamali, S.; Graham, L. Primary Tooth Vital Pulp Therapy: A Systematic Review and Meta-Analysis. *Pediatric Dent.* **2017**, *39*, 16–123.
5. Tedesco, T.K.; Reis, T.M.; Mello-Moura, A.C.V.; Da Silva, G.S.; Scarpini, S.; Floriano, I.; Gimenez, T.; Mendes, F.M.; Raggio, D.P. Management of Deep Caries Lesions with or without Pulp Involvement in Primary Teeth: A Systematic Review and Network Meta-Analysis. *Braz. Oral Res.* **2020**, *35*, 1–14. [CrossRef] [PubMed]
6. Smaïl-Faugeron, V.; Porot, A.; Muller-Bolla, M.; Courson, F. Indirect Pulp Capping versus Pulpotomy for Treating Deep Carious Lesions Approaching the Pulp in Primary Teeth: A Systematic Review. *Eur. J. Paediatr. Dent.* **2016**, *17*, 107–112.
7. Page, M.J.; McKenzie, J.E.; Bossuyt, P.M.; Boutron, I.; Hoffmann, T.C.; Mulrow, C.D.; Shamseer, L.; Tetzlaff, J.M.; Akl, E.A.; Brennan, S.E.; et al. The PRISMA 2020 statement: An updated guideline for reporting systematic reviews. *BMJ* **2021**, *372*, n71. [CrossRef]
8. Shea, B.J.; Reeves, B.C.; Wells, G.; Thuku, M.; Hamel, C.; Moran, J.; Moher, D.; Tugwell, P.; Welch, V.; Kristjansson, E.; et al. AMSTAR 2: A Critical Appraisal Tool for Systematic Reviews That Include Randomised or Non-Randomised Studies of Healthcare Interventions, or Both. *BMJ* **2017**, *358*, j4008. [CrossRef] [PubMed]
9. Duarte, M.L.; Pires, P.M.; Ferreira, D.M.; Pintor, A.V.B.; de Almeida Neves, A.; Maia, L.C.; Primo, L.G. Is There Evidence for the Use of Lesion Sterilization and Tissue Repair Therapy in the Endodontic Treatment of Primary Teeth? A Systematic Review and Meta-Analyses. *Clin. Oral Investig.* **2020**, *24*, 2959–2972. [CrossRef]
10. Peng, L.; Ye, L.; Guo, X.; Tan, H.; Zhou, X.; Wang, C.; Li, R. Evaluation of Formocresol versus Ferric Sulphate Primary Molar Pulpotomy: A Systematic Review and Meta-Analysis. *Int. Endod. J.* **2007**, *40*, 751–757. [CrossRef] [PubMed]
11. Stringhini Junior, E.; dos Santos, M.G.C.; Oliveira, L.B.; Mercadé, M. MTA and Biodentine for Primary Teeth Pulpotomy: A Systematic Review and Meta-Analysis of Clinical Trials. *Clin. Oral Investig.* **2019**, *23*, 1967–1976. [CrossRef] [PubMed]
12. Ansari, G.; Safi Aghdam, H.; Taheri, P.; Ghazizadeh Ahsaie, M. Laser Pulpotomy—An Effective Alternative to Conventional Techniques—A Systematic Review of Literature and Meta-Analysis. *Lasers Med. Sci.* **2018**, *33*, 1621–1629. [CrossRef] [PubMed]
13. Asgary, S.; Shirvani, A.; Fazlyab, M. MTA and Ferric Sulfate in Pulpotomy Outcomes of Primary Molars: A Systematic Review and Meta-Analysis. *J. Clin. Pediatric Dent.* **2014**, *39*, 1–8. [CrossRef] [PubMed]
14. Barcelos, R.; Santos, M.P.A.; Primo, L.G.; Luiz, R.R.; Maia, L.C. ZOE Paste Pulpectomies Outcome in Primary Teeth: A Systematic Review. *J. Clin. Pediatric Dent.* **2011**, *35*, 241–248. [CrossRef] [PubMed]

15. Bossù, M.; Iaculli, F.; Di Giorgio, G.; Salucci, A.; Polimeni, A.; Di Carlo, S. Different Pulp Dressing Materials for the Pulpotomy of Primary Teeth: A Systematic Review of the Literature. *J. Clin. Med.* **2020**, *9*, 838. [CrossRef]
16. Chandran, V.; Ramanarayanan, V.; Menon, M.; Varma, R.B.; Sanjeevan, V. Effect of LASER Therapy Vs. Conventional Techniques on Clinical and Radiographic Outcomes of Deciduous Molar Pulpotomy: A Systematic Review and Meta-Analysis. *J. Clin. Exp. Dent.* **2020**, *12*, e588–e596. [CrossRef]
17. Chugh, V.K.; Patnana, A.K.; Chugh, A.; Kumar, P.; Wadhwa, P.; Singh, S. Clinical Differences of Hand and Rotary Instrumentations during Biomechanical Preparation in Primary Teeth—A Systematic Review and Meta-Analysis. *Int. J. Paediatr. Dent.* **2021**, *31*, 131–142. [CrossRef]
18. Garrocho-Rangel, A.; Esparza-Villalpando, V.; Pozos-Guillen, A. Outcomes of Direct Pulp Capping in Vital Primary Teeth with Cariously and Non-Cariously Exposed Pulp: A Systematic Review. *Int. J. Paediatr. Dent.* **2020**, *30*, 536–546. [CrossRef]
19. Manchanda, S.; Sardana, D.; Yiu, C.K.Y. A Systematic Review and Meta-Analysis of Randomized Clinical Trials Comparing Rotary Canal Instrumentation Techniques with Manual Instrumentation Techniques in Primary Teeth. *Int. Endod. J.* **2020**, *53*, 333–353. [CrossRef]
20. Nagendrababu, V.; Pulikkotil, S.J.; Veettil, S.K.; Jinatongthai, P.; Gutmann, J.L. Efficacy of Biodentine and Mineral Trioxide Aggregate in Primary Molar Pulpotomies—A Systematic Review and Meta-Analysis With Trial Sequential Analysis of Randomized Clinical Trials. *J. Evid.-Based Dent. Pract.* **2019**, *19*, 17–27. [CrossRef]
21. Nuvvula, S.; Bandi, M.; Mallineni, S.K. Efficacy of Ferric Sulphate as a Pulpotomy Medicament in Primary Molars: An Evidence Based Approach. *Eur. Arch. Paediatr. Dent.* **2018**, *19*, 439–447. [CrossRef]
22. Da Rosa, W.L.O.; Lima, V.P.; Moraes, R.R.; Piva, E.; da Silva, A.F. Is a Calcium Hydroxide Liner Necessary in the Treatment of Deep Caries Lesions? A Systematic Review and Meta-Analysis. *Int. Endod. J.* **2019**, *52*, 588–603. [CrossRef]
23. Shirvani, A.; Asgary, S. Mineral Trioxide Aggregate versus Formocresol Pulpotomy: A Systematic Review and Meta-Analysis of Randomized Clinical Trials. *Clin. Oral Investig.* **2014**, *18*, 1023–1030. [CrossRef]
24. Shirvani, A.; Hassanizadeh, R.; Asgary, S. Mineral Trioxide Aggregate vs. Calcium Hydroxide in Primary Molar Pulpotomy: A Systematic Review. *Iran. Endod. J.* **2014**, *9*, 83–88. [CrossRef] [PubMed]
25. Subramanyam, D.; Somasundaram, S. Clinical and Radiographic Outcome of Herbal Medicine versus Standard Pulpotomy Medicaments in Primary Molars: A Systematic Review. *J. Clin. Diagn. Res.* **2017**, *11*, ZE12–ZE16. [CrossRef]
26. Fallahinejad Ghajari, M.; Mirkarimi, M.; Vatanpour, M.; Kharrazi Fard, M.J. Comparison of Pulpotomy with Formocresol and MTA in Primary Molars: A Systematic Review and Meta-Analysis. *Iran. Endod. J.* **2008**, *3*, 45–49. [CrossRef] [PubMed]
27. De Coster, P.; Rajasekharan, S.; Martens, L. Laser-Assisted Pulpotomy in Primary Teeth: A Systematic Review. *Int. J. Paediatr. Dent.* **2013**, *23*, 389–399. [CrossRef]
28. Lin, P.Y.; Chen, H.S.; Wang, Y.H.; Tu, Y.K. Primary Molar Pulpotomy: A Systematic Review and Network Meta-Analysis. *J. Dent.* **2014**, *42*, 1060–1077. [CrossRef]
29. Marghalani, A.A.; Omar, S.; Chen, J.W. Clinical and Radiographic Success of Mineral Trioxide Aggregate Compared with Formocresol as a Pulpotomy Treatment in Primary Molars: A Systematic Review and Meta-Analysis. *J. Am. Dent. Assoc.* **2014**, *145*, 714–721. [CrossRef] [PubMed]
30. Najjar, R.S.; Alamoudi, N.M.; El-Housseiny, A.A.; Al Tuwirqi, A.A.; Sabbagh, H.J. A Comparison of Calcium Hydroxide/Iodoform Paste and Zinc Oxide Eugenol as Root Filling Materials for Pulpectomy in Primary Teeth: A Systematic Review and Meta-Analysis. *Clin. Exp. Dent. Res.* **2019**, *5*, 294–310. [CrossRef] [PubMed]
31. Nematollahi, H.; Sarraf Shirazi, A.; Mehrabkhani, M.; Sabbagh, S. Clinical and Radiographic Outcomes of Laser Pulpotomy in Vital Primary Teeth: A Systematic Review and Meta-Analysis. *Eur. Arch. Paediatr. Dent.* **2018**, *19*, 205–220. [CrossRef]
32. Pintor, A.V.B.; Dos Santos, M.R.M.; Ferreira, D.M.; Barcelos, R.; Primo, L.G.; Maia, L.C. Does Smear Layer Removal Influence Root Canal Therapy Outcome? A Systematic Review. *J. Clin. Pediatric Dent.* **2016**, *40*, 1–6. [CrossRef]
33. Pozos-Guillen, A.; Garcia-Flores, A.; Esparza-Villalpando, V.; Garrocho-Rangel, A. Intracanal Irrigants for Pulpectomy in Primary Teeth: A Systematic Review and Meta-Analysis. *Int. J. Paediatr. Dent.* **2016**, *26*, 412–425. [CrossRef]
34. Schwendicke, F.; Brouwer, F.; Schwendicke, A.; Paris, S. Different Materials for Direct Pulp Capping: Systematic Review and Meta-Analysis and Trial Sequential Analysis. *Clin. Oral Investig.* **2016**, *20*, 1121–1132. [CrossRef] [PubMed]
35. Shafaee, H.; Alirezaie, M.; Rangrazi, A.; Bardideh, E. Comparison of the Success Rate of a Bioactive Dentin Substitute with Those of Other Root Restoration Materials in Pulpotomy of Primary Teeth: Systematic Review and Meta-Analysis. *J. Am. Dent. Assoc.* **2019**, *150*, 676–688. [CrossRef] [PubMed]
36. Boutsiouki, C.; Frankenberger, R.; Krämer, N. Relative Effectiveness of Direct and Indirect Pulp Capping in the Primary Dentition. *Eur. Arch. Paediatr. Dent.* **2018**, *19*, 297–309. [CrossRef] [PubMed]

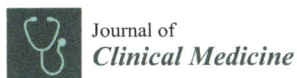

Review

Postoperative Pain following Root Canal Filling with Bioceramic vs. Traditional Filling Techniques: A Systematic Review and Meta-Analysis of Randomized Controlled Trials

Elina Mekhdieva [1], Massimo Del Fabbro [2,3], Mario Alovisi [1], Allegra Comba [1], Nicola Scotti [1], Margherita Tumedei [2,4], Massimo Carossa [1], Elio Berutti [1] and Damiano Pasqualini [1,*]

1. Endodontics and Restorative Dentistry, CIR Dental School, Department of Surgical Sciences, University of Turin, 10126 Turin, Italy; elina.mekhdieva@unito.it (E.M.); mario.alovisi@unito.it (M.A.); allegra.comba@unito.it (A.C.); nicola.scotti@unito.it (N.S.); massimo.carossa@unito.it (M.C.); elio.berutti@unito.it (E.B.)
2. Department of Biomedical, Surgical and Dental Sciences, University of Milan, 20122 Milan, Italy; massimo.delfabbro@unimi.it (M.D.F.); margytumedei@yahoo.it (M.T.)
3. IRCCS Orthopedic Institute Galeazzi, 20161 Milan, Italy
4. Department of Medical, Oral and Biotechnological Sciences, University "G. d'Annunzio" of Chieti-Pescara, 65122 Chieti, Italy
* Correspondence: damiano.pasqualini@unito.it; Tel.: +39-335-451070 or +39-011-6331569

Citation: Mekhdieva, E.; Del Fabbro, M.; Alovisi, M.; Comba, A.; Scotti, N.; Tumedei, M.; Carossa, M.; Berutti, E.; Pasqualini, D. Postoperative Pain following Root Canal Filling with Bioceramic vs. Traditional Filling Techniques: A Systematic Review and Meta-Analysis of Randomized Controlled Trials. *J. Clin. Med.* **2021**, *10*, 4509. https://doi.org/10.3390/jcm10194509

Academic Editors: Alfredo Iandolo, Massimo Amato and Giuseppe Pantaleo

Received: 12 September 2021
Accepted: 27 September 2021
Published: 29 September 2021

Publisher's Note: MDPI stays neutral with regard to jurisdictional claims in published maps and institutional affiliations.

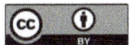

Copyright: © 2021 by the authors. Licensee MDPI, Basel, Switzerland. This article is an open access article distributed under the terms and conditions of the Creative Commons Attribution (CC BY) license (https://creativecommons.org/licenses/by/4.0/).

Abstract: This meta-analysis aimed to evaluate postoperative pain (POP) following root canal filling (RCF) with gutta-percha/bioceramic sealer (BCS) vs. gutta-percha/traditional sealer (TS) techniques. Electronic databases were searched for randomized trials. Subgroup analyses were performed for analgesic intake, flare-ups, postoperative time (24/48 h), pulp status, and retreatment. The search yielded 682 records, and nine studies were selected. BCS was associated with significantly lower POP vs. TS at 24 h ($P = 0.04$) and 48 h ($P = 0.0005$). In addition, non-significant trends favoring BCS for analgesic intake at 24 h ($P = 0.14$), flare-ups ($P = 0.24$) and obturation techniques at 24 h ($P = 0.41$) and 48 h ($P = 0.33$), non-significant trends for lower POP with TS vs. BCS 24 h and 48 h in vital teeth ($P = 0.50$, $P = 0.18$, respectively), and for lower POP with BCS vs. TS in non-vital teeth at 24 h and 48 h ($P = 0.16$, $P = 0.84$, respectively). POP was numerically lower with TS vs. BCS at 24 h ($P = 0.65$) and 48 h after retreatment ($P = 0.59$). Moreover, POP did not vary between fillers when the treatment was over single ($P = 0.28$) or multiple visits ($P = 0.50$). BCS was associated with significantly lower short-term POP, and with a trend for lower analgesic intake and flare-up incidence, as compared to TS.

Keywords: meta-analysis; root canal filling; postoperative pain; bioceramic sealer; analgesic intake; flare-up

1. Introduction

Postoperative pain (POP) after root canal filling (RCF) affects up to 40% of patients [1]. The intensity and duration of POP vary according to multiple prognostic factors [2–4]. The filling technique is considered among the most relevant, in which warm vertical and cold lateral compaction as well as single cone are most traditionally utilized with resin-based or zinc-oxyde eugenol sealers [5,6]. The intensity and duration of postoperative pain are subjective and can be affected by many factors. In particular, by the severity of preoperative pain according to the medical history of the present diagnosis, tooth type, age, gender, etc. [2]. The intraoperative factors are also various, such as physical properties of the endodontic instrument used for the initial treatment, features of the irrigation protocol such as chemical solutions and concentrations, microbiological stability and resistance, histopathological state of the tissues surrounding the tooth, etc. [1–4]. At the final stage of root canal treatment during the obturation step, the endodontic sealer locally and directly contacts with the altered periapical tissues through the apical foramen and additional lateral canals. Accordingly, the physical and chemical properties of the sealer, such as pH-level, consistency, etc., also affect the intensity of postoperative endodontic pain [1,2]. The gutta-percha/bioceramic sealer (BCS) filling technique has gained popularity among endodontists due to features that include biocompatibility (due to their similarity with biological hydroxyapatite) and bioactive stimulation of periapical healing [7]. The setting time (30 min for working time), sealing ability, and antimicrobial properties are all key to the performance of endodontic sealers [8]. Premixed injectable formulations, preloaded syringes, and moldable putty forms are all available, facilitating ease of use [9]. However, there are no robust data evaluating any potential impact of BCS vs. traditional filling techniques on POP among randomized controlled trials (RCTs). The aim of this systematic review and meta-analysis was to assess the effect of the BCS filling technique compared with traditional filling techniques on POP in adult patients following RCF.

2. Materials and Methods

2.1. Study Design

This analysis considered all the studies that evaluated POP in adult patients, following RCF with BCS or traditional filling techniques.

Review question: How does the BCS filling technique affect the intensity of POP compared with the resin-based sealers (RBS) filling technique in patients undergoing a root canal treatment?

This study complies with the Preferred Reporting Items for Systematic Reviews and Meta-Analysis Statement (PRISMA), and was carried out on the basis of the Cochrane PICOS formula, defined as follows: *Population*, adult patients of both genders (not receiving analgesic or antibiotic medications, without long-term use of medications, not pregnant) with pulpal and/or periapical disease (without procedural errors, e.g., overfilling), who received an endodontic treatment in permanent teeth; *Intervention*, RCF with BCS; *Comparison*, RBS; *Outcome*, the primary outcome was the quality of life measured by the self-reported POP score; and *Study type*, RCTs. The systematic review protocol was registered with the International Prospective Register of Systematic Reviews (PROSPERO) a priori, ID: CRD42021227248.

2.2. Search Strategy and Inclusion Criteria

A comprehensive search strategy was designed to access biomedical databases (PubMed, Springer Link, DOSS, Scopus, Nature, Wiley Online Library, Web of Science Core Collection, BMJ, Cochrane Library, Oxford scholarship online, CINAHL complete, Access medicine, Science direct), grey literature (SIGLE—information on grey literature in Europe), and a clinical trials register (clinical trial.gov). A manual search of the main endodontic journals was also carried out (Journal of Endodontics, European Endodontic Journal, International Endodontic Journal). The search terms were "postoperative pain" AND "endodontic sealer" OR "root canal treatment" in studies published from January 2010 to January 2021 in English or German. The inclusion criteria were RCTs that assessed POP after RCF using the BCS filling technique in permanent teeth with pulpal and/or periapical disease. The selected studies compared the impact of BCS vs. TS on POP scores following RCF. POP scores could be reported using any self-recorded pain scale. We excluded the studies that did not compare the individual effect of endodontic sealer on the POP level; studies that additionally assessed the impact of anti-inflammatory medicines and laser applications; assessed the POP level after canal overfilling; or assessed the POP level after different root canal preparation techniques.

2.3. Study Selection

After the removal of duplicate records, the titles and abstracts of the identified studies were independently screened for eligibility by three reviewers (E.M., D.P., and M.D.F.). Consensus was achieved through discussion, where there was discordance in study selection.

2.4. Data Extraction

Three reviewers (E.M., D.P., and M.D.F.) independently extracted data from studies that met the inclusion criteria, using a standardized data collection table consisting of strings: References (title, authors, year of publication, country), study design, sample size, age/sex groups, inclusion and exclusion criteria, diagnosis, pre-op status, operator, quantity of visits, glidepath, instrumentation, irrigation protocols, obturation technique and materials, restoration, POP assessment time and scale, analgesics intake, flare-up, etc. If multiple treatment groups were presented, the data conforming to PICO were collected. Moreover, if any information was missed, the authors were contacted through personal communication via e-mail. Furthermore, if there was no response for up to 5 weeks, the study was not included in the meta-analysis.

2.5. Quality Assessment

The quality of each RCT was assessed according to the Cochrane Risk of Bias Tool. All the domains (random sequence generation, allocation concealment, performance bias, blinding of outcome, attrition bias, reporting bias) were rated as "high", "low" or "unclear" risk of bias. We set an additional risk of bias according to the "Operator" (expert endodontist: Low risk; undergraduate student: High risk). Studies were classified as overall high risk if they contained one or more domains rated as high risk; overall moderate risk if they contained no high-risk domain and one or more were judged as unclear; and overall low risk if all the domains were judged at a low risk of bias.

2.6. Meta-Analysis

The general methodology of this review followed the directions of the Cochrane Handbook for Systematic Reviews of Interventions [10]. If possible, the odds ratio (OR)/risk ratio (RR) or standardized mean differences (SMD) and their 95% confidence intervals (CI) were calculated for the quantitative data extracted from each RCT. Results from comparable groups of studies were pooled into a meta-analysis using Review Manager (RevMan) Software (version 5.4.1, The Cochrane Collaboration, 2020). The findings are presented in a narrative form, if statistical pooling was not possible. The subgroup analysis was conducted on parameters reported by at least two studies. The significance of any variation and degree of heterogeneity was determined by I^2 and chi-square statistics, respectively. Publication bias tests were not conducted due to the low number of studies included.

In some cases, the included studies will present with peculiar features (for example, different inclusion criteria with respect to other studies, presence of patients with systemic conditions or asymptomatic patients). Moreover, the sensitivity analysis will be performed to assess if the exclusion of the study will affect the outcome of the analysis.

3. Results

3.1. Study Selection

The search strategy identified 695 records, including 13 duplicates. The remaining 682 records were screened by the title and abstract (Figure 1). In total, 656 records were considered irrelevant and removed, leaving 26 studies that were assessed for eligibility by full-text reviewing. At this stage, 17 studies were excluded [11–27], most commonly since they did not include a BCS (Supplementary Materials Table S1). Finally, nine studies were included for systematic review. Although each of the selected studies evaluated the POP level following different filling techniques, the variability within the study designs and the materials and methods employed required specific consideration during the analysis.

3.2. Study Characteristics

The characteristics of the selected RCTs are presented in Table 1. All the studies were published single-center RCTs that reported the characteristics of teeth, pre-operative status, diagnosis, instrumentation details and irrigation protocols, endodontic sealers and filling techniques used, analgesic intake, incidence of flare-ups, number of visits, and pulp and periapical status.

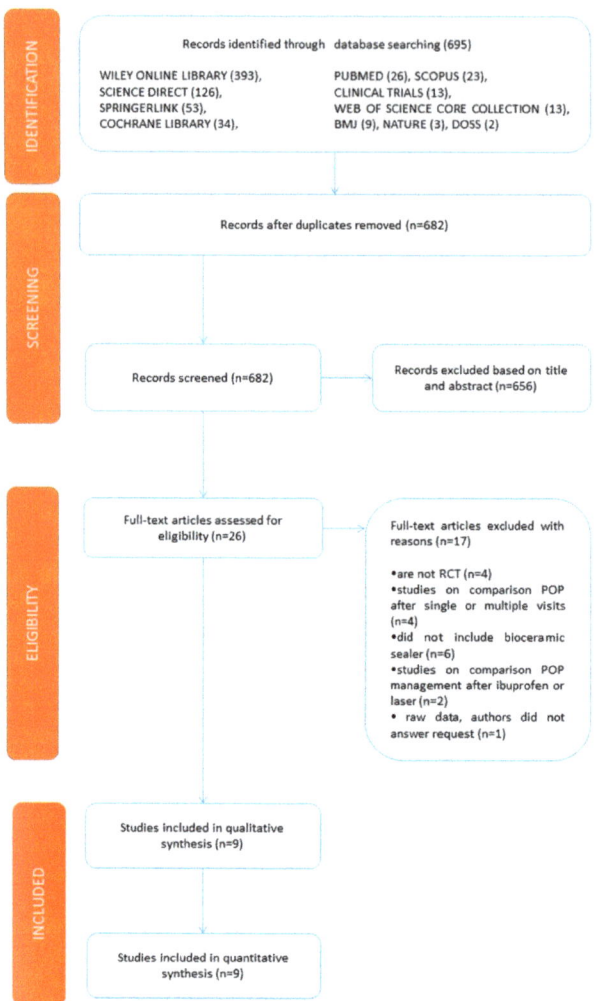

Figure 1. The preferred reporting items for systematic reviews and meta-analysis flow diagram of the search results.

Table 1. Cochrane PICO formula.

Patients	Intervention	Comparison	Outcome
With pulp / periapical disease	Filling with bioceramic technique	Filling with traditional technique	Postoperative pain

All the selected studies included teeth with pulp or periapical pathologies, without signs of radiolucency, requiring a primary endodontic treatment. However, only three studies included teeth that needed retreatment [28–30]. Four studies included teeth that were asymptomatic pre-operatively [30–33], two studies only included symptomatic teeth [28,34], and three studies examined asymptomatic and symptomatic teeth [29,35,36]. Only one study managed an endodontic treatment without local anesthesia [31]. Furthermore, three studies assessed POP in anterior single-rooted teeth only [31–33].

The instrumentation and irrigation protocols were similar across the studies, but the filling techniques varied: Warm vertical condensation (WVC) was utilized in five studies, single-cone technique (SCT) in three studies, carrier-based obturation in one study, and lateral condensation in one study. The resin-based sealer (RBS) was utilized as a control group in all the included studies. One study deliberately carried out the filling procedure during a second visit to exclude the influence of instrumentation stage on POP. The other eight studies evaluated POP in the context of a single visit treatment.

A variety of pain rating scales were used, including variations of the Visual Analog Scale and Verbal Rating Scale, as well as the Heft and Parker Pain Rating Scales of 0–10, 0–100, 0–170 or verbal (no pain/mild pain/moderate pain/severe pain). The data were reported as either means or percentages. Four studies reported an analgesic intake and three studies reported an incidence of flare-ups.

Remarkably, none of the included studies identified significant differences in the POP level, analgesic intake or incidence of flare-ups between different endodontic sealers.

3.3. Risk of Bias

The risk of bias in the nine RCTs is summarized in Table 2. One study was scored as having an overall "low" risk of bias, six studies as having an overall "moderate" risk, and two studies as having an overall "high" risk of bias, since the treatment was managed by undergraduate students.

Table 2. Summary of the risk of bias of the included studies.

Study	Risk of Bias							
	A	B	C	D	E	F	G	Overall
GRAUNAITE et al. 2018 [31]	+	+	?	+	+	+	+	?
PAZ et al. 2018 [28]	?	?	?	+	+	+	-	-
ATES et al. 2019 [35]	+	?		+	+	+	+	?
FERREIRA et al. 2019 [33]	+	+	+	+	+	+	?	?
FONSECA et al. 2019 [32]	+	+	+			+	+	+
NABI et al. 2019 [34]	?	?	+	+	+	+	?	?
SHARMA et al. 2019 [36]	?	?	?	?	+	+	?	?
TAN et al. 2020 [30]	+	+	+	+	+	+	+	+
YU 2020 [29]	+	+	?	?	?	+	?	?

"+": low risk of bias, "?": unclear risk of bias, "-": high risk of bias. (**A**) Random sequence generation (selection bias). (**B**) Allocation concealment (selection bias). (**C**) Blinding of participants and personnel (performance bias). (**D**) Blinding of outcome assessment (detection bias). (**E**) Incomplete outcome data (attrition bias). (**F**) Selective reporting (reporting bias). (**G**) Other bias.

3.4. Meta-Analysis

Pooled POP data (mean ± standard deviation [SD]) experienced by patients 24 h and 48 h after RCF with BCS or RBS are presented in Figures 2 and 3, respectively. Six studies did not report the mean POP ± SD 48 h after RCF and these were not included in the respective forest plot [28,30,33–36]. Since in the study by Graunaite et al. 2018 [31] asymptomatic patients were treated, as opposed to all the other studies in which patients were symptomatic, the sensitivity analysis was performed in all analyses where that study was considered, to see if the results changed with the exclusion of asymptomatic subjects. Pooled data analyses indicate that POP was significantly lower in patients who underwent RCF with BCS compared with RBS at 24 h (SMD = −0.20; $P = 0.04$) and 48 h (SMD = −0.26; $P = 0.0005$) after treatment. After the sensitivity analysis, by excluding Graunaite et al. 2018, the results did not change significantly.

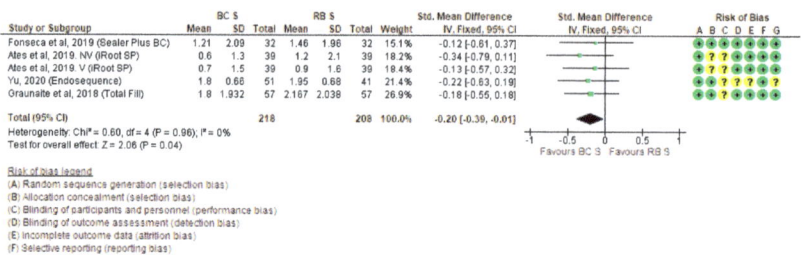

Figure 2. Forest plot of POP level 24 h after RCF with BCS vs. RBS.

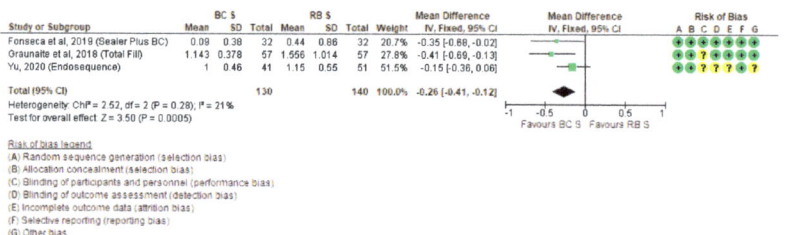

Figure 3. Forest plot of POP level 48 h after RCF with BCS vs. RBS.

The analgesic intake did not significantly differ between the BCS and RBS groups 24 h after RCF (RR = 0.46; P = 0.14; Figure 4). Five studies were not included in this forest plot due to a lack of available data [11–13,33,36]. The incidence of flare-up was also not significantly different between the BCS and RBS groups (OR = 0.32; P = 0.24; Supplementary Materials Figure S1). After the sensitivity analysis, by excluding Graunaite et al. 2018, the results did not change significantly.

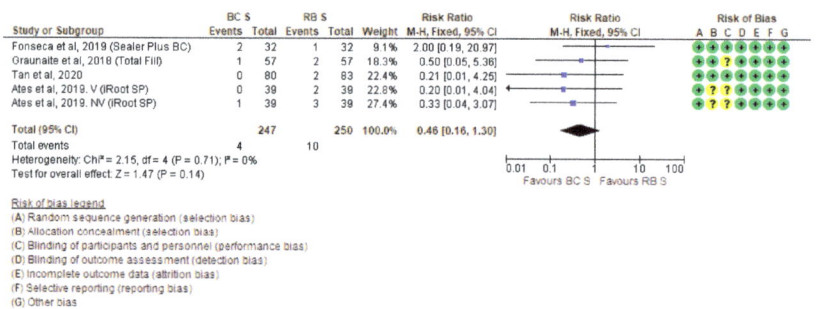

Figure 4. Forest plot of analgesic intake 24 h after RCF with BCS vs. RBS.

The next two diagrams underline the pain prevalence and severity of the BCS group over the RBS group in 24 h (Supplementary Materials Figure S2) and 48 h (Supplementary Materials Figure S3) after RCF.

The probability of "No pain" 24 h after treatment was 1.12× higher in the BCS group vs. the RBS group (OR = 1.12; 95% CI, 0.77–1.64; P = 0.86), while the same was observed for "Moderate pain" probability (OR = 1.21; 95% CI, 0.61–2.38; P = 0.59). There was no heterogeneity in the study effect for the BCS and RBS groups (I^2 = 0%; P = 0.86, and I^2 = 0%; P = 0.89, respectively), indicating perfect consistency in the results. The probability of "Mild pain" and "Severe pain" was 1.2× and 1.7× higher in the RBS group vs. the BCS group, respectively (OR = 0.83; 95% CI, 0.54–1.25; P = 0.37, and OR = 0.59; 95% CI, 0.08–4.58; P = 0.62). There was also no heterogeneity in the study effect in either group (I^2 = 0%; P = 0.97, and I^2 = 0%; P = 0.61, respectively; Supplementary Materials Figure S2).

A diagram of pain characteristics in the BCS and RBS groups 48 h after treatment is presented in Supplementary Materials Figure S3. The studies that did not report pain characteristics 48 h after treatment were excluded. The probability of "No pain" 48 h after treatment was 1.21× higher in the BCS group vs. the RBS group (OR = 1.21; 95% CI, 0.60–2.42; $P = 0.60$; heterogeneity: $I^2 = 18\%$; $P = 0.30$). "Mild pain" was more commonly reported in the RBS group vs. the BCS group 48 h after treatment (OR = 0.82; 95% CI, 0.40–1.68; $P = 0.59$; heterogeneity: $I^2 = 1\%$; $P = 0.40$), while "Moderate pain" was equally likely in both groups 48 h after treatment (OR = 1.00; 95% CI, 0.14–7.27; $P = 1.00$; heterogeneity: $I^2 = 0\%$; $P = 0.33$). "Severe pain" was reported only once in both groups (Supplementary Materials Figure S3). After the sensitivity analysis, by excluding Graunaite et al. 2018, the results did not change significantly neither for data after 24 h nor for 48 h after RCT.

The effect of the obturation technique (WVT vs. SCT) on POP based on data 24 h and 48 h after RCF is presented in Supplementary Materials Figures S4 and S5. The studies that did not report 48-h data were excluded. There was a numerical difference in POP in favor of BCS for both WVT and SCT subgroups 24 h after RCF (OR = 0.85; $P = 0.41$). The probability of POP was numerically higher in the RBS subgroup that underwent the WVT technique ($P = 0.49$) in 1.2× and lower in the BCS subgroup that underwent the SCT technique ($P = 0.64$; Supplementary Materials Figure S4). There was evidence of lower POP in both WVT and SCT subgroups of the BCS group 48 h after RCF ($P = 0.33$). The probability of POP did not differ according to the obturation technique in the BCS group, but was 1.3× higher in the RBS group 48 h after RCF (OR = 0.78; $P = 0.33$; Supplementary Materials Figure S5).

The probability of POP by the pulp status (vital [V] and non-vital [NV] pulp) 24 h and 48 h after RCF is presented in Supplementary Materials Figures S6 and S7, respectively. The studies that did not report 48-h data were excluded. There was evidence of a non-significant difference in POP in favor of RBS in the V subgroup ($P = 0.50$) and a trend for lower POP in NV teeth within the BCS group 24 h after RCF ($P = 0.16$). However, there was no statistically significant overall effect of V vs. NV pulp on POP (OR = 0.84; $P = 0.45$; Supplementary Materials Figure S6). The probability of POP was 2× higher in the V pulp of the BCS group, and there was evidence of lower POP in the V subgroup of the RBS group 48 h after RCF (OR = 2.01; $P = 0.18$). There was also a non-significant trend for lower POP in NV teeth within the BCS group (OR = 0.92; $P = 0.84$; Supplementary Materials Figure S7). After the sensitivity analysis, by excluding Graunaite et al. 2018, the results did not change significantly.

Pooled data from the three studies that reported the retreatment show a trend for a difference in POP in favor of RBS (OR = 1.20; $P = 0.65$) 24 h after RCF (Supplementary Materials Figure S8). The meta-analysis determined that there was a 48% level of heterogeneity within the included nine studies. Only one study had analyzed a consistent number of cases [31]. Supplementary Materials Figure S9 presents POP in retreatment groups 48 h after RCF. Unfortunately, the limited numbers of studies and retreated cases are insufficient to determine any effect of BCS vs. RBS on POP (OR = 1.34).

There was no significant difference in POP between the BCS and RBS groups when the treatment was carried out over single (OR = 0.77; $P = 0.28$) or multiple visits 24 h after RCF (OR = 0.81; $P = 0.50$; Supplementary Materials Figure S10). A lack of data precluded the equivalent analysis of POP 48 h after RCF.

4. Discussion

This meta-analysis of nine pooled RCTs indicates that POP was significantly lower after RCF with BCS compared with RBS. However, none of the RCTs individually reported any significant effect of BSC vs. RBS on POP [28–36].

In this analysis, we found that BCS was non-significantly correlated with reduced analgesic intake vs. RBS, an observation that was also reported by one of the included studies [35] using the warm-obturator filling technique. However, two of the other included RCTs [32,33] demonstrated comparable analgesic intake in the control and experimental groups after RCF using SCT.

This systematic review found a non-significant trend of reduced flare-up in the BCS group vs. the RBS group. This is supported by one of the included RCTs that reported a significant reduction of flare-up following RCF with BCS vs. RBS [35]. However, another reported an equal occurrence between groups [31].

Regarding the warm and cold filling techniques, SCT with BCS has previously been associated with higher POP, while WVT with RBS has been associated with the lowest POP scores [28]. However, our pooled analysis suggests that there is a non-significant trend in favor of BCS.

Our results indicate that POP was lower in the V pulp when filled with RBS and in the NV pulp when filled with BCS. However, we found no additional background literature to place this in context.

Our results also evidence a non-significant difference in POP in favor of RBS at retreatment. Moreover, the only RCT [31] included to report this parameter indicates no difference between filling techniques in POP, following the retreatment procedures.

According to our results, the trend for lower POP following RCF with BCS vs. RBS filling technique was observed across single and multiple visit treatments. However, there are no studies in the literature to provide additional context.

The main limitations of this review are inter-study variability and inconsistency, as well as a lack of clinically relevant outcomes. Furthermore, as mentioned, different scales for pain measurement were used in different studies. Though the authors made efforts to resize all the scales to a 1–10 scale, it is difficult to understand if this had a relevance in the results. Of course, for future studies, it is recommended to use only scales for which there is an overall consensus. Therefore, the findings presented here need to be confirmed by further well-designed studies and should be interpreted with caution.

5. Conclusions

Our findings suggest that the BCS filling technique may positively affect POP, while there was a trend of a beneficial effect for analgesic intake, incidence of flare-up, pulp status, and number of visits when using BCS, compared with RBS. However, due to several limitations in these analyses, further well-designed clinical studies are warranted to supplement our results.

Supplementary Materials: The following are available online at https://www.mdpi.com/article/10.3390/jcm10194509/s1, Table S1: Excluded studies with reasons for exclusion, Figure S1: Forest plot of flare-up after RCF with BCS vs. RBS, Figure S2: Diagram of pain characteristics summary in a subgroup of BCS and RBS traditional filling technique groups 24 h after RCF, Figure S3: Diagram of pain characteristics summary in a subgroup of BCS and RBS traditional filling technique groups 48 h after RCF, Figure S4: Forest plot of POP in patients treated with warm and cold filling techniques 24 h after RCF with BCS vs. RBS, Figure S5: Forest plot of POP in patients treated with warm and cold techniques 48 h after RCF with BCS vs. RBS, Figure S6: Forest plot of POP in vital and non-vital pulp 24 h after RCF with BCS vs. RBS, Figure S7: Forest plot of POP in vital and non-vital pulp 48 h after RCF with BCS vs. RBS, Figure S8: Forest plot of POP following retreatment 24 h after RCF with BCS vs. RBS, Figure S9: Forest plot of POP following retreatment 48 h after RCF with BCS vs. RBS, Figure S10: Forest plot of POP 24 h after RCF with BCS vs. RBS following a single or multiple visit treatment.

Author Contributions: Conceptualization, D.P., M.D.F. and E.B.; methodology, D.P., M.D.F. and E.B.; software, E.M., M.A., N.S., A.C., M.C. and M.T.; data analysis, E.M., M.A., N.S., A.C., M.C. and M.T.; visualization, E.M., M.A., N.S., A.C., M.C. and M.T.; supervision and project administration, D.P., M.D.F. and E.B.; writing, E.M., D.P. and M.D.F.; reviewing and editing, D.P., M.D.F., E.M., M.A. and E.B. All authors have read and agreed to the published version of the manuscript.

Funding: This research received no external funding.

Institutional Review Board Statement: Not applicable.

Informed Consent Statement: Not applicable.

Conflicts of Interest: The authors declare no conflict of interest.

References

1. Nosrat, A.; Dianat, O.; Verma, P.; Nixdorf, D.R.; Law, A.S. Postoperative Pain: An Analysis on Evolution of Research in Half-Century. *J. Endod.* **2020**, *47*, 358–365. [CrossRef]
2. Nagendrababu, V.; Gutmann, J.L. Factors associated with postobturation pain following single-visit nonsurgical root canal treatment: A systematic review. *Quintessence Int.* **2017**, *48*, 193–208. [CrossRef] [PubMed]
3. Comparin, D.; Moreira, E.J.L.; Souza, E.M.; De-Deus, G.; Arias, A.; Silva, E.J.N.L. Postoperative Pain after Endodontic Retreatment Using Rotary or Reciprocating Instruments: A Randomized Clinical Trial. *J. Endod.* **2017**, *43*, 1084–1088. [CrossRef] [PubMed]
4. Demenech, L.S.; de Freitas, J.V.; Tomazinho, F.S.F.; Baratto-Filho, F.; Gabardo, M.C.L. Postoperative Pain after Endodontic Treatment under Irrigation with 8.25% Sodium Hypochlorite and Other Solutions: A Randomized Clinical Trial. *J. Endod.* **2020**, *47*, 696–704. [CrossRef] [PubMed]
5. Moreira, M.S.; Anuar, A.S.N.-S.; Tedesco, T.K.; dos Santos, M.; Morimoto, S. Endodontic Treatment in Single and Multiple Visits: An Overview of Systematic Reviews. *J. Endod.* **2017**, *43*, 864–870. [CrossRef] [PubMed]
6. Sathorn, C.; Parashos, P.; Messer, H. The prevalence of postoperative pain and flare-up in single- and multiple-visit endodontic treatment: A systematic review. *Int. Endod. J.* **2008**, *41*, 91–99. [CrossRef]
7. Raghavendra, S.S.; Jadhav, G.R.; Gathani, K.M.; Kotadia, P. Bioceramics in endodontics—A review. *J. Istanb. Univ. Fac. Dent.* **2017**, *51*, S128–S137. [CrossRef]
8. Komabayashi, T.; Colmenar, D.; Cvach, N.; Bhat, A.; Primus, C.; Imai, Y. Comprehensive review of current endodontic sealers. *Dent. Mater. J.* **2020**, *39*, 703–720. [CrossRef] [PubMed]
9. Vouzara, T.; Dimosiari, G.; Koulaouzidou, E.A.; Economides, N. Cytotoxicity of a New Calcium Silicate Endodontic Sealer. *J. Endod.* **2018**, *44*, 849–852. [CrossRef] [PubMed]
10. Higgins, J.P.T.; Thomas, J.; Chandler, J.; Cumpston, M.; Li, T.; Page, M.J.; Welch, V.A. *Cochrane Handbook for Systematic Reviews of Interventions*, 2nd ed.; John Wiley & Sons: Chichester, UK, 2019.
11. Niang, S.O.; Bane, K.; Sarr, M.; Tourè, B.; Machtou, P. Technical quality and postoperative pain of single visit endodontic treatment of chronic apical periodontitis filled by bioceramic sealer. *IP Indian J. Conserv. Endod.* **2018**, *3*, 92–97. [CrossRef]
12. Filipov, I.; Zagorchev, P.; Dimitrova, S.; Manchorova-Veleva, N. Postoperative pain in cold and warm endo-techniques using bioceramic sealer. In Proceedings of the IADR Poster Session, London, UK, 25–28 July 2018.
13. Reeru, S.; Shresha, D.; Kayasatha, R. Postoperative pain and associated factors in patients undergoing single visit root canal treatment on teeth with vital pulp. *Kathmandu Univ. Med.* **2018**, *16*, 220–223.
14. Arias, A.; de la Macorra, J.C.; Hidalgo, J.J.; Azabal, M. Predictive models of pain following root canal treatment: A prospective clinical study. *Int. Endod. J.* **2013**, *46*, 784–793. [CrossRef]
15. Wang, C.; Xu, P.; Ren, L.; Dong, G.; Ye, L. Comparison of post-obturation pain experience following one-visit and two-visit root canal treatment on teeth with vital pulps: A randomized controlled trial. *Int. Endod. J.* **2010**, *43*, 692–697. [CrossRef] [PubMed]
16. Sadaf, D.; Ahmad, M.Z. Factors associated with postoperative pain in endodontic therapy. *Int. J. Biomed. Sci.* **2014**, *10*, 243–247.
17. Prashanth, M.B.; Tavane, P.N.; Abraham, S.; Chacko, L. Comparative evaluation of pain, tenderness and swelling followed by radiographic evaluation of periapical changes at various intervals of time following single and multiple visit endodontic therapy: An in vivo study. *J. Contemp. Dent. Pract.* **2011**, *12*, 187–191. [CrossRef] [PubMed]
18. Shashirekha, G.; Jena, A.; Pattanaik, S.; Rath, J. Assessment of pain and dissolution of apically extruded sealers and their effect on the periradicular tissues. *J. Conserv. Dent.* **2018**, *21*, 546–550. [PubMed]
19. Nunes, E.C.; Herkrath, F.J.; Suzuki, E.H.; Gualberto, E.C., Jr.; Marques, A.A.F.; Sponchiado, E.C., Jr. Comparison of the effect of photobiomodulation therapy and Ibuprofen on postoperative pain after endodontic retreatment: Randomized, controlled clinical study. *Lasers Med. Sci.* **2020**, *35*, 971–978. [CrossRef] [PubMed]
20. Asgary, S.; Eghbal, M.J. The effect of pulpotomy using a Calcium-enriched mixture cement versus one-visit root canal therapy on postoperative pain relief in irreversible pulpitis: A randomized clinical trial. *Odontology* **2010**, *98*, 125–133. [CrossRef] [PubMed]
21. Rao, K.N.; Kandaswamy, R.; Umashetty, G.; Rathore, V.P.S.; Hotkar, C.; Patil, B.S. Post-obturation pain following one-visit and two-visits root canal treatment in necrotic anterior teeth. *J. Int. Oral Health* **2014**, *6*, 28–32. [CrossRef] [PubMed]
22. Yoshinari, F.M.S.; Pereira, S.; Beraldo, D.Z.; da Silva, J.C.L.; Zafalon, E.J.; da Silva, P.G. Influence of photodynamic therapy in the control of postoperative pain in endodontic treatment: A cross-sectional randomized clinical trial. *Pesqui. Bras. Odontopediatria Clínica Integr.* **2019**, *19*, e4369. [CrossRef]
23. Hepsenoglu, Y.E.; Tan, F.E.; Ozcan, M. Postoperative pain intensity after single- versus two-visit nonsurgical endodontic retreatment: A randomized clinical trial. *J. Endod.* **2018**, *44*, 1339–1346. [CrossRef] [PubMed]
24. Demirci, G.K.; Chalishkan, M.K. A prospective randomized comparative study of cold lateral condensattion versus core/gutta-percha in teeth with periapical lesions. *J. Endod.* **2016**, *42*, 206–210. [CrossRef]
25. Yaylali, I.E.; Kurnaz, S.; Tunca, Y.M. Maintaining apical patency does not increase postoperative pain in molars with necrotic pulp and apical periodontitis: A randomized controlled trial. *J. Endod.* **2018**, *44*, 335–340. [CrossRef] [PubMed]
26. Dhyani, V.K.; Chhabra, S.; Sharma, V.K.; Dhyani, A. A randomized controlled trial to evaluate the incidence of postoperative pain and flare-ups in single and multiple visits root canal treatment. *Med. J. Armed Forces India* **2020**. [CrossRef]

27. Gudlavalleti, B.; Patil, A.A. Comparative evaluation of postoperative pain after root canal treatment using three different sealers, Viz., Tubli-Seal EWT, Apexit Plus, AH Plus: An in-vivo study. *J. Clin. Diag. Res.* **2020**, *14*, ZC04–ZC09. [CrossRef]
28. Paz, A.; Vasconcelos, I.; Ginjeira, A. Evaluation of postoperative pain after using bioceramic materials as endodontic sealers. *EC Dent. Sci.* **2018**, *17*, 1739–1748.
29. Yu, Y.-H.; Kushnir, L.; Kohli, M.; Karabucak, B. Comparing the incidence of postoperative pain after root canal filling with warm vertical obtuation with resin-based sealer and sealer-based obturation with calcium silicate-based sealer: A prospective clinical trial. *Clin. Oral Investig.* **2021**, *25*, 5033–5042. [CrossRef] [PubMed]
30. Tan, H.S.G.; Lim, K.C.; Lui, J.N.; Lai, W.M.C.; Yu, V.S.H. Postobturation Pain Associated with Tricalcium Silicate and Resin-based Sealer Techniques: A Randomized Clinical Trial. *J. Endod.* **2021**, *47*, 169–177. [CrossRef] [PubMed]
31. Graunaite, I.; Skucaite, N.; Lodiene, G.; Agentiene, I.; Machiulskiene, V. Effect of resin-based and bioceramic root canal sealers on postoperative pain. *J. Endod.* **2018**, *44*, 689–693. [CrossRef]
32. Fonseca, B.; Coelho, M.S.; da Bueno, C.E.S.; Fontana, C.E.; De Martin, A.S.; Rocha, D.G.P. Assessment of extrusion and postoperative pain of a bioceramic and resin-based root canal sealer. *Eur. J. Dent.* **2019**, *13*, 343–348. [CrossRef]
33. De Ferreira, N.S.; Gollo, E.K.F.; Boscato, N.; Arias, A.; da Silva, E.J.N.L. Postoperative pain after root canal filling with different endodontic sealers: A randomized clinical trial. *Braz. Oral Res.* **2020**, *34*, e069. [CrossRef] [PubMed]
34. Nabi, S.; Farooq, R.; Purra, A.; Ahmed, F. Comparison of various sealers on postoperative pain in single-visit endodontics: A randomized clinical study. *Indian J. Dent. Sci.* **2019**, *11*, 99–102. [CrossRef]
35. Ates, A.A.; Dumani, A.; Yoldas, O.; Unal, I. Post-obturation pain following the use of carrier-based system with AH Plus or iRoot SP sealers: A randomized controlled clinical trial. *Clin. Oral Investig.* **2019**, *23*, 3053–3061. [CrossRef] [PubMed]
36. Sharma, N.; Mandhotra, P.; Kumari, S.; Chandel, N. A study to compare various sealers on postoperative pain in single visit endodontics. *Ann. Int. Med. Dent. Res.* **2019**, *6*, 40–42.

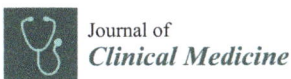

Systematic Review

Clinical Outcome and Comparison of Regenerative and Apexification Intervention in Young Immature Necrotic Teeth—A Systematic Review and Meta-Analysis

Pratima Panda [1], Lora Mishra [1,*,†], Shashirekha Govind [1], Saurav Panda [2] and Barbara Lapinska [3,*,†]

1. Department of Conservative Dentistry and Endodontics, Institute of Dental Sciences, Siksha 'O' Anusandhan University, Bhubaneswar 751003, Odisha, India; pandapratima085@gmail.com (P.P.); shashirekhag@soa.ac.in (S.G.)
2. Department of Periodontics and Oral Implantology, Institute of Dental Sciences, Siksha 'O' Anusandhan University, Bhubaneswar 751003, Odisha, India; sauravpanda@soa.ac.in
3. Department of General Dentistry, Medical University of Lodz, 92-213 Lodz, Poland
* Correspondence: loramishra@soa.ac.in (L.M.); barbara.lapinska@umed.lodz.pl (B.L.); Tel.: +91-889-526-6363 (L.M.); +85-42-675-74-61 (B.L.)
† These authors contributed equally to this work.

Abstract: This systematic review aimed to evaluate interventions individually and compare the clinical outcome of young, immature teeth treated with regenerative endodontic therapy (RET) and apexification procedure. The protocol was registered with PROSPERO (International Prospective Register of Systematic Reviews), bearing the registration number CRD42021230284. A bibliographic search in the biomedical databases was conducted in four databases—PubMed, CENTRAL, EMBASE and ProQuest—using searching keywords and was limited to studies published between January 2000 and April 2022 in English. The search was supplemented by manual searching, citation screening and scanning of all reference lists of selected paper. The study selection criteria were randomized clinical trial, prospective clinical studies and observational studies. The search found 32 eligible articles, which were included in the study. The quality assessment of the studies was performed using the Cochrane risk of bias tool for randomized control trials and non-randomized clinical studies. The meta-analysis was performed using Review Manager software (REVMAN, version 5). The results indicated that a clinicians' MTA apexification procedure was more successful compared to calcium hydroxide. In RET, apical closure and overall success rate is statistically same for both apical platelet concentrates (APCs) and blood clots (BC). Both interventions have similar survival rates; however, RET should be preferred in cases where the root development is severely deficient, there is insufficient dentine and the tooth's prognosis is hopeless even with an apexification procedure.

Keywords: apexification; endodontic therapy; immature permanent tooth; pulp; regeneration

1. Introduction

In permanent dentition, traumatic dental injuries (TDI) are a worldwide health issue and the most frequent cause of pulpal necrosis [1]. In 85% of TDIs, patients have injuries to the oral region [2]. Globally, around one billion people are affected by trauma [3], and one-third of these patients have injuries to their immature teeth that might cause pulp necrosis [4].

Pulp necrosis due to trauma or caries in children and adolescents may hinder permanent tooth root growth, resulting in thin dentinal walls, wide-open apices, and an insufficient crown:root ratio [5]. According to Cvek, the classification of root development in an immature necrotic permanent tooth can be at stage 1, where less than half of the root formation with open apex is present; stage 2 is where half of root formation with open apex is present; and stage 3 is when 2/3 of root development with open apex is present [6].

In conventional root canal fillings, immature permanent teeth with necrotic pulps are difficult candidates and have an increased susceptibility to root fractures after treatment [7]. Hence, early intervention for non-vital immature teeth is critical. However, it is incredibly challenging, time-consuming and technically complex [8]. Apexification and regeneration are interventions routinely practiced in such cases [9]. RET is recommended in short roots with thin canal walls, a wide-open apex and for teeth lacking the potential for root formation, whereas apexification is done in the tooth which has nearly completed root formation with an open apex [5].

Apexification is a method to encourage the development of an apical barrier to close the open apex of an immature necrotic permanent tooth in which filling materials can be placed within the root canal space [10].

In contrast, RET or regenerative endodontic procedures (REPS) are biologically based procedures designed to replace damaged structures, such as the root and dentin, along with cells of the pulp–dentin complex [11]. The main aim of REPS is to establish a suitable environment (biomimetic microenvironment) in the root canal to facilitate mesenchymal stem cells such as osteo/odontoprogenitor stem cells, pulp tissue regeneration and continued root development.

The basic principles underlying both interventions involve removing necrotic pulp, debridement of the canal and control of infection with or without antiseptic medicament. Total treatment time may vary in multi-visit apexification, depending on the medicament used, the initial presence of periapical pathology [6], the frequency of medicament replacement [12], and the age of the patient [13].

This present review compares and assesses both interventions individually to manage immature necrotic young permanent teeth. This review aims to critically evaluate the outcome of regeneration and apexification procedure, which will impact clinical discussion making.

2. Materials and Methods

The review protocol was registered at PROSPERO (International Prospective Register of Systematic Reviews), bearing registration number CRD42021230284. This review followed the Preferred Reporting Items for Systematic Reviews and Meta-analyses (PRISMA) statement guidelines [14].

2.1. Search Strategy

The following PICO components were established: Population (P)—systematically healthy patients with necrotic young, immature permanent tooth; Intervention (I)—regeneration procedure; Comparison (C)—apexification procedure; Outcomes (O)—clinical and radiographical successful outcome. The research question was: "Which intervention between and within the two that is regenerative and apexification, has a more successful outcome in the young permanent non-vital tooth?"

The electronic search strategy is described in Table 1. A comprehensive electronic search for relevant articles was performed in the PubMed, CENTRAL, EMBASE and ProQuest databases using the search keywords and combining the keywords using "AND" and "OR". For all these databases, Boolean operators (OR, AND) were used to combine and narrow down searches that included appropriate MeSH terms, keywords, and other terms following the syntax rules of each database. All references selected in the search were saved in Mendeley Desktop software to remove the duplicates.

A manual search was performed in the following dental journals: *International Endodontic Journal*; *British Dental Journal*; *Journal of Endodontics*; *Oral Surgery, Oral Medicine, Oral Pathology, and Oral Radiology*; and *Endodontics*. The search was supplemented by manual searching, citation screening and scanning all reference lists of the selected paper. Additional studies that were likely suitable for inclusion were screened from the bibliographies of potentially eligible clinical trials, case reports, case studies, and systematic reviews.

Table 1. Search strategy.

Search Strategy
#1 immature teeth/immature tooth/immature permanent tooth/immature permanent teeth/young permanent tooth/young permanent dentition
#2 pulp revascularization/pulp regeneration/pulp revitalization/PRF/PRP/blood clot
#3 apexification/calcific barrier/apical closure/root end closure/root apex closure/root end formation/root apex closure/apical plug/MTA plug
#4 survival rate/dentinal thickness/pulp vitality/root completion/successful rate/periapical healing/decrease in apical foramen width

2.2. Study Selection

The literature search was limited to articles available in English and to those published between January 2000 and April 2022. Each article was assessed carefully and in detail. Two independent reviewers (P.P. and L.M.) read abstracts and titles, and studies not about the research question were excluded. The remaining relevant studies' full texts were read and analyzed independently. In this selection, a third reviewer (S.G.) was called to achieve a consensus if there was a disagreement of opinions.

The selection of studies was performed with no restrictions on place or year of publication. However, a language restriction was applied, and only those articles written in English were included. Titles and abstracts were analyzed to determine whether they fulfilled the inclusion criteria. The inclusion and exclusion criteria are depicted in Table 2.

Table 2. Inclusion and exclusion criteria for selecting studies in the systematic review.

Inclusion Criteria	Exclusion Criteria
Study design: Randomized controlled trials, clinical studies, observational studies (Retrospective study)	Case reports, comments, conference proceedings
Patients with immature necrotic permanent teeth	Studies experimenting on vital teeth
Studies in which either one of the interventions or both are compared	Animal studies, case reports, in vitro studies, laboratory studies
Articles published in English language	

The relevant data of the included trials were extracted in detail using an Excel spreadsheet (Microsoft, Redmond, WA, USA) independently by two review authors (P.P., L.M.) and recorded in spreadsheets. In case of missing or unclear information, the authors of the included reports were contacted by email to provide clarification regarding data given or any missing information. The data of all included studies were entered in the characteristics of included studies tables in Review Manager (RevMan, Version 5).

2.3. Study Quality Assessment

Two review authors (P.P., L.M.) independently assessed the risk of bias in the included studies. In case of disagreement, a third review author (S.G.) was consulted. For the randomized control trials, the assessment was conducted following the instructions and the approach described in the Cochrane Handbook for Systematic Reviews of Interventions [15].

For each study, the following domains were considered: selection bias (random sequence generation and allocation concealment), performance bias (blinding of participants and personnel), detection bias (blinding of outcome assessment), attrition bias (incomplete outcome data addressed), and reporting bias (selective reporting).

For the non-randomized controlled trial, the risk of bias in included studies was assessed using the ROBINS-I risk of bias tool. The bias tool considered: bias due to confounding, selection of participants, classification of interventions, deviations from intended interventions, missing data, measurement of outcomes and selection of reported results.

The overall risk for individual studies was assessed as low, moderate, serious or critical based on the following criteria: low or moderate risk of bias if all domains were at low risk of bias; serious risk of bias if at least one domain was at serious risk of bias but not at critical risk of bias in any domain; critical risk of bias if one domain was at critical risk of bias.

3. Results

3.1. Selection of Studies

The search in the selected databases allowed for the identification of 1430 articles (Figure 1). After eliminating duplicates, the included articles were selected from a pool of 814 articles obtained from digital sources and a manual search. The full text was read for 53 articles, and 21 studies were omitted for the reasons specified in Appendix A (Table A1). A total of 18 randomized clinical trials and 14 non-randomized clinical trials were included in this systematic review to assess the successful outcomes in managing immature young necrotic permanent teeth.

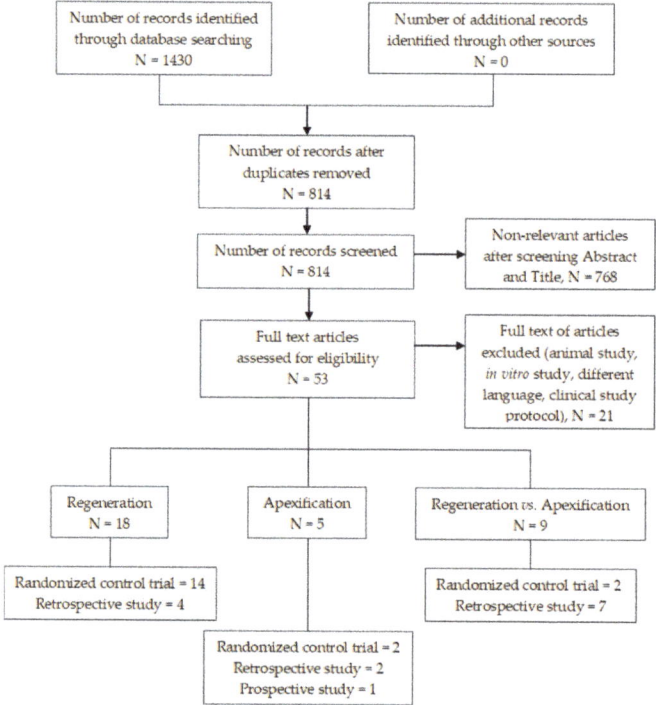

Figure 1. PRISMA 2020 flow diagram for systematic review that includes searches of databases.

3.2. Characteristics of Studies

3.2.1. Design

Thirty-two articles were included in this study (Table 3). Eighteen articles [16–33] evaluated the clinical outcome of regenerative endodontic procedures (REP) and five articles [34–38] on the apexification procedure. Only nine articles [39–47] evaluated and compared the clinical outcome between regeneration and apexification procedure.

Table 3. Data extraction from included studies – the clinical protocol.

Author	Etiology of Pulp Necrosis	Presence of Periapical Lesion	Instrumentation	Irrigation Method	Intracanal Medication	Recall Time (in Weeks)	Preparation Protocol of APC	Access Restoration
Alagl et al., 2017 [16]	Secondary to trauma/caries	Yes	No	2.5% NaOCl (20 mL), sterile saline (20 mL), and 0.12% CHX (10 mL), followed by 17% EDTA after 3 weeks	TAP	3	PRP was prepared according to the description by Dohan et al. [48]. PRP was combined with equal volumes of sterile solution containing 10% calcium chloride and sterile bovine thrombin (100 U/mL) to achieve coagulation.	NR
Bezgin et al., 2015 [17]	Secondary to trauma/caries	Yes	No	2.5% NaOCl (20 mL), sterile saline (20 mL), and 0.12% CHX (10 mL), followed by 5% EDTA (20 mL) after 3 weeks	TAP	3	PRP was prepared according to the description by Dohan et al. [48]. PRP was combined with equal volumes of sterile solution containing 10% calcium chloride and sterile bovine thrombin (100 U/mL) to achieve coagulation.	Final restoration was completed with white MTA (Angelus, Londrina, Brazil), reinforced GI cement (Ketac Molar Easymix; 3M ESPE, Seefeld, Germany) and composite resin (Filtek Supreme XT; 3M ESPE, St. Paul, MN, USA)
Elsheshtawy et al., 2020 [18]	Secondary to trauma and Dens invaginatus	Yes	No	20 mL of 5.25% NaOCl. At recall, 20 mL of 2.5% NaOCl, followed by 20 mL sterile saline and 10 mL of 17% EDTA solution	TAP	NR	PRP was prepared according to Dohan et al. [48], after which concentrated platelet-rich plasma (cPRP) was prepared and introduced inside dry root canals using a sterile 30 G syringe. The canal was then backfilled with cPRP to a level just beneath the CEJ and left to clot for 10 min	MTA, using a layer of reinforced GI (Riva self-cure, SDI limited, Bayswater, Victoria, Australia), followed by resin composite (Filtek Z250 universal restorative, 3 mol L, 3M ESPE, St. Paul, MN, USA)

Table 3. Cont.

Author	Etiology of Pulp Necrosis	Presence of Periapical Lesion	Instrumentation	Irrigation Method	Intracanal Medication	Recall Time (in Weeks)	Preparation Protocol of APC	Access Restoration
Jadhav et al., 2012 [19]	Secondary to trauma/caries	No	Minimal (#60H file)	2.5% NaOCl (copious irrigation)	TAP	NR	PRP: 8 mL of blood drawn by venipuncture of the antecubital vein was collected in a 10 mL sterile glass tube coated with an anticoagulant (acid citrate dextrose) and centrifuged at 2400 rpm for 10 min to separate PRP and platelet-poor plasma (PPP) from the red blood cell fraction. The topmost layer (PRP + PPP) was transferred to another tube and again centrifuged at 3600 rpm for 15 min to separate the PRP to precipitate at the bottom of the glass tube. This was mixed with 1 mL 10% calcium chloride to activate the platelets and to neutralize the acidity of acid citrate dextrose.	Resin-modified GI cement (Photac-Fill; 3M ESPE, St. Paul, MN, USA)
Rizk et al., 2019 [20]	Secondary to trauma	Yes	No	20 mL 2% NaOCl for 5 min, followed by 20 mL 17% EDTA.	TAP	3	PRP was prepared according to the description by Dohan et al. [48]. PRP was combined with equal volumes of sterile solution containing 10% calcium chloride and sterile bovine thrombin (100 U/mL) to achieve coagulation. PRF: 10 mL blood was collected in a sterile tube without anticoagulant and centrifuged immediately for 10 min at a speed of 3000 rpm.	An MTA orifice plug extending 2–3 mm in the canal was used to seal the canal orifice then GI (GC America, Alsip, IL, USA) and composite (Z250, 3M ESPE) were applied to give an effective and durable seal

Table 3. Cont.

Author	Etiology of Pulp Necrosis	Presence of Periapical Lesion	Instrumentation	Irrigation Method	Intracanal Medication	Recall Time (in Weeks)	Preparation Protocol of APC	Access Restoration
Ragab et al., 2019 [21]	Secondary to trauma	Yes	No	20 mL of 5.25% NaOCl followed by 20 mL sterile saline.	DAP	3	PRF was prepared by drawing 12 mL sample of whole blood intravenously from the patient's right antecubital vein and centrifuged at 3000 rpm for 12 min.	MTA plus Light Cure GI cement
Mittal et al., 2019 [22]	Secondary to trauma/caries	Yes	Minimal (#30k file)	2.5% NaOCl (copious irrigation).	DAP	4	PRF was prepared by drawing 5 mL of venous blood from the patient, collected in a dried glass test tube, and centrifuged at 2700 rpm for 12 min.	GI cement followed by composite resin
Shivashankar et al., 2017 [23]	Secondary to trauma/caries	No	Minimal	5.25% NaOCl (copious irrigation).	TAP	3	NR	NR
Hazim Rizk et al., 2020 [24]	Trauma, Caries	Yes	No	20 mL of 2.5% NaOCl followed by 20 mL of 17% EDTA. At recall 20 mL sterile saline followed by 20 mL 17% EDTA solution	TAP	3	PRP and PRF was prepared according to Dohan and Choukroun (2007) [49] method.	MTA, using a layer of GI (GC America, Alsip, IL, USA) followed by composite (Z 250, 3M ESPE)
Jiang et al., 2017 [25]	Trauma, Broken central cusp	Yes	NO	20 mL 1.25% NaOCl. At recall, 20 mL 17% EDTA.	Ca(OH)$_2$ paste	2	NR	A layer of Filtek Z250 composite resin (3M ESPE, Irvine, CA; 3–4 mm) was placed over the capping material for the final restoration.

Table 3. Cont.

Author	Etiology of Pulp Necrosis	Presence of Periapical Lesion	Instrumentation	Irrigation Method	Intracanal Medication	Recall Time (in Weeks)	Preparation Protocol of APC	Access Restoration
Narang et al., 2015 [26]	Secondary to trauma/caries	Yes	Minimal	2.5% NaOCl (copious irrigation)	TAP	4	NR	Resin-modified GI cement was placed extending 3–4 mm in the canal. Access cavity was sealed with composite (Clearfil Majesty, Kuraray Medical Inc., Tokyo, Japan).
Meschi et al., 2021 [27]	Trauma, Caries, Anatomic anomaly (dens invaginatus)	Yes	No	20 mL 1.5% NaOCl and subsequently with 20 mL saline. At recall, 30 mL EDTA 17% 1 mm short of the working length.	DAP	2	Blood samples were centrifuged. Fibrin clots were collected after centrifugation, and 2 of them were transformed into membranes after 5 min of pressure under a sterile glass plate.	Tooth was sealed by means of a GI lining and composite restoration.
Ulusoy et al., 2019 [28]	Secondary to trauma	Yes	No	20 mL 1.25% NaOCl. At recall, 2% CHX, saline and 1 mL 17% EDTA.	TAP	4	PRP: Citrated blood was centrifuged in a standard laboratory centrifuge PK 130 (ALC International; ColognoMonzese, Italy) for 15 min at 1250 rpm to obtain PRP without erythrocytes and leukocytes. PRF: 10 mL blood was collected in a sterile tube without anticoagulant and centrifuged immediately for 10 min at a speed of 3000 rpm (Andreas Hettich Group, Ltd., Tuttlingen, Germany).	MTA coronal barrier was sealed with a thin GI base, and final coronal restorations were placed at the same visit using acid etch composite resin.

Table 3. Cont.

Author	Etiology of Pulp Necrosis	Presence of Periapical Lesion	Instrumentation	Irrigation Method	Intracanal Medication	Recall Time (in Weeks)	Preparation Protocol of APC	Access Restoration
Jayadevan et al., 2021 [33]	Trauma	No	Minimal (#80–120K file)	1.5% NaOCl solution (20 mL) followed by saline and 17% EDTA. Recall session, copious and gentle irrigation with saline and 20 mL of 17% EDTA.	TAP	4	A-PRF or PRF was freshly prepared using a centrifuge (R-8C Laboratory centrifuge, Remi Lab, Mumbai, India). For PRF, 10 mL of intravenous blood was drawn into a tube without anticoagulant and centrifuged at 2700 rpm for 12 min. For A-PRF, 10 mL of intravenous blood was drawn into a tube without anticoagulant and centrifuged at 1500 rpm for 14 min.	GI cement (GC, Fuji IX, GC India) was placed gently in a thickness of about 3–4 mm over the Biodentine and the access was temporized with Cavit. Post regenerative treatment consisted of non-vital bleaching or composite restoration. These procedures were performed after a period of one week.
Peng et al., 2017 [29]	Anatomic, Caries, Trauma	Yes	Minimal (#30K file)	5.25% NaOCl solution (20 mL)	TAP	1–4	NR	Conventional GI cement (Fuji IX, Fuji Corporation, Osaka, Japan) was placed over the blood clot at the level of CEJ, followed by phosphoric acid etching for 30 s, a single-bond adhesive agent, and placement of Filtek Z250 composite resin (3M ESPE, Irvine, CA, USA). Instead of GI cement, mixture of ProRoot MTA (Dentsply Tulsa Dental, Johnson City, TN, USA) with 3 mm thickness was placed at the level of the CEJ.

Table 3. Cont.

Author	Etiology of Pulp Necrosis	Presence of Periapical Lesion	Instrumentation	Irrigation Method	Intracanal Medication	Recall Time (in Weeks)	Preparation Protocol of APC	Access Restoration
Lv et al., 2018 [30]	Dens evaginatus, Tooth fracture	Yes	Minimal (35 K-file)	20 mL of 1% NaOCl followed by 10 mL of 17% EDTA solution	TAP	4	PRF was prepared as described by Choukroun et al. [50]. Immediately before surgery, 5 mL of whole blood was drawn into 10 mL test tubes without anticoagulant reagent and was centrifuged at 400× g for 10 min. The PRF layer was separated using sterile scissors, and PRF clots were pressed into a membranous film with sterile dry gauze.	A 3-mm-thick layer of MTA was placed followed by a moist cotton pellet and Cavit. One week later, the Cavit was removed and replaced with a bonded resin restoration (Filtek Z350 XT: 3M ESPE Dental Products, St. Paul, MN, USA).
Cheng et al., 2022 [31]	Secondary to trauma	No	Minimal or No	0.5–1.5% NaOCl and saline or NaOCl in combination with saline and 17% EDTA	TAP	2	CGF was prepared from the patient's intravenous blood. After immediate differential centrifugation of blood, CGF was represented as the buffy coat in the middle layer. Then the CGF layer was separated using sterile scissors.	Teeth were restored with a bio-ceramic material [i.e., MTA (Dentsply Sirona, Ballaigues, Switzerland) or iRoot BP Plus (Innovative Bioceramix Inc., Vancouver, BC, Canada)] followed by various restorative materials.
Chueh et al., 2009 [32]	Trauma	Yes	No	2.5% NaOCl	$Ca(OH)_2$ paste	1–2	NR	The access was sealed with temporary filling materials or resin.

Table 3. Cont.

Author	Etiology of Pulp Necrosis	Presence of Periapical Lesion	Instrumentation	Irrigation Method	Intracanal Medication	Recall Time (in Weeks)	Preparation Protocol of APC	Access Restoration
Bonte et al., 2014 [34]	Trauma	Yes	No	Active 3% NaOCl	-	-	-	Composite resin
Santhakumar et al., 2018 [35]	Trauma and Dental caries	Yes	No	3% NaOCl followed by saline	TAP	3	A 5 mL blood sample was taken from the patient's anticubital vein. The blood was centrifuged without anticoagulant at 3000 rpm for 10 min, and PRF gel was obtained at the bottom of the test tube and was removed with a sterile tweezer. After obtaining PRF gel, it was squeezed using especially designed PRF compression device to remove the excess fluid. The membrane obtained was cut linearly in the shape of root canal space for ease of placement.	Triple sealed with MTA (ProRoot MTA), type II GI cement (Fugi 2) and composite material (3M ESPE).
Kandemir Demirci et al., 2019 [36]	Trauma, Dens invaginatus, Caries	Yes	No	2.5% NaOCl solution. At recall, 2.5% NaOCl, 17% EDTA followed by 2% CHX	Ca(OH)$_2$ powder mixed with saline	1	-	Bonded composite resin
Tek et al. 2021 [37]	Trauma	Yes	Yes	2.5% NaOCl solution. Recall 2.5% NaOCl solution followed by distilled water	Ca(OH)$_2$ paste	1	-	Resin composite (3M ESPE Filtek Ultimate Seefeld, Germany)
Kinirons et al., 2001 [38]	Trauma	NR	No	NR	-	-	-	NR

Table 3. Cont.

Author	Etiology of Pulp Necrosis	Presence of Periapical Lesion	Instrumentation	Irrigation Method	Intracanal Medication	Recall Time (in Weeks)	Preparation Protocol of APC	Access Restoration
Lin et al., 2017 [39]	Secondary to trauma/Dens evaginatus	Yes	Minimal (#25 K file)	20 mL 1.5% NaOCl, 0.9% physiological saline, 20 mL 17% EDTA	TAP	3	-	GI cement followed by composite resin
Xuan et al., 2018 [40]	Secondary to trauma	Yes	No	NR	NR	4	The pulp tissue for hDPSC isolation was harvested using standard sterile techniques. Autologous hDPSCs were obtained from the patient's maxillary deciduous canine tooth.	NR
Alobaid et al., 2014 [41]	Secondary to Trauma	Yes	No	20 mL 17% EDTA	TAP	3	PRP and PRF were prepared according to the method of Dohan and Choukroun (2007) [49].	An MTA orifice plug extending 2–3 mm in the canal was used to seal the canal orifice then GI (GC America, Alsip, IL, USA) and composite (Z 250, 3 M ESPE) to give an effective and durable seal.
Casey et al., 2022 [42]	Secondary to trauma	Yes	Minimal	Varying concentrations of NaOCl, CHX, and/or EDTA	TAP	2	NR	Resin bonded restoration
Caleza-Jimenez et al., 2022 [43]	Trauma, Caries	Yes	No	1.5–2.5% NaOCl and 17% EDTA	TAP	2	NR	Composite restoration
Pereira et al., 2021 [44]	Trauma	No	Minimal	6% NaOCl, 2% CHX, saline solution, and EDTA 17% or Ca(OH)$_2$ and 2% CHX gel	TAP	3	NR	Resin bonded restoration

Table 3. *Cont.*

Author	Etiology of Pulp Necrosis	Presence of Periapical Lesion	Instrumentation	Irrigation Method	Intracanal Medication	Recall Time (in Weeks)	Preparation Protocol of APC	Access Restoration
Jeeruphan et al., 2012 [45]	Secondary to trauma/Caries	No	Minimal	5.25% NaOCl	TAP	3	NR	NR
Silujjai et al., 2017 [46]	Secondary to trauma/Caries/Dens evaginatus	Yes	No	1.5–2.5% NaOCl followed by 17% EDTA	Ca(OH)$_2$ or TAP	NR	NR	MTA plus bonded restoration
Chen et al., 2016 [47]	Dens evaginatus	Yes	Minimal (#25 K file)	Copious 2.5% NaOCl	NR	NR	NR	NR

Legend: APC = autologous platelet concentrate; NR = not reported; NaOCl = sodium hypochlorite; CHX = chlorhexidine; EDTA = ethylene diamine tetra-acetic acid; DAP = double antibiotic paste; TAP = triple antibiotic paste; Ca(OH)$_2$ = calcium hydroxide; GI = glass ionomer; PRP = platelet-rich plasma; cPRP = concentrated platelet-rich plasma; PPP = platelet-poor plasma; PRF = platelet-rich fibrin; CEJ = cementoenamel junction; MTA = mineral trioxide aggregate; hDPSC = human dental pulp stem cells.

3.2.2. Participants

In total, of the 18 articles [16–33] evaluating regeneration outcomes, 14 articles [16–28,33] were randomized clinical trials, and 4 articles [29–32] were non-randomized clinical articles. In randomized clinical trials, a total of 393 participants and 412 teeth were included. In non-randomized clinical trials, 144 participants and 156 teeth were included.

Five articles [34–38] evaluated apexification outcomes, of which two articles [34,35] were randomized clinical trials and three [36–38] were non-randomized clinical trials. In RCT, a total of 68 participants and 68 teeth were included. In NRCT, a total of 198 participants and 200 teeth were included. One NRCT article was a multicentric study.

Nine articles [39–47] compared the outcome between regeneration and apexification procedure, of which two articles [39,40] were RCTs, and seven articles [41–47] were NRCTs. In the RCTs, a total of 133 participants and 133 teeth were included. In the NRCTs, a total of 439 participants and 446 teeth were included.

3.2.3. Intervention

Of the total eighteen RCTs, four studies [16–28,33] evaluated the revascularization procedure outcomes, two studies [34,35] were on the apexification and two studies [39,40] compared revascularization versus apexification.

Among fourteen NRCTs, four studies [29–32] investigated clinical outcome of the revascularization procedure, three studies [36,38] were on apexification and seven studies [41–47] compared regeneration versus apexification

3.3. Analysis of Quality of the Studies

The risk of bias in included studies is summarized in Figure 2 for RCTs and Figure 3 for NRCTs.

In regeneration RCTs, two studies [18,24] were assessed to be at low risk, whereas twelve studies [16,17,19–23,25–28,33] were at moderate risk of bias. In apexification RCTs, two studies [34,35] were assessed to be at moderate risk of bias. In regeneration versus apexification RCTs, two studies [39,40] were assessed to be at moderate risk of bias.

In most of the randomized clinical trials, there was unclear or no information about allocation concealment, blinding of participants and blinding of outcome evaluation in a few studies. The factors mentioned above resulted in a moderate overall risk assessment in the studies cited above. In most non-randomized control trials, there was unclear or no information on sample selection, exact treatment protocol and deviations from planned interventions in a few studies. The variables mentioned above resulted in a moderate to serious overall risk assessment.

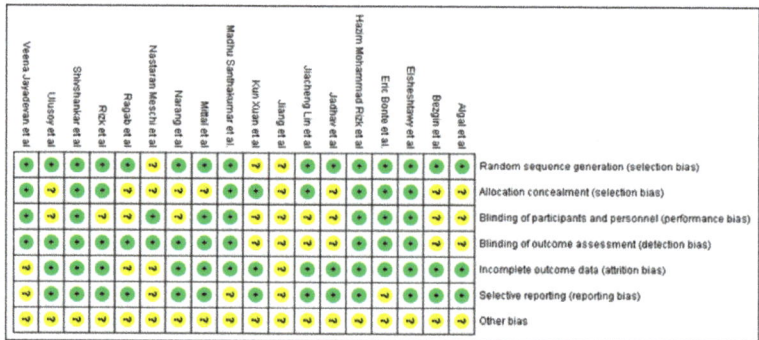

Figure 2. Quality assessment of included RCT studies summary: review authors' judgements about each risk of bias item for each included study.

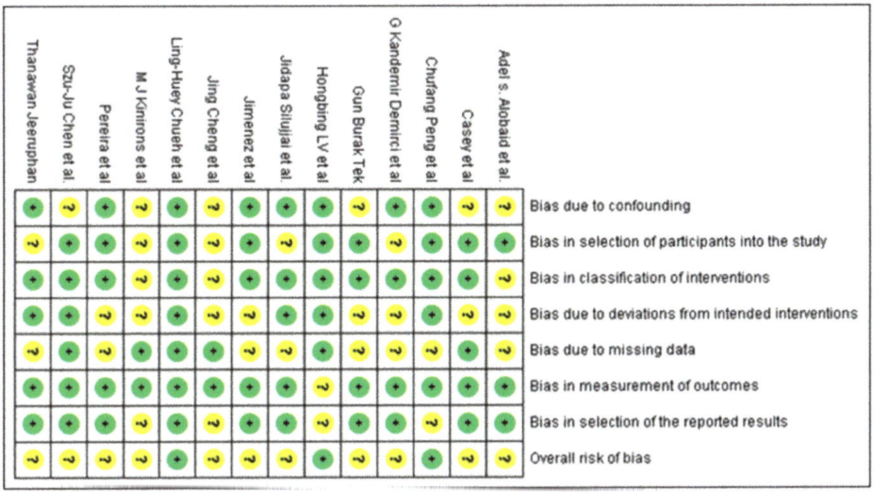

Figure 3. Quality assessment of included NRCT studies summary: review authors' judgements about each risk of bias item for each included study.

In regeneration NRCTs, one study [32] was assessed to be at low risk of bias whereas three studies [29–31] were at moderate risk. In apexification NRCTs, one study [37] was assessed to be at moderate risk of bias and two studies [36,38] were assessed to be at serious risk. In regeneration versus apexification NRCTs, one study [47] was assessed to be a low risk of bias, five studies [42–46] were assessed to be a moderate risk, and one study [41] was at serious risk.

3.4. Synthesis of Results

The meta-analysis (Review Manager, RevMan version 5.3, Copenhagen: Nordic Cochrane Centre, The Cochrane collaboration) was performed with quantitative outcome data extracted from the six included randomised controlled trials in REP, which compared the effectiveness of APCs in comparison to BC for treatment of young, immature, necrotic, permanent teeth. However, it was not possible in case of the NRCTs, as the data from the included studies showed heterogeneity (Table 4).

Table 4. Data extraction from included studies for qualitative analysis – clinical evaluation parameters.

Author	Intervention	Type of Study	Comparative Group	Sample Size	Follow Up Time (in Months)	RA	Parameters to Assess Clinical Evaluation							
							DWT	IRL	AFW	AC	VR	PAH	BD
Alagl et al., 2017 [16]	REP	RCT	BC	15	12	CBCT	-	11.80 ± 3.28 mm	-	53.33%	53.33%	-	445.44 ± 153.54 HU
			PRP	15			-	12.14 ± 3.32 mm	-	93.33%	86.66%	-	485.88 ± 154.15 HU
Bezgin et al., 2015 [17]	REP	RCT	BC	10	18	IOPAR	-	12.6%	-	60%	20%	-	-
			PRP	10			-	9.86%	-	70%	50%	-	-
Elsheshtawy et al., 2020 [18]	REP	RCT	BC	11	12	CBCT	ICC = 1	ICC = 0.998	ICC = 1	-	-	-	-
			PRP	11			ICC = 0.997	ICC = 0.999	ICC = 0.998	-	-	-	-
Jadhav et al., 2012 [19]	REP	RCT	BC	10	12	IOPAR	S = 70% G = 30%	S = 40% G = 60%	-	S = 50% G = 30 E = 20%	-	S = 30%, G = 70%	-
			PRP	10			S = 20%, G = 50%, E = 30%	S = 10% G = 50% E = 40%	-	G = 30%, E = 70%	-	S = 10% G = 40% E = 50%	-
Rizk et al., 2019 [20]	REP	RCT	BC	13	12	IOPAR	-	0.68 ± 0.44 mm	2.2 ± 3.97 mm	-	-	-	58.96 ± 19.95 Grey
			PRP	13			-	1.48 ± 0.37 mm	2.49 ± 3.93 mm	-	-	-	65.08 ± 30.043 Grey
Ragab et al., 2019 [21]	REP	RCT	BC	11	12	IOPAR	-	14.8%	-	45.4%	-	80.5%	-
			PRF	11			-	12.8%	-	63.6%	-	70.2%	-
Mittal et al., 2019 [22]	REP	RCT	BC	4	12	IOPAR	100%	25%	-	25%	-	75%	-
			PRF	4			100%	0	-	100%	-	75%	-

Table 4. Cont.

Author	Intervention	Type of Study	Comparative Group	Sample Size	Follow Up Time (in Months)	RA	Parameters to Assess Clinical Evaluation							
							DWT	IRL	AFW	AC	VR	PAH	BD
Shivashankar et al., 2017 [23]	REP	RCT	BC	15	12	IOPAR	93.3%	86.7%	-	-	13.30%	2.07 ± 0.594 mm	-
			PRP	19			84.2%	73.7%	-	-	15.8%	1.32 ± 0.478 mm	-
			PRF	20			70%	65%	-	-	15%	1.85 ± 1.040 mm	-
Hazim Rizk et al., 2020 [24]	REP	RCT	PRP	13	12	IOPAR	-	1.48 ± 0.37 mm	0.97 ± 0.75 mm	-	-	-	65.08 ± 30.043 Grey
			PRF	12			-	1.24 ± 0.54 mm	1.003 ± 0.392 mm	-	-	-	53.44 ± 22.165 Grey
Jiang et al., 2017 [25]	REP	RCT	Without Bio-Gide	22	6	IOPAR	21.2 ± 19.5%	15.4 ± 13.6%	−55 ± 34%	-	18%	-	-
			With Bio-Gide	21			21.5 ± 22.5%	16.4 ± 13.6%	−65 ± 34%	-	33%	-	-
Narang et al., 2015 [26]	REP	RCT	MTA	5	18	IOPAR	0%	0%	-	0%	-	58%	-
			BC	5			50%	40%	-	66.67%	-	60%	-
			PRP	5			60%	99%	-	40%	-	98%	-
			PRF	5			20%	40%	-	60%	-	80%	-
Meschi et al., 2021 [27]	REP	RCT	REP-LPRF	13	36	CBCT	30%	0%	-	-	-	100%	-
			REP + LPRF	6			10%	10%	-	-	-	100%	-

Table 4. Cont.

Author	Intervention	Type of Study	Comparative Group	Sample Size	Follow Up Time (in Months)	RA	Parameters to Assess Clinical Evaluation							
							DWT	IRL	AFW	AC	VR	PAH	BD
Ulusoy et al., 2019 [28]	REP	RCT	BC	21	Until complete healing 10–49	IOPAR	14.91 ± 3.38 mm	7.15 ± 1.39 mm	-	-	-	-	-
			PRP	18			19.01 ± 4.20 mm	4.74 ± 0.91 mm	-	-	-	-	-
			PRF	17			9.80 ± 3.03 mm	6.00 ± 1.57 mm	-	-	-	-	-
			PP	17			8.55 ± 3.55 mm	4.17 ± 1.33 mm	-	-	-	-	-
Jayadevan et al., 2021 [33]	REP	RCT	PRF	10	12	IOPAR	50%	80%	-	-	-	45.5%	-
			APRF	11			91%	72%	-	-	-	40%	-
Peng et al., 2017 [29]	REP	NRCT	Conventional GIC	32	12	IOPAR	26.3%	10.5%	-	-	-	-	-
			ProRoot MTA	28			30.7%	11.0%	-	-	-	-	-
Lv et al., 2018 [30]	REP	NRCT	BC	5	12	IOPAR	80%	80%	-	80%	100%	100%	-
			PRF	5			80%	80%	-	80%	100%	100%	-
Cheng et al., 2022 [31]	REP	NRCT	BC	32	16	IOPAR	F = 17.4 ± 16.4% L = 52.5 ± 24.8% Ci = 26.0 ± 37.3%	F = 8.3 ± 11.7% L = 23.8 ± 18.1% Ci = 10.3 ± 89.5%	F = 76.4 ± 30.9% L = 69.3 ± 43.9% Ci = 45.0 ± 87.5%	-	-	-	-
			CGF	30			A = 37.0%	A = 12.0%	A = 100.0%	-	-	-	-
Chueh et al., 2009 [32]	REP	NRCT	MTA	8	6–108	IOPAR	-	93.33%	80%	-	-	-	-
			MTA + GP/GP/ Amalgam	15									
Bonte et al., 2014 [34]	APP	RCT	MTA	15	12	IOPAR	-	-	76.5%	-	-	82.4%	-
			CH	15			-	-	50%	-	-	75.0%	-
Santhakumar et al., 2018 [35]	APP	RCT	PRF Gel	19	18	IOPAR	-	94.73%	-	-	100%	-	-
			PRF Membrane	19			-	89.47%	-	-	100%	-	-

210

Table 4. Cont.

Author	Intervention	Type of Study	Comparative Group	Sample Size	Follow Up Time (in Months)	RA	DWT	IRL	AFW	AC	VR	PAH	BD
Kandemir Demirci et al., 2019 [36]	APP	NRCT	MTA	39	12	IOPAR	-	-	74%	-	-	92%	-
			CH	34			-	-	79%	-	-	91%	-
Tek et al., 2021 [37]	APP	NRCT	Apical plug with MTA	10	12	IOPAR	-	-	-	-	-	50%	-
			Collagen sponge + apical plug with MTA	10			-	-	-	-	-	62.5%	-
Kinirons et al., 2001 [38]	APP	NRCT	CH in Newcastle	43	3	IOPAR	-	-	100%	-	-	-	-
			CH in Belfast	64			-	-	100%	-	-	-	-
Lin et al., 2017 [39]	REP vs. APP	RCT	BC	69	12	CBCT	82.60%	81.16%	-	65.21%	-	100%	-
			Vitapex paste	34			0%	26.47%	-	82.35%	-	100%	-
Xuan et al., 2018 [40]	REP vs. APP	RCT	hDPSC	20	12	CBCT	-	5.24 ± 0.92 mm	2.64 ± 0.73 mm	-	43.43 ± 0.86 mm	-	-
			CH	10			-	0.88 ± 0.67 mm	0.62 ± 0.22 mm	-	0.17 ± 0.16 mm	-	-
Alobaid et al., 2014 [41]	REP vs. APP	NRCT	BC	19	15–22	IOPAR	-	20%	10.2 ± −4.0%	-	-	-	-
			CH & MTA	12			-	12.5%	1.4 ± −3.2%	-	-	-	-
Casey et al., 2022 [42]	REP vs. APP	NRCT	BC	93	31–33	IOPAR	-	-	-	-	19%	-	-
			CH & MTA	118			-	-	-	-	0	-	-
Caleza-Jimenez et al., 2022 [43]	REP vs. APP	NRCT	BC	9	6–66	IOPAR	-	12.76%	34.57 ± 16.62%				
			MTA	9			-	0.29%	−3.36 ± 4.13%				

Table 4. *Cont.*

Author	Intervention	Type of Study	Comparative Group	Sample Size	Follow Up Time (in Months)	RA	Parameters to Assess Clinical Evaluation						
							DWT	IRL	AFW	AC	VR	PAH	BD
Pereira et al., 2021 [44]	REP vs. APP	NRCT	BC	22	12–30	IOPAR	0.21 ± 0.35 mm	1.42 ± 1.25 mm	0.88 ± 0.77 mm	-	-	95.45%	-
			MTA	22			0.03 ± 0.07 mm	0.88 ± 0.7 mm	0.6 ± 0.51 mm	-	-	86.36%	-
Jeeruphan et al., 2012 [45]	REP vs. APP	NRCT	BC	20	24	IOPAR	-	14.9%	28.2%	-	-	80%	-
			MTA	19			-	6.1%	0.00%	-	-	68%	-
			CH	22			-	0.4%	1.52%	-	-	77%	-
Silujjai et al., 2017 [46]	REP vs. APP	NRCT	BC	17	12–96	IOPAR	-	9.51 ± 18.14%	13.75 ± 19.91%	-	-	-	-
			MTA	26			-	8.55 ± 8.97%	−3.30 ± 14.14%	-	-	-	-
Chen et al., 2016 [47]	REP vs. APP	NRCT	CH, BC, MTA	17	12	IOPAR	-	94.12%	-	-	-	-	-
			CH, MTA	21			-	85.71%	-	-	-	-	-

Legend: REP = Regenerative Endodontic Procedure; APP = Apexification Procedure; RCT = Randomized clinical trial; NRCT = Non-randomised clinical trial; DWT = Dentin wall thickness; IRL = Increase in root length; AFW = Apical foramen width; AC = apical closure; VR = Vitality response; PAH = Periapical healing; BD = Bone density; BC = Blood clot; PRF = Platelet rich plasma; PRF = Platelet rich fibrin; PP = Platelet plug; MTA = Mineral trioxide aggregate; CH = Calcium hydroxide; hDPSC = Human dental pulp stem cells; RA = radiological assessment; IOPAR = Intraoral periapical radiographs; CBCT = cone-beam computed tomography; S = Satisfactory; G= Good; E= Excellent; ICC= Intraclass Correlation Coefficient; HU= Hounsfield units F= Fracture; L = Luxation; Ci= Combined injuries; A= Avulsion.

Forest plots were plotted individually in a random effect model for dentinal wall thickness (DWT), increase in root length (RL), apical closure (AC), vitality response (VR) and success rate (SR). Meta-analysis was also performed to compare REP and Apexification procedure. The meta-analysis was made from six included trials. Forest plots were plotted for survival rate (SR), success rate (SR), increase in root length (RL) and decrease in foramen width (FW).

3.4.1. DWT in REP with APC Compared to BC in Young Immature Permanent Teeth

Four studies [19,22,23,26] compared the DWT in REP between APC and BC. Data were pooled to assess the dentinal wall thickness (Figure 4). The overall risk ratio is 1.07, at 95% CI [0.77, 1.49] of achieving adequate dentinal wall thickness was found to be insignificant among these two group ($p = 0.68$). The heterogenicity between the study was moderate, at $I^2 = 38\%$.

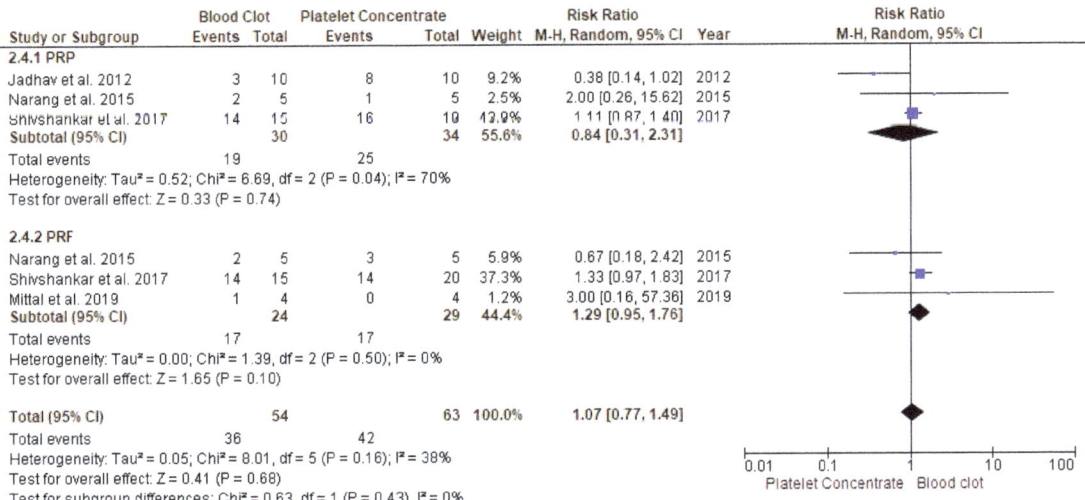

Figure 4. Meta-analysis of dentin wall thickness (DWT) in regenerative endodontic procedure (REP) using APC or BC.

3.4.2. Increased Root Length in REP with APC Compared to BC in Young Immature Permanent Teeth

Four studies [19,22,23,26] compared the effectiveness of APC to BC and assessed the increase in root length (Figure 5). The overall risk ratio was 1.00 with the 95% CI [0.71, 1.39] of achieving excellent/good root length found not to be significant among the two groups $p = 0.95$. The heterogenicity between the study was low, at $I^2 = 38\%$.

3.4.3. Apical Closure Formation in REP with APC Compared to BC in Young Immature Permanent Teeth

Six studies [16,17,19,23,26,28] compared the apical closure of APCs to BC. Both the procedures showed no significant difference between the groups with a RR of 0.97 and 95% CI [0.84, 1.13], $p = 0.19$; this suggested a similar rate of apical closure at the end of follow-up (Figure 6). The heterogeneity between the study was low, at $I^2 = 30\%$.

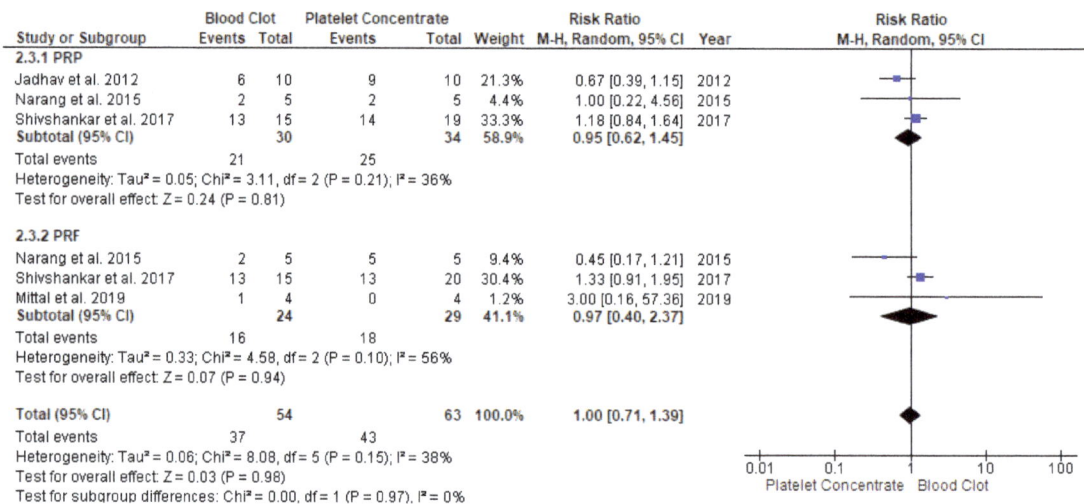

Figure 5. Meta-analysis of increased root length (IRL) in regenerative endodontic procedure (REP) using APC or BC.

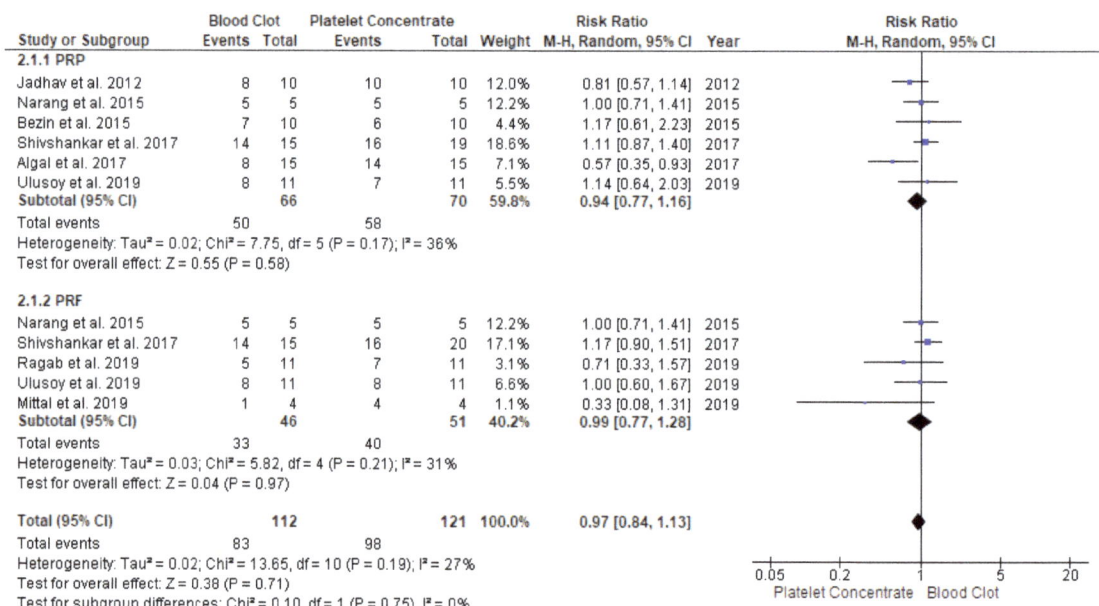

Figure 6. Meta-analysis of apical foramen width (AFW) in regenerative endodontic procedure (REP) using APC or BC.

3.4.4. Vitality Response in REP with APC Compared to BC in Young Immature Permanent Teeth

Three studies [16,17,23] compared the effectiveness of APC and BC. Both procedures had significant difference with RR 0.48, at 95% CI [0.28, 0.84], $p = 0.01$ (Figure 7). These findings suggests that positive vitality response at the end of follow-up was higher in the APC group. The heterogenicity between the studies was low at $I^2 = 16\%$.

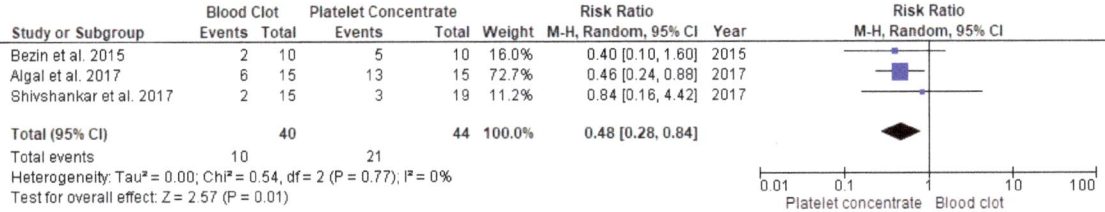

Figure 7. Meta-analysis of vitality response (VR) in regenerative endodontic procedure (REP) using APC or BC.

3.4.5. Success Rate of REP with APC Compared to BC in Young Immature Permanent Teeth

Four studies [16–18,23] were pooled to assess the success rate. The overall risk ratio was 1.00 with a 95% CI [0.92, 1.08] and $p = 0.96$ (Figure 8). The success rate between both groups was found not to be statistically significantly different.

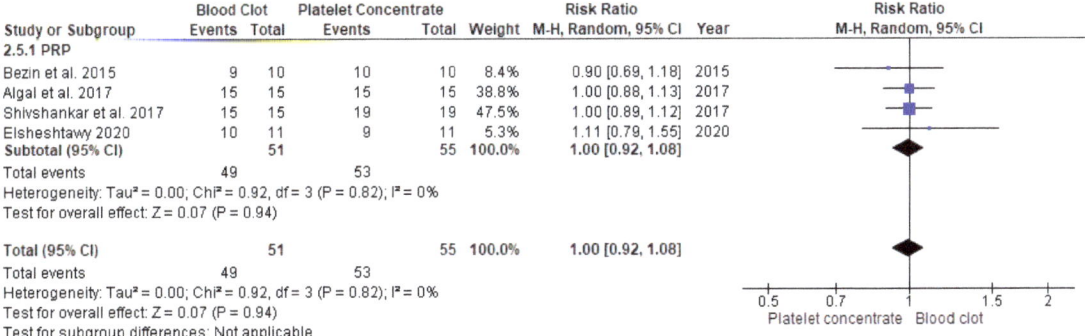

Figure 8. Meta-analysis of success rate in regenerative endodontic procedure (REP) using APC or BC.

3.4.6. Survival Assessment in Young Immature Permanent Teeth Undergone either REP or Apexification Procedure in Young Immature Permanent Teeth

Five studies [39,41,42,45,46] were pooled to assess the survival rate. The procedures showed no significant difference with RR 1.01, at 95% CI [0.97, 1.06], $p = 0.55$ (Figure 9). These values suggest that both interventions led to a statistically similar rate of survival at the end of follow-up. The heterogeneity between the studies was low, at $I^2 = 0$%.

However, a subgroup analysis observation was that apexification with MTA and REP exhibited a similar survival rate at RR 0.99, with 95% CI [0.93, 1.05], $p = 0.76$, $I^2 = 0$%. In the same forest plot it was observed that the $Ca(OH)_2$ apexification procedure had a low success rate compared to the MTA apexification procedure.

The funnel plot suggests low publication bias, with all studies placed within the inverted funnel (Figure 10).

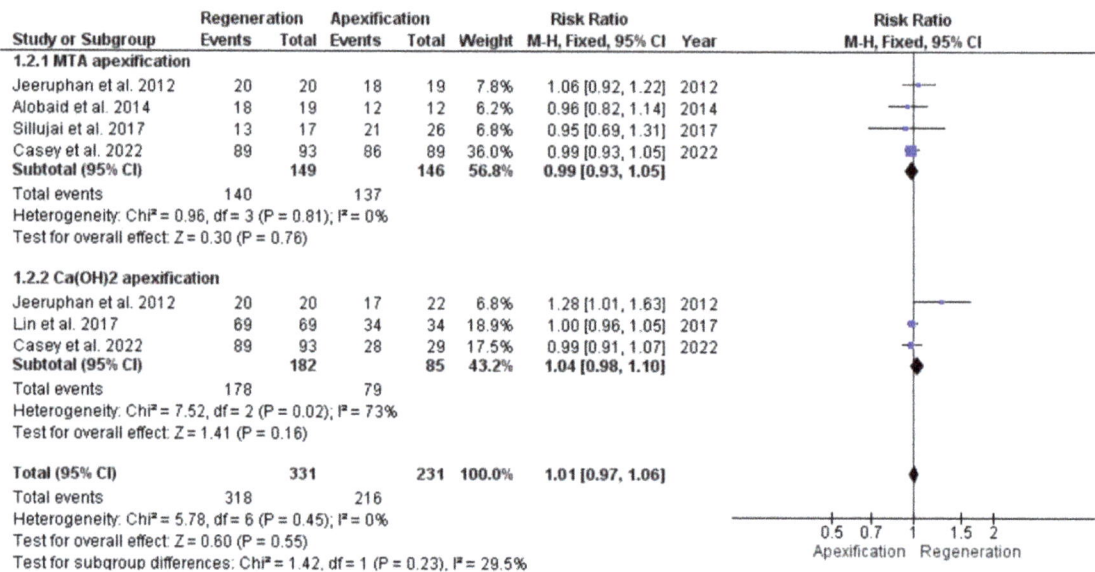

Figure 9. Meta-analysis of survival rate of young immature permanent teeth that underwent regenerative endodontic procedure (REP) or apexification procedure.

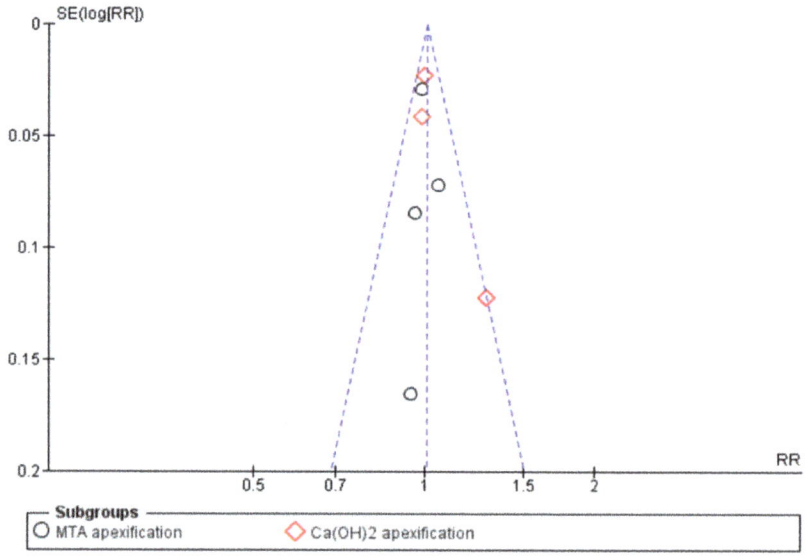

Figure 10. Funnel plot showing publication bias of studies on survival rate of young immature permanent teeth that underwent regenerative endodontic procedure (REP) or apexification procedure.

3.4.7. Comparison of Success Rate in Young Immature Permanent Teeth Treated with REP or Apexification Procedure

Seven studies [39,41,42,44–47] were pooled to assess the success rate between two interventions. However both the procedures showed no significant difference with RR of 0.95, at 95% CI [0.87, 1.04], $p = 0.27$; suggesting similar success rates at the end of follow-up. The heterogeneity between the studies was low, at $I^2 = 33\%$ (Figure 11).

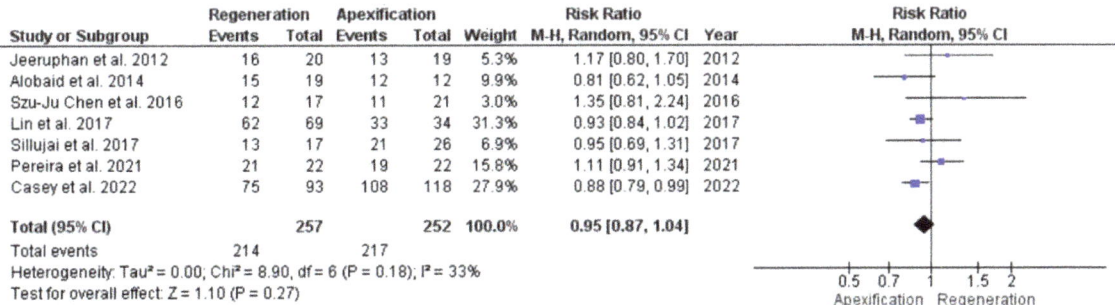

Figure 11. Meta-analysis of success rate in young immature permanent teeth undergoing regenerative endodontic procedure (REP) or apexification procedure.

The funnel plot suggests low publication bias, with all studies placed within the inverted funnel (Figure 12).

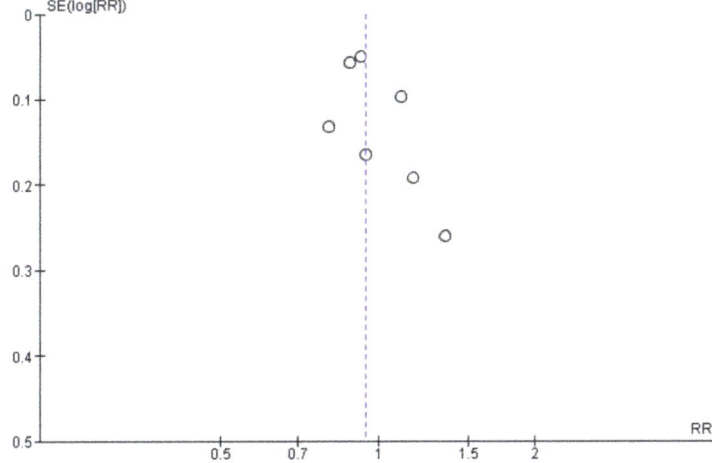

Figure 12. Funnel plot showing publication bias of studies on success rate in young immature permanent teeth undergoing regenerative endodontic procedure (REP) or apexification procedure.

3.4.8. Comparison of Increase in Root Length in Young Immature Permanent Teeth Treated with REP or Apexification Procedure

Three studies [39,40,44] were pooled to assess and compare the increase in root length. The increase in root length was significantly greater in the regenerative procedure compared to apexification, with a mean difference MD 1.98, 95% CI [-0.36, 4.32], $p < 0.00001$ (Figure 13). However, the heterogeneity between the studies was high, at $I^2 = 98\%$, questioning the reliability of the finding.

3.4.9. Comparison of Decrease in Apical Foramen Width in Young Immature Permanent Teeth Treated with REP Or AEP

Three studies [39,40,44] were pooled to assess and compare the decrease in apical foramen width. The decrease in apical foramen width was significantly greater in the REP compared to the apexification procedure with a mean difference (MD) of 0.65 at 95% CI [−0.83, 2.14], $p < 0.00001$ (Figure 14). However, the heterogeneity between the studies was high, at $I^2 = 98\%$, questioning the reliability of the finding.

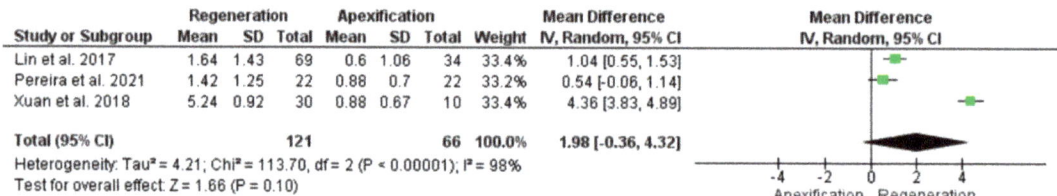

Figure 13. Meta-analysis of increase in root length (IRL) in young immature teeth treated with regenerative endodontic procedure (REP) or apexification procedure.

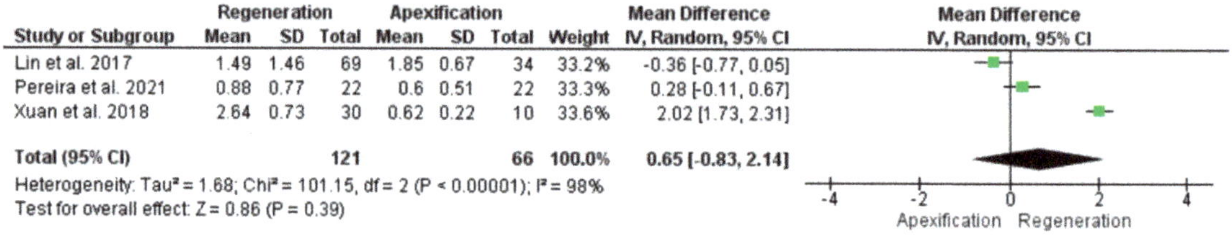

Figure 14. Meta-analysis of apical foramen width (AFW) in young immature teeth treated with regenerative endodontic procedure (REP) or apexification procedure.

4. Discussion

This systematic review was intended to analyze the various parameters that affect the survival of the immature necrotic tooth in the oral cavity after regeneration (REP) or apexification (AEP). The body of evidence for each comparison and outcome was assessed by considering the overall risk of bias in the included studies. The directness of the evidence, the inconsistency of the results, the precision of the estimates and the risk of publication bias were considered.

REP is based on tissue engineering, where a scaffold consisting of stem cells and essential growth factors support the proliferation and differentiation of stem cells [51]. An ideal natural scaffold should have a suitable porosity for cell seeding, potency to transport the nutrients, oxygen and waste, proper physical and mechanical strength, minimal inflammatory response and a similar biodegradable ability compared with the tissue regeneration process [52]. Blood clots (BC) and autologous platelet concentrates (APCs) are routinely used as scaffolds in REP [51]. BC is the process of forming a natural clot where the blood changes from a liquid to a gel. It has several advantages over alternative scaffolds, such as no allergic reaction, reduced cost and visiting time, convenience and comfort for patients. The clotting process involves many blood cells and clotting factors [51].

APCs are blood-derived products with an above-baseline concentration of platelets and an increased number of platelet-derived growth factors [53]. The principle of APC formation is the collection of the most active constituents of a small blood sample, which are plasma, platelets, fibrin, and leukocytes in most cases [54]. APCs are a cost-effective and useful in regenerative endodontics due to their high concentration of growth factors that induce migration, proliferation, and differentiation of stem cells, their dense fibrin matrix that serves as a stable scaffold and their bacteriostatic properties [55].

Platelet-rich plasma (PRP) is a gel with a high concentration of autologous platelets suspended in a small amount of plasma after centrifugation of the patient's blood. The platelets in PRP play an essential role in treating the healing of damaged tissue due to the release of various growth factors such as PDGF, VEGF, IGF-1, FGF and EGF. The granules in platelets contain cytokines, chemokines and many other proteins that help stimulate proliferation and cellular maturation [56]. The platelet rich fibrin (PRF) is achieved with a simplified preparation, with no biochemical manipulation of blood. This technique does not require anticoagulants [57].

The teeth included for RET intervention were those that were affected by either trauma [58], secondary caries [59] or developmental anomalies [58]. Factors that can affect the outcome of RET are irrigation protocol, final rinsing of canal and intracanal medicaments (ICM). Six out of twelve studies [16–18,20,22] of the included clinical trials followed standardized irrigation protocol given by the American Association of Endodontists (AAE) and the European Society of Endodontics (ESE) [60]. The other six studies [16,17,19,21,23,24] did not follow the irrigation protocol religiously. The ideal concentration of NaOCl is 1.25%, but if a higher concentration is used, it reduces the viability of stem cells and their odontogenic/osteogenic differentiation [61]. EDTA reduces the deleterious effect of sodium hypochlorite and improves cell survival and differentiation [61]. It also liberates the growth factors present in dentin that positively affect stem cell adhesion, migration and differentiation [62]. Studies in which EDTA was not used as final irrigant also affected the outcome. The most preferred ICM used in RET is a triple antibiotic paste containing minocycline, ciprofloxacin and metronidazole, followed by calcium hydroxide paste [63]. AAE recommends 0.1 mg of TAP, but at high concentrations, it has a cytotoxic effect on stem cells and reduces mineralization [64] and when minocycline is included, it can cause significant tooth discoloration [65]. Overall, it can be concluded that RET is a successful intervention for the management of immature necrotic permanent teeth with high to moderate certainty.

The meta-analysis conducted in this systematic review concluded that APCs significantly improved apical closure and response to vitality pulp tests. In contrast, no significant difference between APC and BC was observed in root lengthening, dentin wall thickness or the success rate of immature, necrotic teeth treated with regenerative endodontics. This finding agrees with the outcome of other studies by Panda et al. [66]. The possible reasons could be due to intentional induction of bleeding from the periapical region and the formation of a blood clot into the root canal in the revascularization procedure of immature necrotic teeth acts as a scaffold supporting angiogenesis, providing a pathway for the migration of stem cells from the periapical area, and inducing pulp regeneration and maturation of the root [67]. Some vital pulp tissue and Hertwig's Epithelial Root Sheath may remain in teeth with open apices and necrotic pulps. When the canal is sufficiently disinfected, the inflammatory process reverses, and these tissues may proliferate [68]. The second factor is the apex diameter. A tooth with an open apex allows the migration of mesenchymal stem cells into the root canal space, allowing the host cell homing to form new tissue in the root canal space. An apical opening of 1.1 mm in diameter or more is beneficial, with natural regenerative endodontic treatment occurring in approximately 18–34% of teeth with immature roots [68]. The third factor is the patient age. It is directly related to the stage of root formation and apical diameter; it is likely a modifying factor in regenerative endodontic procedures [69]. RET was capable of regenerating the pulp–dentine complex to restore the vitality of tissue damaged in the canal space and increase thee thickness of the canal walls to strengthen the fragile immature permanent teeth [70,71]. The possible reasons that APC performed better than BC in these two parameters could be difficulties in sensible evaluating because of the layered coronal seal over the BC scaffold [72].

Among APC, PRF had better outcomes in terms of AC and VPR. Possible reasons could be that PRF is collection of a dense and stable fibrin network [73] that allows a slower release of growth factors compared to PRP; PRP releases significantly more growth factors when compared to PRF during the first 15–60 min after clot formation. In a short time, high concentrations of bioactive molecules released by PRP could be responsible for the apparent beneficial effects over PRF. From these observations, it could be concluded that there is a trend of PRP showing better results than PRF in regenerative endodontic procedures. However, more clinical studies with large sample sizes are required to confirm or deny this trend over a long follow-up period [74]. The outcome of teeth in Apexification studies evaluated the outcome in terms of calcific barrier [30,32,34], periapical healing [30,34], and success rate [29,30,34]. The material used for apexification is $Ca(OH)_2$ and MTA in both RCTs and NRCTs. The traditional method for the treatment of young, permanent, non-vital teeth is apexification. Traditionally, the approach has been to use calcium hydroxide

(Ca(OH)$_2$) to induce apexification after disinfection of the root canals in a conventional manner [75]. Ca(OH)$_2$ is readily available, easy to use, relatively inexpensive and widely used in clinical procedures [10]. The disadvantages of traditional, long-term Ca(OH)$_2$ therapy include variability in treatment time, the unpredictability of formation of an apical seal, difficulty in following up with patients and delayed treatment [76].

The traditional use of Ca(OH)$_2$ to achieve apexification is being gradually replaced by mineral trioxide aggregate (MTA) as a one-step technique [51,52]. The advantages of using an apical plug include the requirement for fewer appointments to complete the treatment, more predictable apical barrier formation and reduced need for patient follow-up appointments [77].

The results showed that both materials had similar clinical success rates, radiographic success rates and apical barrier formation rates; there was no significant difference between these two groups. To obtain complete closure of the root apex, Ca(OH)$_2$ based apexification procedure requires long-term application of the dressing material (from 3 to 24 months). However, MTA was associated with a significantly shorter time to achieve apical barrier formation than the calcium hydroxide [74]. The clinical protocol for apexification may involve one or multiple monthly appointments to place calcium hydroxide inside the root canal and eliminate the intracanal infection, which stimulates calcification and produces the apical closure [78]. A systematic review [79] evaluated the outcomes of the apexification method using Ca(OH)$_2$ or MTA in young, immature permanent teeth. The authors found that the MTA barrier is a better procedure compared to Ca(OH)$_2$ apexification, because it does not require many appointments and the conformation of the barrier does not require an external factor to develop, as it does with Ca(OH)$_2$ apexification and pulp regeneration. These findings are in agreement with the present systematic review.

Calcium hydroxide can induce underlying tissues to produce large amounts of mineralized matrices. In the matrix attached to calcium, calcified foci induce calcification of the newly formed collagenous matrix. The high pH of calcium hydroxide also plays a vital role in inducing hard tissue formation [80].

The MTA can be placed as an apical plug with previous applications intracanal with Ca(OH)$_2$ to produce the disinfection of the same [53,81], or even the MTA can be used as a material for canal filling. MTA is not bonded to dentin, but the interaction of calcium and hydroxyl ions components with a phosphate-containing synthetic body fluid results in the formation of apatite-like interfacial deposits [82].

This systematic review included studies that compared regeneration procedures and apexification procedures. Both the interventions are aimed at saving immature necrotic teeth. However regeneration is best attempted when the root formation is less than two-thirds [6] according Cvek's classification.

The studies included compared both the interventions, involving the teeth with the apex open more than 1 mm. In this scenario, both regeneration and apexification have a similar outcomes. Overall, both interventions are comparable and successful.

The clinical outcome of teeth in RET versus APT studies was evaluated in terms of increase in root length [39,40], apical foramen width [40,41,45,46], periapical healing [39,45], survival rate [39,41,45,46] and successful rate [39,41,45–47]. The scaffold to initiate regeneration was BC, and apexification was calcium hydroxide or MTA.

Meta-analysis showed that the regeneration procedure resulted in significant improvement in root length and apical foramen width, but there was no significant difference concerning 'overall outcomes' (clinical and radiographic) and survival rate outcomes between revascularization and apexification.

Revascularization generates a new pulp-like tissue inside the root canal to restore the tooth physiology and significantly reduce the risk of tooth loss [10,12,70,71,83]. This could be the reason for revascularization to yield significantly better results in terms of root maturation than apexification, and to be slightly more effective in providing an increasing lateral dentinal wall thickness and promoting the continuation of dentin thickness and root width with a reduction of periapical radiolucency. However, further investigation is required into whether this increase in DWT is truly from dentin deposition or cementum-like and bone-like structures [84]. Another systematic review [85], evaluated the clinical, radiographic and functional retention outcomes in immature necrotic permanent teeth treated either with pulp revascularization or apexification after a minimum of three months to determine which one provides the best results. The authors found that although pulp revascularization procedures may increase root length and width, some attempts should be made to use standard methods to quantify the 'real gain' in root development because some X-ray distortions may overestimate its increase. Moreover, it was concluded that there is still a need to establish proper concentrations for root canal disinfectants that might enhance the survival of SCAP, but also reduce the microbial load and risk of reinfection. Based on their meta-analysis, the results do not favor one treatment modality over the other.

According to AAE [60], irrigation with 1.5% NaOCl followed by 17% EDTA and intracanal medicaments with either TAP in concentrations of 0.1–1 mg/mL or $Ca(OH)_2$ with 1 mg/mL provide a higher survival of stems cells of the apical papilla (SCAP) that may play an essential role in root maturation. However, the treatment protocols adopted in the included studies comparing apexification with RET [53,56,58] did not use this proposed concentration. This could be the reason why reinfection occurred more in RET compared to apexification.

Only one study evaluated the reinfection post intervention and concluded that it was seen more in RET than in apexification. The possible reasons could be the use of higher concentrations of irrigating solutions that may be harming the SCAP, precluding a potential benefit of root maturation in both the interventions. Some failures were observed due to reinfection of the canal, perhaps due to residual bacteria in the root canal as effectively observed in histological analyses [86]. There is still a need for further investigation on this topic because most of the failures observed in these studies were due to persistent infection or reinfection.

In another systematic review [59] evaluating the clinical and radiographic outcomes for nonvital immature permanent teeth treated using RET, the authors found excellent success rates regarding tooth survival and periapical pathology resolution following RET. However, the results for more favorable outcomes, such as continued root growth, were uncertain. This study is also in agreement with our systematic review results.

Discoloration to the tooth was seen more in RET than in apexification [39]. Only one study [39] analyzed crown discoloration in the regeneration procedure. This study reported that 2 out of 19 teeth (10.5%) treated with BC revascularization presented crown staining. The possible reason could be the use of intracanal medication TAP containing minocycline.

Only one study [39] analyzed the root fracture in the apexification procedure. In this study, dens evaginatus (DE) premolar was analyzed, and $Ca(OH)_2$ was used to create the calcific barrier at the apex. Of 21 patients, 2 had cervical fractures, and one had an apical fracture. The possible reason for this outcome could be the fact that DE frequently occurs on the lingual side of the buccal cusp, which is part of the functional cusp, and thus fractures easily when the occlusal force is exercised. In the same study [39], pulp canal obliteration was observed in RET. The possible reason could be internal replacement resorption during the hard tissue regeneration inside the root canal [87]. A longer follow-up period would be required to observe the results and whether this influences the dental treatment. However, this is the only study with a moderate risk of bias. Hence, the inference of this study should be analyzed with caution.

Out of 32 studies included in this review, 17 studies were randomized control trials; 3 had a low risk of bias, and 14 had a moderate risk of bias. Most of the studies failed to ensure concealment of allocation and blinding of the outcome assessment. In addition, due to the nature of the treatment, most studies found it impossible to ensure blinding of the patient and personnel because the patients receiving platelet concentrates knew which groups they were assigned since they were submitted to blood draw. In non-randomized control trials, there was uncertainty in defining the proper selection of participants in most studies, along with the classification of interventions and deviations from intended interventions in a few studies. Therefore, these reasons led to moderate to serious overall risk assessment.

5. Conclusions

Clinicians should consider employing the REP in cases when the root development is severely deficient, with insufficient dentine, and where the tooth's prognosis is hopeless even with an apexification procedure. With moderate to high certainty, APCs used in the REP procedure significantly improved apical closure and response to vitality pulp tests. However, overall both APCs and BC showed similar successful outcomes in the regeneration procedure. In the apexification procedure with moderate certainty, it can be concluded that both MTA and $Ca(OH)_2$ are equally effective in forming the calcific barrier. With moderate certainty, it can be concluded that both regeneration and apexification procedures are equally comparable interventions and result with similar overall outcomes.

Author Contributions: Conceptualization, L.M. and P.P.; methodology, P.P.; software, S.P.; validation, L.M., P.P. and S.G.; formal analysis, B.L.; investigation, P.P.; resources, B.L.; data curation, S.P.; writing—original draft preparation, L.M.; writing—review and editing, L.M. and B.L.; visualization, P.P.; supervision, S.G.; project administration, L.M.; funding acquisition, B.L. All authors have read and agreed to the published version of the manuscript.

Funding: This research received no external funding.

Institutional Review Board Statement: Not applicable for secondary research.

Informed Consent Statement: Not applicable.

Data Availability Statement: Not applicable.

Conflicts of Interest: The authors declare no conflict of interest.

Appendix A

The list of 21 articles [88–108] excluded from the review, with reasons for exclusion, is shown in Table A1.

Table A1. List of excluded studies after reading the full text.

Study	Reason for Exclusion
Alhaddad Alhamoui et al., 2014 [88]	In vitro study
Alkaisi et al., 2013 [89]	Animal study
El Arshy et al., 2016 [90]	Animal study
El-Tayeb et al., 2019 [91]	Animal study
Huang et al., 2013 [92]	Animal study
Peng et al., 2017 [93]	Chinese language
Jamshidi et al., 2018 [94]	In vitro study
Moradi et al., 2016 [95]	Animal study
Ok et al., 2015 [96]	In vitro study
Pagliarin et al., 2016 [97]	Animal study
Rafaei et al., 2020 [98]	In vitro study
Ritter AL et al., 2004 [99]	Animal study
Sogukpinar et al., 2020 [100]	In vitro study
Thibodeau et al., 2007 [101]	In vitro study
Valera et al., 2015 [102]	Animal study

Table A1. *Cont.*

Study	Reason for Exclusion
Yang et al., 2018 [103]	Animal study
Yoo et al., 2014 [104]	Animal study
Zhang et al., 2014 [105]	Animal study
Zuong et al., 2010 [106]	Animal study
Beslot-Neveu et al., 2011 [107]	Study protocol
Bukhari et al., 2016 [108]	Case series

References

1. Wikström, A.; Brundin, M.; Lopes, M.F.; El Sayed, M.; Tsilingaridis, G. What is the best long-term treatment modality for immature permanent teeth with pulp necrosis and apical periodontitis? *Eur. Arch. Paediatr. Dent.* **2021**, *22*, 311–340. [CrossRef] [PubMed]
2. Locker, D. Self-reported dental and oral injuries in a population of adults aged 18–50 years. *Dent. Traumatol.* **2007**, *23*, 291–296. [CrossRef] [PubMed]
3. Petti, S.; Glendor, U.; Andersson, L. World traumatic dental injury prevalence and incidence, a meta-analysis-One billion living people have had traumatic dental injuries. *Off. Publ. Int. Assoc. Dent. Traumatol. Dent. Traumatol.* **2018**, *34*, 71–86. [CrossRef] [PubMed]
4. Hecova, H.; Tzigkounakis, V.; Merglova, V.; Netolický, J. A retrospective study of 889 injured permanent teeth. *Dent. Traumatol.* **2010**, *26*, 466–475. [CrossRef] [PubMed]
5. Kim, S.G.; Malek, M.; Sigurdsson, A.; Lin, L.M.; Kahler, B. Regenerative endodontics: A comprehensive review. *Int. Endod. J.* **2018**, *51*, 1367–1388. [CrossRef] [PubMed]
6. Cvek, M. Prognosis of luxated non-vital maxillary incisors treated with calcium hydroxide and filled with gutta-percha. A retrospective clinical study. *Endod. Dent. Traumatol.* **1992**, *8*, 45–55. [CrossRef]
7. Trope, M. Treatment of the Immature Tooth with a Non–Vital Pulp and Apical Periodontitis. *Dent. Clin. N. Am.* **2010**, *54*, 313–324. [CrossRef]
8. Duggal, M.; Tong, H.J.; Alansary, M.; Twati, W.; Day, P.F.; Nazzal, H. Interventions for the endodontic management of non-vital traumatised immature permanent anterior teeth in children and adolescents: A systematic review of the evidence and guidelines of the European Academy of Paediatric Dentistry. *Eur. Arch. Paediatr. Dent.* **2017**, *18*, 139–151. [CrossRef]
9. Lee, B.-N.; Moon, J.-W.; Chang, H.-S.; Hwang, I.-N.; Oh, W.-M.; Hwang, Y.-C. A review of the regenerative endodontic treatment procedure. *Restor. Dent. Endod.* **2015**, *40*, 179–187. [CrossRef]
10. Rafter, M. Apexification: A review. *Dent. Traumatol.* **2005**, *21*, 1–8. [CrossRef]
11. Murray, P.E.; Garcia-Godoy, F.; Hargreaves, K.M. Regenerative Endodontics: A Review of Current Status and a Call for Action. *J. Endod.* **2007**, *33*, 377–390. [CrossRef]
12. Finucane, D.; Kinirons, M.J. Non-vital immature permanent incisors: Factors that may influence treatment outcome. *Dent. Traumatol.* **1999**, *15*, 273–277. [CrossRef]
13. Mackie, I.C.; Bentley, E.M.; Worthington, H.V. The closure of open apices in non-vital immature incisor teeth. *Br. Dent. J.* **1988**, *165*, 169–173. [CrossRef]
14. Liberati, A.; Altman, D.G.; Tetzlaff, J.; Mulrow, C.; Gøtzsche, P.C.; Ioannidis, J.P.A.; Clarke, M.; Devereaux, P.J.; Kleijnen, J.; Moher, D. The PRISMA Statement for Reporting Systematic Reviews and Meta-Analyses of Studies That Evaluate Healthcare Interventions: Explanation and Elaboration. *BMJ* **2009**, *339*, b2700. [CrossRef] [PubMed]
15. Higgins, J.P.T.; Altman, D.G.; Gøtzsche, P.C.; Jüni, P.; Moher, D.; Oxman, A.D.; Savović, J.; Schulz, K.F.; Weeks, L.; Sterne, J.A.C.; et al. The Cochrane Collaboration's tool for assessing risk of bias in randomised trials. *BMJ* **2011**, *343*, d5928. [CrossRef]
16. Alagl, A.; Bedi, S.; Hassan, K.; AlHumaid, J. Use of platelet-rich plasma for regeneration in non-vital immature permanent teeth: Clinical and cone-beam computed tomography evaluation. *J. Int. Med. Res.* **2017**, *45*, 583–593. [CrossRef] [PubMed]
17. Bezgin, T.; Yilmaz, A.D.; Celik, B.N.; Kolsuz, M.E.; Sonmez, H. Efficacy of Platelet-rich Plasma as a Scaffold in Regenerative Endodontic Treatment. *J. Endod.* **2015**, *41*, 36–44. [CrossRef] [PubMed]
18. ElSheshtawy, A.S.; Nazzal, H.; El Shahawy, O.I.; El Baz, A.A.; Ismail, S.M.; Kang, J.; Ezzat, K.M. The effect of platelet-rich plasma as a scaffold in regeneration/revitalization endodontics of immature permanent teeth assessed using 2-dimensional radiographs and cone beam computed tomography: A randomized controlled trial. *Int. Endod. J.* **2020**, *53*, 905–921. [CrossRef] [PubMed]
19. Jadhav, G.; Shah, N.; Logani, A. Revascularization with and without Platelet-rich Plasma in Nonvital, Immature, Anterior Teeth: A Pilot Clinical Study. *J. Endod.* **2012**, *38*, 1581–1587. [CrossRef]
20. Rizk, H.M.; Al-Deen, M.S.S.; Emam, A.A. Regenerative Endodontic Treatment of Bilateral Necrotic Immature Permanent Maxillary Central Incisors with Platelet-rich Plasma versus Blood Clot: A Split Mouth Double-blinded Randomized Controlled Trial. *Int. J. Clin. Pediatr. Dent.* **2019**, *12*, 332–339. [CrossRef]

21. Ragab, R.A.; El Lattif, A.E.A.; Dokky, N.A.E.W.E. Comparative Study between Revitalization of Necrotic Immature Permanent Anterior Teeth with and without Platelet Rich Fibrin: A Randomized Controlled Trial. *J. Clin. Pediatr. Dent.* **2019**, *43*, 78–85. [CrossRef] [PubMed]
22. Mittal, N.; Parashar, V. Regenerative Evaluation of Immature Roots Using PRF and Artificial Scaffolds in Necrotic Perma-nent Teeth: A Clinical Study. *J. Contemp. Dent. Pract.* **2019**, *20*, 720–726. [CrossRef] [PubMed]
23. Shivashankar, V.Y.; Johns, D.A.; Maroli, R.K.; Sekar, M.; Chandrasekaran, R.; Karthikeyan, S.; Renganathan, S.K. Comparison of the Effect of PRP, PRF and Induced Bleeding in the Revascularization of Teeth with Necrotic Pulp and Open Apex: A Triple Blind Randomized Clinical Trial. *J. Clin. Diagn. Res.* **2017**, *11*, ZC34–ZC39. [CrossRef]
24. Rizk, H.M.; Al-Deen, M.S.M.S.; Emam, A.A. Comparative evaluation of Platelet Rich Plasma (PRP) versus Platelet Rich Fibrin (PRF) scaffolds in regenerative endodontic treatment of immature necrotic permanent maxillary central incisors: A double blinded randomized controlled trial. *Saudi Dent. J.* **2020**, *32*, 224–231. [CrossRef] [PubMed]
25. Jiang, X.; Liu, H.; Peng, C. Clinical and Radiographic Assessment of the Efficacy of a Collagen Membrane in Regenerative Endodontics: A Randomized, Controlled Clinical Trial. *J. Endod.* **2017**, *43*, 1465–1471. [CrossRef]
26. Narang, I.; Mittal, N.; Mishra, N. A comparative evaluation of the blood clot, platelet-rich plasma, and platelet-rich fibrin in regeneration of necrotic immature permanent teeth: A clinical study. *Contemp. Clin. Dent.* **2015**, *6*, 63–68. [CrossRef]
27. Meschi, N.; EzEldeen, M.; Garcia, A.E.T.; Lahoud, P.; Van Gorp, G.; Coucke, W.; Jacobs, R.; Vandamme, K.; Teughels, W.; Lambrechts, P. Regenerative Endodontic Procedure of Immature Permanent Teeth with Leukocyte and Platelet-rich Fibrin: A Multicenter Controlled Clinical Trial. *J. Endod.* **2021**, *47*, 1729–1750. [CrossRef]
28. Ulusoy, A.T.; Turedi, I.; Cimen, M.; Cehreli, Z.C. Evaluation of Blood Clot, Platelet-rich Plasma, Platelet-rich Fibrin, and Platelet Pellet as Scaffolds in Regenerative Endodontic Treatment: A Prospective Randomized Trial. *J. Endod.* **2019**, *45*, 560–566. [CrossRef]
29. Peng, C.; Yang, Y.; Zhao, Y.; Liu, H.; Xu, Z.; Zhao, D.; Qin, M. Long-term treatment outcomes in immature permanent teeth by revascularisation using MTA and GIC as canal-sealing materials: A retrospective study. *Int. J. Paediatr. Dent.* **2017**, *27*, 454–462. [CrossRef]
30. Lv, H.; Chen, Y.; Cai, Z.; Lei, L.; Zhang, M.; Zhou, R.; Huang, X. The efficacy of platelet-rich fibrin as a scaffold in regenerative endodontic treatment: A retrospective controlled cohort study. *BMC Oral Health* **2018**, *18*, 139. [CrossRef]
31. Cheng, J.; Yang, F.; Li, J.; Hua, F.; He, M.; Song, G. Treatment Outcomes of Regenerative Endodontic Procedures in Traumatized Immature Permanent Necrotic Teeth: A Retrospective Study. *J. Endod.* **2022**. *epub ahead of print*. [CrossRef]
32. Chueh, L.-H.; Ho, Y.-C.; Kuo, T.-C.; Lai, W.-H.; Chen, Y.-H.M.; Chiang, C.-P. Regenerative Endodontic Treatment for Necrotic Immature Permanent Teeth. *J. Endod.* **2009**, *35*, 160–164. [CrossRef] [PubMed]
33. Jayadevan, V.; Gehlot, P.-M.; Manjunath, V.; Madhunapantula, S.V.; Lakshmikanth, J.-S. A comparative evaluation of Advanced Platelet-Rich Fibrin (A-PRF) and Platelet-Rich Fibrin (PRF) as a Scaffold in Regenerative Endodontic Treatment of Traumatized Immature Non-vital permanent anterior teeth: A Prospective clinical study. *J. Clin. Exp. Dent.* **2021**, *13*, e463–e472. [CrossRef] [PubMed]
34. Bonte, E.; Beslot, A.; Boukpessi, T.; Lasfargues, J.-J. MTA versus Ca(OH)$_2$ in apexification of non-vital immature permanent teeth: A randomized clinical trial comparison. *Clin. Oral Investig.* **2015**, *19*, 1381–1388. [CrossRef] [PubMed]
35. Santhakumar, M.; Yayathi, S.; Retnakumari, N. A clinicoradiographic comparison of the effects of platelet-rich fibrin gel and platelet-rich fibrin membrane as scaffolds in the apexification treatment of young permanent teeth. *J. Indian Soc. Pedod. Prev. Dent.* **2018**, *36*, 65–70.
36. Demirci, G.K.; Kaval, M.E.; Güneri, P.; Çalışkan, M.K. Treatment of immature teeth with nonvital pulps in adults: A prospective comparative clinical study comparing MTA with Ca(OH)$_2$. *Int. Endod. J.* **2020**, *53*, 5–18. [CrossRef] [PubMed]
37. Tek, G.B.; Keskin, G. Use of Mineral Trioxide Aggregate with or without a Collagen Sponge as an Apical Plug in Teeth with Immature Apices. *J. Clin. Pediatr. Dent.* **2021**, *45*, 165–170. [CrossRef]
38. Kinirons, M.J.; Srinivasan, V.; Welbury, R.R.; Finucane, D. A study in two centres of variations in the time of apical barrier detection and barrier position in nonvital immature permanent incisors. *Int. J. Paediatr. Dent.* **2001**, *11*, 447–451. [CrossRef]
39. Lin, J.; Zeng, Q.; Wei, X.; Zhao, W.; Cui, M.; Gu, J.; Lu, J.; Yang, M.; Ling, J. Regenerative Endodontics Versus Apexification in Immature Permanent Teeth with Apical Periodontitis: A Prospective Randomized Controlled Study. *J. Endod.* **2017**, *43*, 1821–1827. [CrossRef]
40. Xuan, K.; Li, B.; Guo, H.; Sun, W.; Kou, X.; He, X.; Zhang, Y.; Sun, J.; Liu, A.; Liao, L.; et al. Deciduous autologous tooth stem cells regenerate dental pulp after implantation into injured teeth. *Sci. Transl. Med.* **2018**, *10*, eaaf3227. [CrossRef]
41. Alobaid, A.S.; Cortes, L.M.; Lo, J.; Nguyen, T.T.; Albert, J.; Abu-Melha, A.S.; Lin, L.M.; Gibbs, J.L. Radiographic and Clinical Outcomes of the Treatment of Immature Permanent Teeth by Revascularization or Apexification: A Pilot Retrospective Cohort Study. *J. Endod.* **2014**, *40*, 1063–1070. [CrossRef] [PubMed]
42. Casey, S.M.; Fox, D.; Duong, W.; Bui, N.; Latifi, N.; Ramesh, V.; Podborits, E.; Flake, N.M.; Khan, A.A.; Gibbs, J.L. Patient Centered Outcomes among a Cohort Receiving Regenerative Endodontic Procedures or Apexification Treatments. *J. Endod.* **2022**, *48*, 345–354. [CrossRef] [PubMed]
43. Caleza-Jiménez, C.; Ribas-Pérez, D.; Biedma-Perea, M.; Solano-Mendoza, B.; Mendoza-Mendoza, A. Radiographic differences observed following apexification vs revascularization in necrotic immature molars and incisors: A follow-up study of 18 teeth. *Eur. Arch. Paediatr. Dent. Off. J. Eur. Acad. Paediatr. Dent.* **2022**, *23*, 381–389. [CrossRef] [PubMed]

44. Pereira, A.C.; Oliveira, M.L.; Cerqueira-Neto, A.C.C.L.; Vargas-Neto, J.; Nagata, J.Y.; Gomes, B.P.; Ferraz, C.C.R.; de Almeida, J.F.A.; De-Jesus-Soares, A. Outcomes of traumatised immature teeth treated with apexification or regenerative endodontic procedure: A retrospective study. *Aust. Endod. J.* **2020**, *47*, 178–187. [CrossRef]
45. Jeeruphan, T.; Jantarat, J.; Yanpiset, K.; Suwannapan, L.; Khewsawai, P.; Hargreaves, K.M. Mahidol Study 1: Comparison of Radiographic and Survival Outcomes of Immature Teeth Treated with Either Regenerative Endodontic or Apexification Methods: A Retrospective Study. *J. Endod.* **2012**, *38*, 1330–1336. [CrossRef]
46. Silujjai, J.; Linsuwanont, P. Treatment Outcomes of Apexification or Revascularization in Nonvital Immature Permanent Teeth: A Retrospective Study. *J. Endod.* **2017**, *43*, 238–245. [CrossRef]
47. Chen, S.-J.; Chen, L.-P. Radiographic outcome of necrotic immature teeth treated with two endodontic techniques: A retrospective analysis. *Biomed. J.* **2016**, *39*, 366–371. [CrossRef]
48. Dohan, D.M.; Choukroun, J.; Diss, A.; Dohan, S.L.; Dohan, A.J.; Mouhyi, J.; Gogly, B. Platelet-rich fibrin (PRF): A second generation platelet concentrate—part I: Technological concepts and evolution. *Oral Surg. Oral Med. Oral Pathol. Oral Radiol. Endod.* **2006**, *101*, e37–e44. [CrossRef]
49. Dohan, D.M.; Choukroun, J. PRP, cPRP, PRF, PRG, PRGF, FC . . . How to find your way in the jungle of platelet concentrates? *Oral Surg. Oral Med. Oral Pathol. Oral Radiol. Endod.* **2007**, *103*, 305–306. [CrossRef]
50. Choukroun, J.; Diss, A.; Simonpieri, A.; Girard, M.O.; Schoeffler, C.; Dohan, S.L.; Dohan, A.J.; Mouhyi, J.; Dohan, D.M. Platelet-rich fibrin (PRF): A second-generation platelet concentrate. Part V: Histologic evaluations of PRF effects on bone allograft maturation in sinus lift. *Oral Surg. Oral Med. Oral Pathol. Oral Radiol. Endod.* **2006**, *101*, 299–303.
51. Saber, S.E.-D.M. Tissue engineering in endodontics. *J. Oral Sci.* **2009**, *51*, 495–507. [CrossRef]
52. Taweewattanapaisan, P.; Jantarat, J.; Ounjai, P.; Janebodin, K. The Effects of EDTA on Blood Clot in Regenerative Endodontic Procedures. *J. Endod.* **2019**, *45*, 281–286. [CrossRef] [PubMed]
53. Metlerska, J.; Fagogeni, I.; Nowicka, A. Efficacy of Autologous Platelet Concentrates in Regenerative Endodontic Treatment: A Systematic Review of Human Studies. *J. Endod.* **2019**, *45*, 20–30.e1. [CrossRef] [PubMed]
54. Del Fabbro, M.; Lolato, A.; Bucchi, C.; Taschieri, S.; Weinstein, R.L. Autologous Platelet Concentrates for Pulp and Dentin Regeneration: A Literature Review of Animal Studies. *J. Endod.* **2016**, *42*, 250–257. [CrossRef] [PubMed]
55. Ezzatt, O.M. Autologous Platelet Concentrate Preparations in Dentistry. *Biomed. J. Sci. Tech. Res.* **2018**, *8*. [CrossRef]
56. Giannini, S.; Cielo, A.; Bonanome, L.; Rastelli, C.; Derla, C.; Corpaci, F.; Falisi, G. Comparison between PRP, PRGF and PRF: Lights and shadows in three similar but different protocols. *Eur. Rev. Med. Pharmacol. Sci.* **2015**, *19*, 927–930.
57. Goel, D.S.; Sinha, D.D.J.; Singh, D.U.P.; Jaiswal, D.N. Advancements in Regenerative Endodontics: Platelet-Rich Plasma (PRP) And Platelet-Rich Fibrin (PRF). *Int. J. Curr. Res.* **2019**, *11*, 5.
58. Koç, S.; Del Fabbro, M. Does the Etiology of Pulp Necrosis Affect Regenerative Endodontic Treatment Outcomes? A Systematic Review and Meta-analyses. *J. Évid. Based Dent. Pract.* **2020**, *20*, 101400. [CrossRef]
59. Tong, H.J.; Rajan, S.; Bhujel, N.; Kang, J.; Duggal, M.; Nazzal, H. Regenerative Endodontic Therapy in the Management of Nonvital Immature Permanent Teeth: A Systematic Review—Outcome Evaluation and Meta-analysis. *J. Endod.* **2017**, *43*, 1453–1464. [CrossRef]
60. Regenerative Endodontics Clinical Newsletter—AAE. Am. Assoc. Endodontists. Available online: https://www.aae.org/specialty/newsletter/regenerative-endodontics/ (accessed on 26 July 2021).
61. Martin, D.E.; De Almeida, J.F.A.; Henry, M.A.; Khaing, Z.Z.; Schmidt, C.E.; Teixeira, F.B.; Diogenes, A. Concentration-dependent Effect of Sodium Hypochlorite on Stem Cells of Apical Papilla Survival and Differentiation. *J. Endod.* **2014**, *40*, 51–55. [CrossRef]
62. Galler, K.M.; Widbiller, M.; Buchalla, W.; Eidt, A.; Hiller, K.-A.; Hoffer, P.C.; Schmalz, G. EDTA conditioning of dentine promotes adhesion, migration and differentiation of dental pulp stem cells. *Int. Endod. J.* **2016**, *49*, 581–590. [CrossRef] [PubMed]
63. Pai, A.V.; Pai, S.; Thomas, M.S.; Bhat, V. Effect of calcium hydroxide and triple antibiotic paste as intracanal medicaments on the incidence of inter-appointment flare-up in diabetic patients: An in vivo study. *J. Conserv. Dent.* **2014**, *17*, 208–211. [CrossRef] [PubMed]
64. Rahhal, J.G.; Rovai, E.D.S.; Holzhausen, M.; Caldeira, C.L.; Dos Santos, C.F.; Sipert, C.R. Root canal dressings for revascularization influence in vitro mineralization of apical papilla cells. *J. Appl. Oral Sci. Rev. FOB* **2019**, *27*, e20180396. [CrossRef] [PubMed]
65. Kim, J.-H.; Kim, Y.; Shin, S.-J.; Park, J.-W.; Jung, I.Y. Tooth Discoloration of Immature Permanent Incisor Associated with Triple Antibiotic Therapy: A Case Report. *J. Endod.* **2010**, *36*, 1086–1091. [CrossRef]
66. Panda, S.; Mishra, L.; Arbildo-Vega, H.I.; Lapinska, B.; Lukomska-Szymanska, M.; Khijmatgar, S.; Parolia, A.; Bucchi, C.; Del Fabbro, M. Effectiveness of Autologous Platelet Concentrates in Management of Young Immature Necrotic Permanent Teeth—A Systematic Review and Meta-Analysis. *Cells* **2020**, *9*, 2241. [CrossRef]
67. Management of Non-Vital Permanent Teeth with Incomplete Root Formation. Available online: https://ukdiss.com/examples/non-vital-permanent-teeth-incomplete-root.php (accessed on 26 July 2021).
68. Kleier, D.J.; Barr, E.S. A study of endodontically apexified teeth. *Dent. Traumatol.* **1991**, *7*, 112–117. [CrossRef]
69. Hargreaves, K.M.; Diogenes, A.; Teixeira, F.B. Treatment options: Biological basis of regenerative endodontic procedures. *Pediatr. Dent.* **2013**, *35*, 129–140. [CrossRef]
70. Banchs, F.; Trope, M. Revascularization of Immature Permanent Teeth with Apical Periodontitis: New Treatment Protocol? *J. Endod.* **2004**, *30*, 196–200. [CrossRef]

71. Iwaya, S.-I.; Ikawa, M.; Kubota, M. Revascularization of an immature permanent tooth with periradicular abscess after luxation. *Dent. Traumatol.* **2011**, *27*, 55–58. [CrossRef]
72. Tong, H.J.; Sim, Y.F.; Berdouses, E.; Al-Jundi, S.; El Shahawy, O.; Nazzal, H. Regenerative endodontic therapy (RET) for managing immature non-vital teeth: Experiences and opinions of paediatric dental practitioners in the European and Arabian regions. *Eur. Arch. Paediatr. Dent.* **2021**, *22*, 145–155. [CrossRef]
73. Kobayashi, E.; Flückiger, L.; Fujioka-Kobayashi, M.; Sawada, K.; Sculean, A.; Schaller, B.; Miron, R.J. Comparative release of growth factors from PRP, PRF, and advanced-PRF. *Clin. Oral Investig.* **2016**, *20*, 2353–2360. [CrossRef] [PubMed]
74. Savović, J.; Turner, R.M.; Mawdsley, D.; Jones, H.E.; Beynon, R.; Higgins, J.P.T.; Sterne, J.A.C. Association between Risk-of-Bias Assessments and Results of Randomized Trials in Cochrane Reviews: The ROBES Meta-Epidemiologic Study. *Am. J. Epidemiol.* **2018**, *187*, 1113–1122. [CrossRef] [PubMed]
75. Vidal, K.; Martin, G.; Lozano, O.; Salas, M.; Trigueros, J.; Aguilar, G. Apical Closure in Apexification: A Review and Case Report of Apexification Treatment of an Immature Permanent Tooth with Biodentine. *J. Endod.* **2016**, *42*, 730–734. [CrossRef] [PubMed]
76. Shabahang, S. Treatment options: Apexogenesis and apexification. *Pediatr. Dent.* **2013**, *35*, 125–128. [CrossRef]
77. Holden, D.T.; Schwartz, S.A.; Kirkpatrick, T.C.; Schindler, W.G. Clinical Outcomes of Artificial Root-end Barriers with Mineral Trioxide Aggregate in Teeth with Immature Apices. *J. Endod.* **2008**, *34*, 812–817. [CrossRef]
78. Apexification—An Overview | ScienceDirect Topics. Available online: https://www.sciencedirect.com/topics/medicine-and-dentistry/apexification (accessed on 21 June 2021).
79. Guerrero, F.; Mendoza, A.; Ribas, D.; Aspiazu, K. Apexification: A systematic review. *J. Conserv. Dent.* **2018**, *21*, 462–465. [CrossRef]
80. Mohammadi, Z.; Dummer, P.M.H. Properties and applications of calcium hydroxide in endodontics and dental traumatology. *Int. Endod. J.* **2011**, *44*, 697–730. [CrossRef]
81. Kunert, M.; Lukomska-Szymanska, M. Bio-Inductive Materials in Direct and Indirect Pulp Capping—A Review Article. *Materials* **2020**, *13*, 1204. [CrossRef]
82. Sood, R.; Hans, M.K.; Shetty, S. Apical barrier technique with mineral trioxide aggregate using internal matrix: A case report. *Compend. Contin. Educ. Dent.* **2012**, *33*, e88–e90.
83. Shokouhinejad, N.; Khoshkhounejad, M.; Alikhasi, M.; Bagheri, P.; Camilleri, J. Prevention of coronal discoloration induced by regenerative endodontic treatment in an ex vivo model. *Clin. Oral Investig.* **2018**, *22*, 1725–1731. [CrossRef]
84. Sharma, V.; Srinivasan, A.; Nikolajeff, F.; Kumar, S. Biomineralization process in hard tissues: The interaction complexity within protein and inorganic counterparts. *Acta Biomater.* **2021**, *120*, 20–37. [CrossRef] [PubMed]
85. Nicoloso, G.F.; Goldenfum, G.M.; Pizzol, T.D.S.D.; Scarparo, R.K.; Montagner, F.; Rodrigues, J.D.A.; Casagrande, L. Pulp Revascularization or Apexification for the Treatment of Immature Necrotic Permanent Teeth: Systematic Review and Meta-Analysis. *J. Clin. Pediatr. Dent.* **2019**, *43*, 305–313. [CrossRef] [PubMed]
86. Becerra, P.; Ricucci, D.; Loghin, S.; Gibbs, J.L.; Lin, L.M. Histologic Study of a Human Immature Permanent Premolar with Chronic Apical Abscess after Revascularization/Revitalization. *J. Endod.* **2014**, *40*, 133–139. [CrossRef] [PubMed]
87. Chen, M.Y.-H.; Chen, K.-L.; Chen, C.-A.; Tayebaty, F.; Rosenberg, P.A.; Lin, L.M. Responses of immature permanent teeth with infected necrotic pulp tissue and apical periodontitis/abscess to revascularization procedures. *Int. Endod. J.* **2012**, *45*, 294–305. [CrossRef] [PubMed]
88. Alhamoui, F.A.; Steffen, H.; Splieth, C.H. The sealing ability of ProRoot MTA when placed as an apical barrier using three different techniques: An in-vitro apexification model. *Quintessence Int. Berl. Ger. 1985* **2014**, *45*, 821–827. [CrossRef]
89. Alkaisi, A.; Ismail, A.R.; Mutum, S.S.; Ahmad, Z.A.R.; Masudi, S.; Razak, N.H.A. Transplantation of Human Dental Pulp Stem Cells: Enhance Bone Consolidation in Mandibular Distraction Osteogenesis. *J. Oral Maxillofac. Surg.* **2013**, *71*, 1758.e1–1758.e13. [CrossRef]
90. El Ashry, S.H.; Abu-Seida, A.M.; Bayoumi, A.A.; Hashem, A.A. Regenerative potential of immature permanent non-vital teeth following different dentin surface treatments. *Exp. Toxicol. Pathol.* **2016**, *68*, 181–190. [CrossRef]
91. El-Tayeb, M.M.; Abu-Seida, A.M.; El Ashry, S.; El-Hady, S.A. Evaluation of antibacterial activity of propolis on regenerative potential of necrotic immature permanent teeth in dogs. *BMC Oral Health* **2019**, *19*, 174. [CrossRef]
92. Huang, R.; Liu, P.; Xiao, M.; Zhou, Z. A comparative study on apexification using different kinds of materials in dogs. *Hua Xi Kou Qiang Yi Xue Za Zhi = Huaxi Kouqiang Yixue Zazhi = WNort. China J. Stomatol.* **2013**, *31*, 377–388.
93. Peng, C.F.; Zhao, Y.M.; Yang, Y.; Liu, H.; Qin, M. Retrospective analysis of pulp revascularization in immature permanent teeth with diffuse pulpitis. *Zhonghua Kou Qiang Yi Xue Za Zhi = Zhonghua Kouqiang Yixue Zazhi = Chin. J. Stomatol.* **2017**, *52*, 10–15.
94. Jamshidi, D.; Homayouni, H.; Majd, N.M.; Shahabi, S.; Arvin, A.; Ranjbaromidi, B. Impact and Fracture Strength of Simulated Immature Teeth Treated with Mineral Trioxide Aggregate Apical Plug and Fiber Post Versus Revascularization. *J. Endod.* **2018**, *44*, 1878–1882. [CrossRef] [PubMed]
95. Moradi, S.; Talati, A.; Forghani, M.; Jafarian, A.H.; Naseri, M.; Shojaeian, S. Immunohistological Evaluation of Revascularized Immature Permanent Necrotic Teeth Treated by Platelet-Rich Plasma: An Animal Investigation. *Cell J.* **2016**, *18*, 389–396. [CrossRef] [PubMed]
96. Ok, E.; Altunsoy, M.; Tanriver, M.; Çapar, I.D. Effectiveness of different irrigation protocols on calcium hydroxide removal from simulated immature teeth after apexification. *Acta Biomater. Odontol. Scand.* **2015**, *1*, 1–5. [CrossRef] [PubMed]

97. Pagliarin, C.M.L.; Londero, C.D.L.D.; Felippe, M.C.S.; Felippe, W.T.; Danesi, C.C.; Barletta, F.B. Tissue characterization following revascularization of immature dog teeth using different disinfection pastes. *Braz. Oral Res.* **2016**, *30*. [CrossRef]
98. Jahromi, M.Z.; Refaei, P.; Moughari, A.A.K. Comparison of the microleakage of mineral trioxide aggregate, calcium-enriched mixture cement, and Biodentine orthograde apical plug. *Dent. Res. J.* **2020**, *17*, 66. [CrossRef]
99. Ritter, A.L.D.S.; Ritter, A.V.; Murrah, V.; Sigurdsson, A.; Trope, M. Pulp revascularization of replanted immature dog teeth after treatment with minocycline and doxycycline assessed by laser Doppler flowmetry, radiography, and histology. *Dent. Traumatol.* **2004**, *20*, 75–84. [CrossRef]
100. Sogukpinar, A.; Arikan, V. Comparative evaluation of four endodontic biomaterials and calcium hydroxide regarding their effect on fracture resistance of simulated immature teeth. *Huaxi Kouqiang Yixue Zazhi W. Chin. J. Stomatol.* **2020**, *21*, 23–28. [CrossRef]
101. Thibodeau, B.; Teixeira, F.; Yamauchi, M.; Caplan, D.J.; Trope, M. Pulp Revascularization of Immature Dog Teeth with Apical Periodontitis. *J. Endod.* **2007**, *33*, 680–689. [CrossRef]
102. Valera, M.C.; Albuquerque, M.T.P.; Yamasaki, M.C.; Vassallo, F.N.S.; da Silva, D.; Nagata, J.Y. Fracture resistance of weakened bovine teeth after long-term use of calcium hydroxide. *Dent. Traumatol.* **2015**, *31*, 385–389. [CrossRef]
103. Yang, J.; Wang, W.J.; Jia, W.Q.; Zhao, Y.M.; Ge, L.H. Effect of exogenous stem cells from apical papillae in the pulp re-vascularization treatment for the immature permanent tooth with periapical periodontitis. *Zhonghua Kou Qiang Yi Xue Za Zhi = Zhonghua Kouqiang Yixue Zazhi = Chin. J. Stomatol.* **2018**, *53*, 459–465. [CrossRef]
104. Yoo, Y.-J.; Lee, W.; Cho, Y.-A.; Park, J.-C.; Shon, W.-J.; Baek, S.-H. Effect of Conditioned Medium from Preameloblasts on Regenerative Cellular Differentiation of the Immature Teeth with Necrotic Pulp and Apical Periodontitis. *J. Endod.* **2014**, *40*, 1355–1361. [CrossRef] [PubMed]
105. Zhang, D.-D.; Chen, X.; Bao, Z.-F.; Chen, M.; Ding, Z.-J.; Zhong, M. Histologic Comparison between Platelet-rich Plasma and Blood Clot in Regenerative Endodontic Treatment: An Animal Study. *J. Endod.* **2014**, *40*, 1388–1393. [CrossRef] [PubMed]
106. Zuong, X.-Y.; Yang, Y.-P.; Chen, W.-X.; Zhang, Y.-J.; Wen, C.-M. [Pulp revascularization of immature anterior teeth with apical periodontitis]. *Hua Xi Kou Qiang Yi Xue Za Zhi = Huaxi Kouqiang Yixue Zazhi = W. Chin. J. Stomatol.* **2010**, *28*, 672–674.
107. Beslot-Neveu, A.; Bonte, E.; Baune, B.; Serreau, R.; Aissat, F.; Quinquis, L.; Grabar, S.; Lasfargues, J.-J. Mineral trioxyde aggregate versus calcium hydroxide in apexification of non vital immature teeth: Study protocol for a randomized controlled trial. *Trials* **2011**, *12*, 174. [CrossRef] [PubMed]
108. Bukhari, S.; Kohli, M.R.; Setzer, F.; Karabucak, B. Outcome of Revascularization Procedure: A Retrospective Case Series. *J. Endod.* **2016**, *42*, 1752–1759. [CrossRef] [PubMed]

MDPI
St. Alban-Anlage 66
4052 Basel
Switzerland
Tel. +41 61 683 77 34
Fax +41 61 302 89 18
www.mdpi.com

Journal of Clinical Medicine Editorial Office
E-mail: jcm@mdpi.com
www.mdpi.com/journal/jcm

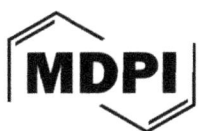